State-Level Data Book on Health Care Access and Financing

Pamela Loprest and
Michael Gates

THE URBAN INSTITUTE
Washigton, D.C.

THE URBAN INSTITUTE PRESS

2100 M Street, N.W.
Washington, D.C. 20037

Library of Congress Cataloging in Publication Data

State-Level Data book on Health Care Access and Financing / Pamela Loprest and Michael Gates.

1. Medical economics—United States—States—Statistics. 2. Insurance, Health—United States—States—Statistics. 3. Medically uninsured persons—United States—States—Statistics. 4. Health status indicators—United States—States—Statistics. 5. United States—Statistics, Medical. I. Gates, Michael.

[DNLM: 1. Insurance, Health—economics—United States—tables. 2. Health Services Accessibility—economics—United States—tables. 3. Health Services—economics—United States—tables. 4. Health Status Indicators—United States—tables.
W 16 L864s 1993.]

RA410.53.L67	1993	93-14692
362.1'0973—dc20		CIP

ISBN 0-87766-596-6
ISBN 0-87766-597-4 (paperback)

Printed in the United States of America.

Distributed by University Press of America

4720 Boston Way	3 Henrietta Street
Lanham, MD 20706	London WC2E 8LU
	ENGLAND

THE URBAN INSTITUTE is a nonprofit policy research and educational organization established in Washington, D.C. in 1968. Its staff investigates the social and economic problems confronting the nation and public and private means to alleviate them. The Urban Institute has three goals for its research and dissemination activities: to sharpen thinking about societal problems and efforts to solve them, to improve government decisions and performance, and to increase citizen awareness of important public choices.

Through work that ranges from broad conceptual studies to administrative and technical assistance, Institute researchers contribute to the stock of knowledge and the analytic tools available to guide decision making in the public interest.

The Institute disseminates its research and the research of others through The Urban Institute Press, which makes publication decisions based on referees' reports solicited from recognized experts in the field.

Conclusions or opinions expressed are those of the authors and do not necessarily reflect the views of staff members, officers, trustees, advisory groups, or funders of the Institute.

Acknowledgments

The authors gratefully acknowledge John Holahan, Paul Johnson, Colin Winterbottom, and Sheila Zedlewski at The Urban Institute. Funding for this project was provided by The Robert Wood Johnson Foundation under the State Initiatives in Health Care Financing Reform program. Opinions expressed are those of the authors and do not necessarily represent the views of The Urban Institute or its sponsors.

CONTENTS

Introduction

Despite recent federal initiatives that have expanded health insurance coverage for low-income children, the number of Americans without health insurance remains high, at more than 35 million people in 1990. In addition, rapidly increasing health care costs are having large impacts on employers providing coverage to workers, on state and federal governments funding public insurance, and on individuals buying private policies. Increases in health care costs have led to recent declines in employment-based coverage and to some employers scaling back the generosity of their coverage. Federal and state governments already confronting budget problems must find funds to provide public insurance to the poor and elderly. The private sector, the public sector, and individuals all bear the cost of providing uncompensated care to individuals without health insurance. In the face of more individuals with less coverage, policymakers need to find ways to expand health care coverage for the uninsured and to provide more secure coverage for everyone, while devising ways to contain increases in health care costs.

While debate continues over health care reform at the federal level, there is uncertainty about whether major national initiatives will be enacted in the near future. Consequently, state-based health care reform initiatives have intensified as states continue to bear a large share of the cost for the uninsured and expanding Medicaid programs. Responses to the Robert Wood Johnson Foundation's recent health care financing reform initiative provide evidence of the level of health system reform activity in the states. Despite severe budget constraints in many states, the foundation received 35 applications for planning grants from states considering major health care financing reform initiatives.

As some states undertake innovative health care reform initiatives and others debate possible strategies, each state will need a comprehensive picture of its own current health system. Information on health insurance status, the cost of different health system components, the availability of various health system resources, and the demographic and economic profile of each state's population will be required. This monograph compiles state-level data on a variety of indicators from many sources as a reference for state policymakers and researchers working on state health care reform. Although many of the statistics presented here are drawn from resources readily available from the Health Care Financing Administration and other federal statistical agencies, other data are drawn from more unique and difficult-to-access resources. In addition, we have developed profiles of state populations by combining annual survey data from the U.S. Bureau of the Census across three years to increase the reliability of state-level estimates.

We include measures for every state and, where available, for the District of Columbia. We also report totals for the entire United States and averages for the nine Census regions. The information is organized into the following seven sections:

A. *Health Insurance Coverage:* A profile of insurance coverage of nonelderly persons in the states by age, sex, race, family type, and work status.

B. *Health Insurance Coverage of Workers:* A profile of insurance coverage of workers by full-time or part-time status, firm size, sector, and industry.

C. *Characteristics of the Uninsured:* A profile of persons in the states who have no apparent, regular source of health insurance coverage by age, sex, race, family type, work status, firm size, and sector.

D. *Medicaid:* The number and characteristics of persons eligible for and enrolled in Medicaid, as well as current Medicaid expenditures and how fees for various services relate to private and Medicare fees.

E. *Indices of Health Status:* A profile of the health status of the population including infant mortality, AIDS-related statistics, and adult disability indicators.

F. Health Care Costs, Access, and Utilization: Indicators of health care costs including hospital costs, physician costs, Medicare spending, and access and utilization, including number of hospital and nursing home beds, length of hospital stays, number of physicians, and health maintenance organizations (HMOs).

G. State Demographic and Economic Profiles: A profile of the states' population characteristics, worker characteristics, number of establishments and worker pay by establishment size, and state financing and expenditure indices.

The beginning of each section contains a short introduction discussing the measures included. Each section also highlights a few results to provide some contextual basis for the data presented. However, since this monograph is intended to serve primarily as a data reference, we do not attempt to analyze all the differences in these measures across states or to draw policy conclusions.

DATA SOURCES

Many of the tables included in this monograph are drawn from the March Current Population Survey (CPS). The CPS provides data on work status and income, demographic characteristics, health insurance coverage, and other individual characteristics of interest. The CPS sample is based on the civilian noninstitutionalized population of the United States. In one year the survey interviews approximately 57,000 households, or 160,000 individuals, nationally. However, the sample size for a given state can be relatively small, leading to less-reliable estimates of state population characteristics.

To report more-reliable statistics, we merged three consecutive March CPS files, from 1989, 1990, and 1991. As noted in more detail in Appendix One, this procedure approximately doubled state sample sizes. Since households were interviewed in two consecutive years and we only wanted to included each household once, we include all of the observations from the March 1990 survey, plus approximately half from the 1989 and 1991 surveys. The CPS collects information from households for the previous calendar year, so the CPS-based estimates presented in this volume represent an average value for the 1988-90 period.

In a number of cases data from the Current Population Survey have been augmented by estimates derived from the Urban Institute's microsimulation model, called the Transfer Income Model (TRIM2).[1] TRIM2 has been used by various government agencies over the last 20 years to provide more information about the tax, health benefit, and income transfer system in the United States. For example, it includes modules that simulate the program rules for Medicaid, Aid to Families with Dependent Children (AFDC), and Supplemental Security Income (SSI). These modules correct for underreporting of benefits on the Current Population Survey (see Appendix Two), and they generate estimates of the size of the population eligible for benefits. (Some persons are eligible for benefits under government assistance programs but never apply for benefits. The ratio of persons actually enrolled in a program to the total number eligible provides an estimate of the "participation rate.") Where appropriate, we use this information from TRIM2 to augment the various state profiles.

Information from data sources other than the CPS is also included in this monograph. All tables use the most recently available data. Tables are included on health costs, status, access, and utilization from a variety of sources. We also include background data on states and summary information on state finances and spending. Sources for information presented and explanatory notes defining variables and concepts are presented at the end of each section.

Reliability of estimates

To help the user in determining the precision of the estimates, we provide standard errors on all of the estimates reported from the CPS. The CPS sample estimate and the standard error can be used to construct a confidence interval. For example, a confidence interval defined as the estimate plus or minus 1.96 times its standard error indicates that the true estimate is within that interval with 95 percent probability. If we estimate that 10 percent of a given population are uninsured with a standard error of 1 percent, a user can say with a 95 percent certainty that the true percentage of uninsured falls somewhere between 8 percent and 12 percent. The standard errors are also important for determining whether two estimates are statistically different. For example, the standard errors can be used to compare whether the percentage of uninsured is significantly different in two states, or whether it differs significantly from the percentage on Medicaid in a single state.

Appendix One describes how to use standard errors to make these comparisons.

Even given the increased number of observations in the merged sample used here, there are some limitations to the state-level estimates. The CPS is designed to provide state and national estimates; however, the survey does not interview individuals from every county in a state. The sample is located in 729 sample areas comprising 1,973 counties and independent cities. Therefore the CPS cannot provide accurate substate estimates. In addition, certain state subsamples, such as the nonwhite population may still be small in the merged CPS sample, and therefore estimates based on this subsample may be unreliable. For this reason, we do not report estimates based on less than 100 unweighted sample observations.[2]

Notes, Introduction

1. Linda Giannarelli, 1992, *An Analyst's Guide to TRIM2* (Washington, D.C.: Urban Institute Press).

2. For further information on data reliability, see the Current Population Survey, March 1989, 1990, and 1991, and "The Current Population Survey: Design and Methodology," CPS Technical Paper No. 40, U.S. Bureau of the Census.

Health Insurance Coverage

The tables in this section show health insurance coverage for various subsets of the nonelderly population. Persons appear in only one health insurance category, even though some report more than one source of coverage on the Current Population Survey. We use a hierarchy to assign each person to one category. First we show the percentage of the population insured through their own employer's group health plan and the percentage insured through another worker's employer group plan. The latter group includes dependents who do not work and dependents who work but receive coverage through their spouse's employer group plan. Then we show the percentage of persons enrolled in Medicaid, other government insurance programs (CHAMPUS and Medicare), other private insurance plans, and the percentage without health insurance.

In the Current Population Survey, persons are asked to report their insurance status for the last year. In fact, some had spells of uninsurance interspersed with spells of employer group insurance. The fact that we define "uninsurance" as the residual category in this hierarchy means that we will understate the number of persons who experienced a spell of uninsurance during the year. See Appendix Two for a fuller description of these measurement issues.

TYPES OF INSURANCE COVERAGE

About 66 percent of the nonelderly population in the United States are insured through employer group plans. Thirty-three percent have coverage through their own employers, and 33 percent have coverage as dependents on another family member's employer group policy (table A1). The extent of employer group coverage varies geographically. In general, persons in the New England, Middle Atlantic, and East North Central regions are more likely to have coverage through an employer group plan than persons living elsewhere in the country. As we show later in sections B and G, this probably reflects the higher concentration of large manufacturing employers in these areas, which are more likely to provide insurance. These data also show important variations in coverage across states within geographic regions. For example, within the South Atlantic region, the percentage of persons with insurance through their own employers' plans ranges from 29 percent in West Virginia to 39 percent in Maryland.

Medicaid coverage is more common in the East South Central and Pacific regions than elsewhere. In addition, the percentage of the population insured through Medicaid varies considerably across the states. For example, Medicaid insures 15 percent of Mississippi's population compared to 3 percent of New Hampshire's population. Higher rates of Medicaid coverage can reflect both relatively lower incomes of some states' populations as well as the states' Medicaid coverage policies. (Data in section D further illuminate differences in Medicaid eligibility and enrollment across states.)

About 16 percent of the nonelderly population are without health insurance. The extent of uninsurance varies widely across states, however, and, not surprisingly, it varies inversely with the extent of employer group coverage. The New England, Middle Atlantic and North Central regions have the lowest rates of uninsurance (about 11–12 percent), and the southern, Mountain, and Pacific regions have the highest rates of uninsurance (19–23 percent). However, there are some notable exceptions to these general regional patterns. For example, within the Mountain region, Utah has a relatively low rate of uninsurance (11 percent).

DEMOGRAPHIC CHARACTERISTICS

We show insurance coverage separately for children (under age 18) and adults (18 and older) in tables A2 and A3, respectively. (Only one category is shown for employer group insurance for children because nearly all receive coverage as dependents on a parent's health plan.) The geographic patterns in insurance coverage are similar to those for the general population, with the exception that more children have Medicaid coverage than do adults. In some states (Mississippi, Louisiana, and California), approximately one-quarter of all children are enrolled in Medicaid, whereas the percentage of adults enrolled in Medicaid rarely exceeds 8 percent in any state. Recent federal changes in the Medicaid program have increased the proportion of children relative to adults in the program. During 1988 to 1990, the period covered by these tables, states were required to provide Medicaid coverage to children under age 6 in families with income below 133 percent of poverty, and many states took advantage of optional coverage rules that permitted coverage for older low-income children in families with income up to the poverty threshold.

Tables A4 through A7 show insurance coverage by sex and race (white and nonwhite). We then show the insurance status of nonelderly persons by the type of family in which they live—married couples with children, married couples without children, single parents with children, and single persons without children (tables A8 through A11, respectively). These tables demonstrate some important differences in access to health insurance for families. A large share of persons living in married-couple families with children (table A8) are covered by employer group insurance (76 percent). However, more of these are covered as dependents (51 percent) than as workers covered under their own employer's plan (25 percent). Medicaid covers 5 percent of persons in this family group because some two-parent families qualify for Aid to Families with Dependent Children (AFDC) and some low-income children now qualify for Medicaid even though both parents are present. California stands out with the highest rate of Medicaid coverage among two-parent families with children (11 percent), reflecting its generous eligibility standards.

Nearly half of all persons living in married couple families with no children have coverage through their own employer's group policy, and another 23 percent are insured as dependents on their spouse's policy, bringing coverage under employer group insurance for this type of family unit to 72 percent. On the other hand, only 2 percent of persons in this group have Medicaid coverage; most likely these are persons qualifying under the program's disability provisions.

Medicaid is the largest insurer for persons living in single-parent families with children (table A10). The program covers 40 percent of persons in single-parent families, ranging from less than 30 percent in states like Connecticut, Virginia, and Delaware to about 50 percent in

Mississippi and Louisiana. Broad levels of Medicaid coverage keep the rate of uninsurance for this group at 15 percent, about the national average for all persons.

Single adults without children (table A11) have the highest rate of uninsurance (27 percent) among all family types. Nationwide, about one-half have employer group insurance, 6 percent have Medicaid, and 14 percent have other types of private insurance such as individually purchased, nongroup insurance policies. In many states, more than one in three single adults have no source of health insurance. This includes Alabama, Mississippi, all of the states in the West South Central Region, and many of the Mountain states (Nevada, New Mexico, and Wyoming).

FAMILY INCOME

The next set of tables (A12 through A14) shows insurance status by income relative to the poverty line (below poverty, 100-199 percent of poverty, and 200 percent or higher), respectively. These data show important differences in coverage across income levels. They also roughly indicate the population's ability to pay for additional health care coverage. Relatively few persons with incomes below the poverty threshold have employer group coverage (table A12). Nearly half are covered under Medicaid, and 29 percent have no health insurance. Coverage for persons in families with incomes above 200 percent of poverty stands in stark contrast to that for the poor—81 percent have coverage through employer group plans (42 percent are covered as workers and 39 percent as dependents), and 9 percent have no health insurance.

Some important differences in coverage by income level emerge across states following patterns noted earlier. For example, persons in the southern states are less likely to have employer group insurance coverage across all income groups. However, more generous Medicaid coverage policies in some states make up a larger share of the insurance gap than in others. For example, only 12 percent of persons in the West South Central and 11 percent of persons in the Pacific region with incomes below poverty have employer group coverage. However, the percentage of uninsured poor persons is 43 percent in the West South Central region and 28 percent in the Pacific region. Medicaid provides coverage to 54 percent of all poor persons in the Pacific region compared to 38 percent in the West South Central.

WORK STATUS OF THE FAMILY HEAD AND SPOUSE

The last group of tables (A15–A17) in this section highlights the importance of work status for families' insurance coverage. We categorize people by whether the family head *or* spouse works full-time (35 hours or more), part-time (less than 35 hours), or does not work. Table A15 shows that 75 percent of persons in families where either the head or spouse had a full-time job have employer group insurance (37 percent through their own employer and 38 percent as dependents). As discussed earlier, however, the prevalence of employer-group coverage does vary across the states, leading to significant variation in rates of uninsurance. For example, about 81 percent of families with a full-time worker have employer group coverage in New Jersey and Pennsylvania, and 9 percent are uninsured. On the other hand, in Louisiana and Oklahoma only 68 percent of persons in families where the head or spouse works full-time have employer group insurance, and 19 percent are uninsured.

Persons in families where the head or spouse only works part-time and neither works full-time (table A16) are much less likely to have employer group insurance. More than one in four persons in part-time worker families are uninsured, partly owing to the low rates of Medicaid coverage (18 percent). In some states (for example, Georgia, Indiana, Louisiana, and Texas), more than 40 percent of people in part-time worker families are uninsured. In contrast, families where both the head and spouse are not working are less likely to be uninsured (table A17). Broader Medicaid coverage of this group (46 percent) is responsible for holding their uninsured rate to 20 percent. Note that employer group coverage among persons in families with no workers includes persons with retiree health benefits, as well as persons covered under the provisions of the Consolidated Budget Reconciliation Act of 1986 (COBRA), which requires employers to extend employer group insurance for 18 months after job termination (while allowing employers to require the terminating worker to pay the full cost of the insurance). In addition, some children may have employer group coverage from a working parent not living with the family.

TABLE A1
TOTAL POPULATION UNDER AGE 65: BY TYPE OF HEALTH INSURANCE COVERAGE

	Number (000s)	Employer (own)	Employer (other)	Medicaid	Other Government	Other Private	Uninsured
UNITED STATES	213,580	33% (0.10)	33% (0.10)	9% (0.06)	2% (0.03)	7% (0.06)	16% (0.08)
NEW ENGLAND	11,157	38% (0.36)	36% (0.36)	7% (0.19)	1% (0.08)	7% (0.19)	11% (0.23)
Connecticut	2,761	41% (1.03)	37% (1.01)	5% (0.43)	1% (0.20)	6% (0.49)	10% (0.62)
Maine	1,055	33% (0.87)	36% (0.89)	10% (0.55)	2% (0.26)	8% (0.51)	11% (0.59)
Massachusetts	5,062	37% (0.48)	36% (0.47)	8% (0.27)	1% (0.11)	7% (0.25)	10% (0.30)
New Hampshire	972	36% (0.97)	36% (0.97)	3% (0.34)	1% (0.23)	8% (0.56)	16% (0.75)
Rhode Island	823	38% (1.00)	36% (0.99)	7% (0.52)	1% (0.22)	7% (0.52)	11% (0.64)
Vermont	485	36% (0.97)	35% (0.96)	7% (0.50)	1% (0.23)	9% (0.58)	11% (0.64)
MIDDLE ATLANTIC	32,415	36% (0.24)	35% (0.24)	9% (0.15)	1% (0.05)	7% (0.13)	12% (0.17)
New Jersey	6,631	40% (0.47)	35% (0.46)	6% (0.24)	1% (0.08)	7% (0.25)	11% (0.30)
New York	15,507	34% (0.36)	33% (0.36)	12% (0.25)	1% (0.08)	7% (0.19)	14% (0.26)
Pennsylvania	10,277	36% (0.45)	38% (0.45)	8% (0.25)	1% (0.10)	7% (0.24)	10% (0.28)
SOUTH ATLANTIC	36,005	35% (0.26)	31% (0.25)	8% (0.14)	2% (0.08)	7% (0.14)	17% (0.20)
Delaware	574	38% (0.96)	33% (0.93)	5% (0.45)	2% (0.27)	6% (0.49)	16% (0.72)
District of Columbia	493	37% (1.02)	18% (0.81)	15% (0.77)	2% (0.26)	8% (0.57)	20% (0.86)
Florida	10,334	32% (0.43)	28% (0.41)	7% (0.23)	3% (0.15)	9% (0.26)	22% (0.38)
Georgia	5,475	34% (0.85)	31% (0.82)	9% (0.51)	2% (0.26)	6% (0.43)	17% (0.67)
Maryland	3,977	39% (0.95)	35% (0.93)	8% (0.53)	2% (0.24)	5% (0.44)	11% (0.61)
North Carolina	5,469	38% (0.46)	30% (0.43)	7% (0.25)	2% (0.15)	7% (0.25)	15% (0.34)
South Carolina	2,932	36% (0.80)	32% (0.77)	7% (0.44)	3% (0.28)	6% (0.38)	16% (0.60)
Virginia	5,166	36% (0.78)	34% (0.77)	6% (0.38)	2% (0.26)	6% (0.39)	16% (0.60)
West Virginia	1,586	29% (0.83)	35% (0.87)	13% (0.61)	2% (0.27)	6% (0.42)	14% (0.63)
EAST SOUTH CENTRAL	13,214	30% (0.42)	32% (0.42)	11% (0.28)	3% (0.15)	7% (0.23)	17% (0.34)
Alabama	3,570	30% (0.82)	33% (0.84)	8% (0.48)	3% (0.32)	6% (0.43)	20% (0.71)
Kentucky	3,123	31% (0.85)	33% (0.87)	12% (0.60)	3% (0.31)	7% (0.46)	14% (0.64)
Mississippi	2,285	25% (0.74)	29% (0.77)	15% (0.61)	3% (0.31)	7% (0.44)	20% (0.68)
Tennessee	4,236	33% (0.82)	33% (0.82)	10% (0.53)	2% (0.25)	7% (0.44)	15% (0.63)
WEST SOUTH CENTRAL	23,455	28% (0.32)	30% (0.32)	8% (0.20)	3% (0.12)	7% (0.19)	23% (0.30)
Arkansas	2,103	27% (0.79)	32% (0.83)	9% (0.52)	4% (0.33)	8% (0.47)	20% (0.71)
Louisiana	3,701	25% (0.81)	30% (0.86)	13% (0.63)	3% (0.32)	7% (0.48)	22% (0.77)
Oklahoma	2,679	28% (0.82)	31% (0.84)	8% (0.50)	3% (0.32)	9% (0.51)	21% (0.74)
Texas	14,973	29% (0.42)	30% (0.42)	7% (0.24)	2% (0.14)	7% (0.24)	24% (0.39)

TOTAL POPULATION UNDER AGE 65: BY TYPE OF HEALTH INSURANCE COVERAGE

	Number (000s)	Employer (own)	Employer (other)	Medicaid	Other Government	Other Private	Uninsured
EAST NORTH CENTRAL	**36,786**	**34%** (0.25)	**37%** (0.25)	**9%** (0.15)	**1%** (0.06)	**7%** (0.13)	**11%** (0.16)
Illinois	10,171	35% (0.45)	34% (0.45)	10% (0.29)	1% (0.11)	8% (0.25)	12% (0.31)
Indiana	4,773	34% (0.89)	36% (0.91)	5% (0.43)	2% (0.26)	8% (0.51)	14% (0.65)
Michigan	8,201	33% (0.44)	37% (0.46)	12% (0.30)	1% (0.10)	6% (0.23)	10% (0.28)
Ohio	9,537	34% (0.44)	39% (0.45)	9% (0.27)	1% (0.11)	6% (0.22)	10% (0.28)
Wisconsin	4,104	36% (0.83)	40% (0.85)	6% (0.42)	1% (0.18)	8% (0.46)	9% (0.49)
WEST NORTH CENTRAL	**15,279**	**32%** (0.38)	**36%** (0.39)	**7%** (0.21)	**2%** (0.10)	**12%** (0.27)	**12%** (0.26)
Iowa	2,386	31% (0.82)	37% (0.86)	6% (0.43)	1% (0.21)	15% (0.64)	9% (0.50)
Kansas	2,078	32% (0.83)	38% (0.87)	7% (0.45)	1% (0.19)	11% (0.55)	10% (0.55)
Minnesota	3,849	34% (0.87)	34% (0.87)	8% (0.51)	1% (0.21)	12% (0.59)	11% (0.58)
Missouri	4,475	34% (0.88)	36% (0.90)	7% (0.47)	2% (0.25)	8% (0.50)	14% (0.64)
Nebraska	1,361	31% (0.80)	36% (0.83)	6% (0.40)	1% (0.21)	14% (0.61)	12% (0.56)
North Dakota	546	25% (0.74)	35% (0.82)	6% (0.40)	2% (0.24)	23% (0.72)	10% (0.51)
South Dakota	585	26% (0.73)	33% (0.77)	6% (0.38)	2% (0.25)	17% (0.62)	16% (0.60)
MOUNTAIN	**11,712**	**30%** (0.36)	**34%** (0.37)	**6%** (0.19)	**2%** (0.12)	**8%** (0.22)	**19%** (0.30)
Arizona	3,016	32% (0.87)	31% (0.87)	7% (0.48)	3% (0.30)	8% (0.50)	20% (0.75)
Colorado	2,836	32% (0.90)	35% (0.92)	6% (0.46)	3% (0.31)	7% (0.50)	18% (0.74)
Idaho	896	27% (0.76)	36% (0.82)	4% (0.35)	2% (0.25)	12% (0.56)	18% (0.66)
Montana	711	27% (0.78)	32% (0.82)	8% (0.48)	2% (0.27)	13% (0.60)	18% (0.67)
Nevada	1,010	38% (0.91)	31% (0.87)	4% (0.36)	2% (0.27)	7% (0.47)	19% (0.74)
New Mexico	1,302	24% (0.75)	30% (0.81)	8% (0.47)	3% (0.31)	7% (0.46)	28% (0.79)
Utah	1,525	27% (0.77)	46% (0.86)	6% (0.41)	1% (0.19)	9% (0.48)	11% (0.54)
Wyoming	414	29% (0.94)	38% (1.01)	6% (0.49)	2% (0.32)	10% (0.63)	14% (0.73)
PACIFIC	**33,556**	**31%** (0.29)	**29%** (0.29)	**12%** (0.21)	**2%** (0.08)	**7%** (0.17)	**19%** (0.25)
Alaska	435	29% (0.80)	30% (0.80)	8% (0.48)	4% (0.33)	6% (0.42)	23% (0.73)
California	25,588	30% (0.35)	27% (0.33)	13% (0.25)	1% (0.09)	7% (0.20)	20% (0.30)
Hawaii	850	41% (0.99)	31% (0.93)	9% (0.56)	2% (0.29)	6% (0.48)	11% (0.62)
Oregon	2,464	34% (0.93)	35% (0.94)	7% (0.50)	1% (0.23)	7% (0.49)	15% (0.70)
Washington	4,219	35% (0.86)	33% (0.85)	8% (0.50)	3% (0.29)	8% (0.49)	13% (0.60)

Source: Three-year merged March CPS, 1989, 1990, and 1991.

TABLE A2
CHILDREN UNDER AGE 18: BY TYPE OF HEALTH INSURANCE COVERAGE

	Number (000s)	Employer	Medicaid	Other	Uninsured
UNITED STATES	63,262	64% (0.19)	17% (0.15)	5% (0.09)	14% (0.14)
NEW ENGLAND	2,994	73% (0.64)	14% (0.49)	4% (0.28)	9% (0.41)
Connecticut	740	79% (1.64)	10% (1.18)	3% (0.66)	9% (1.14)
Maine	308	70% (1.58)	17% (1.28)	6% (0.79)	8% (0.92)
Massachusetts	1,331	71% (0.87)	17% (0.72)	4% (0.36)	8% (0.51)
New Hampshire	271	69% (1.77)	5% (0.80)	6% (0.91)	20% (1.54)
Rhode Island	216	77% (1.69)	13% (1.37)	3% (0.72)	6% (0.97)
Vermont	130	71% (1.77)	12% (1.26)	9% (1.10)	9% (1.09)
MIDDLE ATLANTIC	9,153	69% (0.45)	19% (0.38)	4% (0.19)	8% (0.27)
New Jersey	1,776	73% (0.82)	14% (0.64)	5% (0.39)	9% (0.52)
New York	4,430	64% (0.69)	24% (0.61)	4% (0.26)	9% (0.40)
Pennsylvania	2,947	72% (0.78)	15% (0.63)	4% (0.36)	8% (0.48)
SOUTH ATLANTIC	10,038	63% (0.49)	15% (0.37)	5% (0.22)	16% (0.38)
Delaware	157	69% (1.75)	13% (1.26)	3% (0.68)	15% (1.35)
District of Columbia	124	46% (2.11)	35% (2.02)	4% (0.78)	15% (1.49)
Florida	2,815	57% (0.87)	15% (0.62)	6% (0.42)	22% (0.73)
Georgia	1,610	62% (1.59)	18% (1.26)	5% (0.73)	15% (1.17)
Maryland	1,042	73% (1.69)	17% (1.44)	2% (0.48)	8% (1.04)
North Carolina	1,470	65% (0.87)	15% (0.65)	6% (0.42)	14% (0.64)
South Carolina	845	65% (1.47)	14% (1.07)	5% (0.65)	17% (1.15)
Virginia	1,497	67% (1.43)	10% (0.93)	5% (0.65)	18% (1.16)
West Virginia	476	63% (1.59)	21% (1.35)	5% (0.71)	11% (1.02)
EAST SOUTH CENTRAL	4,001	59% (0.81)	20% (0.66)	5% (0.36)	16% (0.60)
Alabama	1,100	62% (1.57)	14% (1.12)	5% (0.70)	19% (1.27)
Kentucky	890	62% (1.67)	21% (1.40)	5% (0.72)	12% (1.14)
Mississippi	772	50% (1.46)	29% (1.33)	6% (0.68)	16% (1.07)
Tennessee	1,239	60% (1.57)	20% (1.28)	5% (0.68)	15% (1.16)
WEST SOUTH CENTRAL	7,493	55% (0.62)	16% (0.46)	6% (0.30)	23% (0.52)
Arkansas	693	57% (1.53)	17% (1.17)	6% (0.70)	20% (1.24)
Louisiana	1,173	50% (1.66)	24% (1.41)	6% (0.77)	21% (1.36)
Oklahoma	796	55% (1.65)	17% (1.26)	8% (0.90)	19% (1.32)
Texas	4,831	56% (0.80)	14% (0.56)	6% (0.38)	24% (0.69)

CHILDREN UNDER AGE 18: BY TYPE OF HEALTH INSURANCE COVERAGE

	Number (000s)	Employer	Medicaid	Other	Uninsured
EAST NORTH CENTRAL	**10,951**	**70%**	**18%**	**5%**	**8%**
		(0.44)	**(0.36)**	**(0.20)**	**(0.26)**
Illinois	2,997	65%	22%	5%	8%
		(0.84)	(0.72)	(0.38)	(0.48)
Indiana	1,382	67%	11%	8%	14%
		(1.64)	(1.08)	(0.94)	(1.21)
Michigan	2,446	69%	21%	3%	7%
		(0.80)	(0.70)	(0.31)	(0.43)
Ohio	2,920	73%	17%	3%	7%
		(0.75)	(0.63)	(0.30)	(0.42)
Wisconsin	1,205	78%	11%	6%	5%
		(1.33)	(1.00)	(0.75)	(0.72)
WEST NORTH CENTRAL	**4,731**	**68%**	**13%**	**9%**	**10%**
		(0.69)	**(0.49)**	**(0.42)**	**(0.45)**
Iowa	731	72%	11%	11%	6%
		(1.44)	(1.00)	(1.01)	(0.75)
Kansas	634	73%	13%	6%	8%
		(1.43)	(1.09)	(0.77)	(0.87)
Minnesota	1,192	65%	15%	9%	10%
		(1.57)	(1.19)	(0.96)	(0.98)
Missouri	1,375	68%	12%	6%	14%
		(1.57)	(1.10)	(0.79)	(1.16)
Nebraska	433	68%	10%	12%	10%
		(1.43)	(0.94)	(1.00)	(0.91)
North Dakota	180	61%	10%	20%	8%
		(1.46)	(0.91)	(1.21)	(0.80)
South Dakota	186	61%	10%	13%	16%
		(1.42)	(0.86)	(0.99)	(1.08)
MOUNTAIN	**3,841**	**64%**	**11%**	**7%**	**18%**
		(0.66)	**(0.43)**	**(0.34)**	**(0.53)**
Arizona	939	59%	14%	5%	22%
		(1.65)	(1.18)	(0.72)	(1.38)
Colorado	898	65%	11%	5%	19%
		(1.64)	(1.07)	(0.77)	(1.34)
Idaho	314	65%	7%	12%	16%
		(1.38)	(0.75)	(0.94)	(1.06)
Montana	231	57%	14%	13%	16%
		(1.53)	(1.07)	(1.03)	(1.14)
Nevada	285	68%	8%	7%	17%
		(1.65)	(0.97)	(0.91)	(1.32)
New Mexico	424	53%	14%	5%	29%
		(1.54)	(1.06)	(0.70)	(1.39)
Utah	617	76%	9%	7%	8%
		(1.17)	(0.79)	(0.68)	(0.75)
Wyoming	133	69%	10%	10%	11%
		(1.69)	(1.10)	(1.09)	(1.15)
PACIFIC	**10,061**	**56%**	**22%**	**5%**	**16%**
		(0.57)	**(0.48)**	**(0.26)**	**(0.42)**
Alaska	140	59%	17%	6%	17%
		(1.52)	(1.16)	(0.76)	(1.16)
California	7,718	53%	24%	5%	18%
		(0.68)	(0.59)	(0.30)	(0.52)
Hawaii	224	66%	18%	4%	11%
		(1.85)	(1.51)	(0.81)	(1.22)
Oregon	750	68%	13%	5%	14%
		(1.65)	(1.19)	(0.75)	(1.24)
Washington	1,229	68%	17%	7%	9%
		(1.56)	(1.24)	(0.84)	(0.94)

Source: **Three-year merged March CPS, 1989, 1990, and 1991.**

TABLE A3

ADULTS AGES 18-65: BY TYPE OF HEALTH INSURANCE COVERAGE

	Number (000s)	Employer (own)	Employer (other)	Medicaid	Other	Uninsured
UNITED STATES	150,318	47% (0.13)	20% (0.10)	6% (0.06)	11% (0.08)	16% (0.10)
NEW ENGLAND	8,163	52% (0.44)	23% (0.37)	4% (0.18)	10% (0.26)	12% (0.28)
Connecticut	2,022	56% (1.21)	22% (1.01)	3% (0.39)	8% (0.67)	10% (0.74)
Maine	747	47% (1.10)	22% (0.91)	7% (0.55)	12% (0.72)	13% (0.73)
Massachusetts	3,731	51% (0.57)	23% (0.48)	5% (0.25)	10% (0.34)	11% (0.36)
New Hampshire	701	49% (1.20)	23% (1.00)	2% (0.34)	11% (0.75)	15% (0.84)
Rhode Island	607	51% (1.20)	22% (0.99)	5% (0.50)	9% (0.70)	13% (0.80)
Vermont	355	50% (1.18)	22% (0.98)	5% (0.50)	11% (0.74)	12% (0.77)
MIDDLE ATLANTIC	23,262	50% (0.30)	22% (0.25)	6% (0.14)	9% (0.18)	14% (0.21)
New Jersey	4,855	54% (0.56)	21% (0.45)	4% (0.21)	9% (0.33)	12% (0.36)
New York	11,077	47% (0.45)	20% (0.37)	7% (0.23)	9% (0.26)	16% (0.33)
Pennsylvania	7,330	51% (0.55)	24% (0.47)	5% (0.24)	9% (0.32)	11% (0.35)
SOUTH ATLANTIC	25,967	48% (0.32)	18% (0.25)	5% (0.13)	11% (0.20)	17% (0.24)
Delaware	417	52% (1.16)	19% (0.91)	3% (0.40)	10% (0.70)	16% (0.85)
District of Columbia	369	49% (1.23)	8% (0.68)	9% (0.69)	11% (0.78)	22% (1.02)
Florida	7,518	44% (0.54)	17% (0.40)	4% (0.21)	13% (0.37)	22% (0.44)
Georgia	3,865	49% (1.06)	18% (0.82)	5% (0.47)	10% (0.63)	18% (0.82)
Maryland	2,936	53% (1.13)	22% (0.93)	5% (0.47)	9% (0.64)	12% (0.74)
North Carolina	3,998	52% (0.55)	17% (0.42)	5% (0.24)	12% (0.35)	15% (0.39)
South Carolina	2,087	51% (0.98)	19% (0.77)	5% (0.42)	10% (0.60)	15% (0.71)
Virginia	3,669	51% (0.97)	20% (0.77)	4% (0.37)	10% (0.58)	16% (0.70)
West Virginia	1,110	42% (1.07)	23% (0.91)	10% (0.64)	9% (0.64)	16% (0.79)
EAST SOUTH CENTRAL	9,213	44% (0.54)	20% (0.44)	7% (0.28)	12% (0.35)	17% (0.41)
Alabama	2,469	44% (1.07)	20% (0.86)	5% (0.48)	11% (0.69)	20% (0.86)
Kentucky	2,233	44% (1.08)	21% (0.90)	9% (0.62)	12% (0.70)	15% (0.77)
Mississippi	1,513	38% (1.02)	18% (0.81)	8% (0.58)	13% (0.71)	22% (0.87)
Tennessee	2,997	46% (1.03)	21% (0.84)	6% (0.50)	11% (0.64)	15% (0.75)
WEST SOUTH CENTRAL	15,962	41% (0.42)	19% (0.33)	5% (0.18)	12% (0.28)	23% (0.36)
Arkansas	1,410	40% (1.06)	20% (0.86)	6% (0.50)	14% (0.75)	20% (0.87)
Louisiana	2,528	36% (1.09)	21% (0.93)	8% (0.61)	12% (0.74)	22% (0.94)
Oklahoma	1,882	40% (1.06)	20% (0.87)	5% (0.46)	13% (0.74)	22% (0.89)
Texas	10,142	43% (0.55)	17% (0.42)	4% (0.22)	12% (0.36)	24% (0.48)

TABLE A3 (continued)
ADULTS AGES 18-65: BY TYPE OF HEALTH INSURANCE COVERAGE

	Number (000s)	Employer (own)	Employer (other)	Medicaid	Other	Uninsured
EAST NORTH CENTRAL	25,836	49% (0.31)	23% (0.26)	6% (0.14)	10% (0.18)	12% (0.20)
Illinois	7,174	49% (0.57)	22% (0.47)	6% (0.27)	10% (0.35)	13% (0.38)
Indiana	3,391	48% (1.12)	24% (0.95)	3% (0.40)	11% (0.69)	14% (0.78)
Michigan	5,755	48% (0.56)	24% (0.48)	8% (0.30)	9% (0.32)	12% (0.36)
Ohio	6,617	49% (0.56)	24% (0.48)	5% (0.25)	9% (0.32)	12% (0.36)
Wisconsin	2,898	51% (1.03)	25% (0.89)	4% (0.41)	10% (0.62)	10% (0.62)
WEST NORTH CENTRAL	10,548	47% (0.49)	21% (0.41)	4% (0.20)	15% (0.36)	12% (0.33)
Iowa	1,655	45% (1.06)	22% (0.88)	4% (0.42)	19% (0.84)	10% (0.64)
Kansas	1,444	47% (1.07)	23% (0.90)	4% (0.43)	14% (0.74)	12% (0.68)
Minnesota	2,657	49% (1.10)	20% (0.88)	5% (0.49)	15% (0.78)	12% (0.72)
Missouri	3,100	49% (1.12)	22% (0.93)	4% (0.45)	11% (0.72)	14% (0.78)
Nebraska	927	45% (1.04)	21% (0.86)	3% (0.38)	18% (0.80)	13% (0.70)
North Dakota	366	37% (1.01)	22% (0.87)	4% (0.39)	27% (0.93)	11% (0.66)
South Dakota	399	39% (0.97)	20% (0.80)	4% (0.38)	22% (0.83)	15% (0.72)
MOUNTAIN	7,871	45% (0.47)	20% (0.38)	4% (0.18)	13% (0.32)	19% (0.37)
Arizona	2,078	46% (1.12)	19% (0.88)	4% (0.42)	13% (0.76)	19% (0.88)
Colorado	1,938	47% (1.17)	20% (0.94)	4% (0.44)	12% (0.76)	17% (0.88)
Idaho	582	42% (1.04)	20% (0.85)	3% (0.35)	16% (0.77)	19% (0.83)
Montana	480	40% (1.05)	19% (0.85)	5% (0.47)	17% (0.81)	18% (0.83)
Nevada	725	52% (1.11)	16% (0.82)	3% (0.38)	9% (0.65)	20% (0.90)
New Mexico	878	36% (1.03)	19% (0.84)	5% (0.47)	13% (0.72)	28% (0.96)
Utah	909	46% (1.12)	26% (0.98)	4% (0.44)	12% (0.72)	12% (0.74)
Wyoming	281	42% (1.25)	24% (1.08)	4% (0.48)	14% (0.88)	16% (0.92)
PACIFIC	23,495	45% (0.38)	17% (0.29)	8% (0.20)	11% (0.23)	20% (0.30)
Alaska	295	43% (1.05)	17% (0.79)	4% (0.42)	11% (0.67)	25% (0.92)
California	17,870	43% (0.45)	16% (0.33)	8% (0.25)	10% (0.27)	21% (0.37)
Hawaii	626	55% (1.16)	19% (0.92)	5% (0.52)	10% (0.69)	11% (0.72)
Oregon	1,714	49% (1.17)	21% (0.96)	4% (0.48)	10% (0.70)	16% (0.85)
Washington	2,990	49% (1.07)	19% (0.84)	5% (0.46)	13% (0.71)	14% (0.75)

Source: Three-year merged March CPS, 1989, 1990, and 1991.

TABLE A4

MALES UNDER AGE 65: BY TYPE OF HEALTH INSURANCE COVERAGE

	Number (000s)	Employer (own)	Employer (other)	Medicaid	Other	Uninsured
UNITED STATES	105,945	40% (0.15)	27% (0.14)	7% (0.08)	9% (0.09)	17% (0.12)
NEW ENGLAND	5,562	45% (0.53)	30% (0.48)	5% (0.23)	8% (0.29)	12% (0.35)
Connecticut	1,381	49% (1.47)	30% (1.35)	4% (0.58)	6% (0.69)	11% (0.93)
Maine	523	39% (1.28)	31% (1.22)	8% (0.72)	10% (0.78)	12% (0.86)
Massachusetts	2,516	45% (0.69)	29% (0.63)	6% (0.33)	9% (0.39)	11% (0.44)
New Hampshire	483	44% (1.43)	27% (1.28)	2% (0.40)	10% (0.87)	17% (1.07)
Rhode Island	419	43% (1.43)	31% (1.33)	5% (0.63)	7% (0.74)	14% (0.99)
Vermont	241	42% (1.41)	30% (1.31)	5% (0.64)	10% (0.87)	13% (0.95)
MIDDLE ATLANTIC	16,017	43% (0.36)	28% (0.33)	8% (0.19)	8% (0.19)	13% (0.25)
New Jersey	3,292	47% (0.68)	28% (0.61)	5% (0.30)	8% (0.37)	12% (0.44)
New York	7,668	41% (0.54)	27% (0.48)	9% (0.32)	8% (0.29)	15% (0.39)
Pennsylvania	5,057	45% (0.66)	30% (0.61)	6% (0.33)	7% (0.35)	11% (0.42)
SOUTH ATLANTIC	17,739	41% (0.38)	25% (0.33)	6% (0.18)	9% (0.22)	19% (0.30)
Delaware	284	45% (1.40)	26% (1.24)	4% (0.55)	9% (0.80)	16% (1.02)
District of Columbia	237	38% (1.48)	14% (1.08)	13% (1.02)	11% (0.96)	24% (1.31)
Florida	5,086	36% (0.63)	22% (0.55)	5% (0.30)	11% (0.42)	24% (0.56)
Georgia	2,702	40% (1.24)	27% (1.12)	7% (0.65)	8% (0.67)	19% (0.99)
Maryland	1,900	49% (1.41)	26% (1.24)	6% (0.66)	7% (0.71)	12% (0.92)
North Carolina	2,740	43% (0.66)	25% (0.58)	6% (0.32)	10% (0.41)	16% (0.48)
South Carolina	1,479	40% (1.14)	27% (1.04)	6% (0.55)	9% (0.67)	18% (0.89)
Virginia	2,533	43% (1.16)	27% (1.04)	3% (0.42)	9% (0.67)	17% (0.89)
West Virginia	778	39% (1.26)	26% (1.14)	12% (0.84)	8% (0.69)	15% (0.93)
EAST SOUTH CENTRAL	6,465	36% (0.62)	26% (0.57)	9% (0.37)	10% (0.38)	19% (0.51)
Alabama	1,723	36% (1.24)	25% (1.12)	7% (0.64)	10% (0.77)	22% (1.07)
Kentucky	1,533	38% (1.28)	27% (1.16)	10% (0.79)	10% (0.78)	16% (0.96)
Mississippi	1,127	31% (1.12)	23% (1.03)	13% (0.81)	10% (0.74)	22% (1.01)
Tennessee	2,082	38% (1.21)	28% (1.11)	8% (0.69)	9% (0.71)	17% (0.92)
WEST SOUTH CENTRAL	11,621	34% (0.47)	24% (0.43)	7% (0.25)	10% (0.30)	25% (0.43)
Arkansas	1,046	31% (1.16)	28% (1.13)	7% (0.65)	11% (0.77)	23% (1.05)
Louisiana	1,790	33% (1.27)	24% (1.15)	10% (0.82)	9% (0.79)	23% (1.13)
Oklahoma	1,368	35% (1.21)	24% (1.08)	7% (0.63)	12% (0.83)	23% (1.06)
Texas	7,417	34% (0.62)	24% (0.55)	6% (0.31)	10% (0.39)	26% (0.57)

	Number (000s)	Employer (own)	Employer (other)	Medicaid	Other	Uninsured
EAST NORTH CENTRAL	18,257	43% (0.37)	29% (0.33)	7% (0.19)	8% (0.20)	12% (0.24)
Illinois	5,104	43% (0.67)	26% (0.59)	8% (0.37)	8% (0.37)	14% (0.46)
Indiana	2,340	43% (1.33)	29% (1.22)	4% (0.52)	11% (0.84)	13% (0.91)
Michigan	4,111	43% (0.66)	29% (0.61)	9% (0.39)	7% (0.35)	11% (0.42)
Ohio	4,642	43% (0.66)	31% (0.62)	7% (0.34)	8% (0.35)	11% (0.42)
Wisconsin	2,061	45% (1.21)	32% (1.13)	5% (0.51)	9% (0.71)	9% (0.70)
WEST NORTH CENTRAL	7,601	38% (0.57)	30% (0.53)	5% (0.27)	14% (0.40)	12% (0.39)
Iowa	1,198	38% (1.22)	31% (1.16)	4% (0.52)	17% (0.94)	9% (0.73)
Kansas	1,017	40% (1.25)	32% (1.19)	5% (0.56)	12% (0.83)	11% (0.81)
Minnesota	1,924	39% (1.27)	29% (1.17)	7% (0.66)	14% (0.89)	12% (0.83)
Missouri	2,213	40% (1.30)	30% (1.22)	5% (0.59)	10% (0.79)	15% (0.94)
Nebraska	678	36% (1.18)	29% (1.12)	5% (0.54)	16% (0.90)	14% (0.84)
North Dakota	278	29% (1.09)	30% (1.10)	5% (0.53)	26% (1.05)	11% (0.74)
South Dakota	293	30% (1.07)	29% (1.06)	4% (0.44)	19% (0.92)	17% (0.88)
MOUNTAIN	5,842	36% (0.53)	29% (0.50)	5% (0.24)	11% (0.34)	20% (0.44)
Arizona	1,503	36% (1.27)	27% (1.18)	6% (0.62)	10% (0.79)	21% (1.08)
Colorado	1,396	37% (1.33)	30% (1.26)	4% (0.54)	10% (0.82)	19% (1.08)
Idaho	449	34% (1.15)	29% (1.09)	3% (0.43)	15% (0.85)	19% (0.94)
Montana	360	32% (1.15)	27% (1.10)	7% (0.64)	16% (0.92)	18% (0.94)
Nevada	511	41% (1.31)	26% (1.16)	3% (0.45)	9% (0.76)	21% (1.08)
New Mexico	653	30% (1.14)	24% (1.06)	6% (0.58)	11% (0.77)	30% (1.13)
Utah	759	35% (1.17)	38% (1.19)	5% (0.55)	9% (0.71)	13% (0.82)
Wyoming	210	37% (1.41)	30% (1.34)	4% (0.58)	13% (0.97)	16% (1.07)
PACIFIC	16,841	37% (0.43)	23% (0.38)	10% (0.27)	9% (0.26)	21% (0.36)
Alaska	227	33% (1.14)	26% (1.06)	6% (0.58)	9% (0.70)	25% (1.05)
California	12,829	36% (0.51)	22% (0.44)	11% (0.33)	9% (0.30)	22% (0.44)
Hawaii	431	48% (1.41)	26% (1.24)	7% (0.72)	7% (0.74)	11% (0.89)
Oregon	1,240	41% (1.36)	28% (1.25)	5% (0.61)	9% (0.79)	16% (1.02)
Washington	2,114	41% (1.25)	28% (1.15)	6% (0.61)	10% (0.78)	14% (0.88)

Source: Three-year merged March CPS, 1989, 1990, and 1991.

TABLE A5
FEMALES UNDER AGE 65: BY TYPE OF HEALTH INSURANCE COVERAGE

	Number (000s)	Employer (own)	Employer (other)	Medicaid	Other	Uninsured
UNITED STATES	107,634	26% (0.14)	39% (0.15)	11% (0.10)	9% (0.09)	14% (0.11)
NEW ENGLAND	5,595	31% (0.49)	43% (0.52)	9% (0.30)	8% (0.29)	10% (0.31)
Connecticut	1,381	33% (1.39)	45% (1.46)	6% (0.70)	8% (0.79)	8% (0.82)
Maine	532	28% (1.17)	40% (1.28)	11% (0.81)	11% (0.82)	10% (0.79)
Massachusetts	2,545	30% (0.64)	42% (0.68)	11% (0.43)	8% (0.37)	9% (0.40)
New Hampshire	489	27% (1.28)	44% (1.42)	4% (0.56)	9% (0.82)	16% (1.04)
Rhode Island	404	33% (1.37)	42% (1.45)	9% (0.83)	9% (0.82)	8% (0.81)
Vermont	243	31% (1.31)	41% (1.40)	8% (0.77)	10% (0.87)	10% (0.86)
MIDDLE ATLANTIC	16,398	28% (0.32)	41% (0.35)	11% (0.23)	8% (0.19)	11% (0.22)
New Jersey	3,339	33% (0.63)	42% (0.66)	8% (0.36)	8% (0.37)	10% (0.40)
New York	7,839	27% (0.48)	39% (0.53)	14% (0.38)	8% (0.29)	13% (0.36)
Pennsylvania	5,221	28% (0.59)	45% (0.65)	9% (0.38)	8% (0.37)	9% (0.38)
SOUTH ATLANTIC	18,266	29% (0.34)	36% (0.36)	9% (0.22)	9% (0.22)	15% (0.27)
Delaware	290	31% (1.29)	39% (1.36)	6% (0.68)	8% (0.74)	16% (1.02)
District of Columbia	256	36% (1.41)	21% (1.20)	18% (1.13)	8% (0.80)	17% (1.11)
Florida	5,247	28% (0.58)	33% (0.61)	8% (0.36)	11% (0.41)	19% (0.51)
Georgia	2,773	29% (1.14)	35% (1.19)	11% (0.78)	9% (0.72)	16% (0.91)
Maryland	2,077	30% (1.24)	43% (1.34)	10% (0.80)	7% (0.68)	10% (0.81)
North Carolina	2,729	33% (0.63)	35% (0.64)	9% (0.38)	10% (0.39)	14% (0.46)
South Carolina	1,453	32% (1.10)	37% (1.14)	9% (0.68)	8% (0.65)	14% (0.81)
Virginia	2,633	29% (1.04)	39% (1.12)	8% (0.62)	8% (0.63)	15% (0.82)
West Virginia	808	20% (1.01)	44% (1.26)	14% (0.89)	8% (0.71)	13% (0.87)
EAST SOUTH CENTRAL	6,749	25% (0.55)	38% (0.62)	13% (0.42)	9% (0.37)	15% (0.46)
Alabama	1,847	25% (1.07)	40% (1.22)	9% (0.72)	9% (0.71)	18% (0.95)
Kentucky	1,590	25% (1.12)	39% (1.26)	14% (0.91)	10% (0.76)	12% (0.84)
Mississippi	1,158	19% (0.95)	34% (1.14)	17% (0.91)	11% (0.75)	18% (0.91)
Tennessee	2,154	27% (1.09)	37% (1.18)	12% (0.79)	9% (0.69)	14% (0.85)
WEST SOUTH CENTRAL	11,834	22% (0.41)	36% (0.48)	10% (0.30)	10% (0.30)	21% (0.41)
Arkansas	1,057	23% (1.05)	36% (1.20)	12% (0.80)	12% (0.81)	18% (0.96)
Louisiana	1,911	17% (0.98)	36% (1.25)	15% (0.94)	11% (0.81)	21% (1.06)
Oklahoma	1,310	21% (1.06)	38% (1.26)	10% (0.79)	12% (0.83)	19% (1.02)
Texas	7,556	24% (0.55)	36% (0.62)	8% (0.36)	10% (0.38)	22% (0.54)

FEMALES UNDER AGE 65: BY TYPE OF HEALTH INSURANCE COVERAGE

	Number (000s)	Employer (own)	Employer (other)	Medicaid	Other	Uninsured
EAST NORTH CENTRAL	**18,529**	**26%** (0.32)	**45%** (0.36)	**11%** (0.23)	**8%** (0.20)	**10%** (0.22)
Illinois	5,067	26% (0.60)	43% (0.67)	13% (0.45)	9% (0.39)	9% (0.40)
Indiana	2,434	26% (1.15)	43% (1.31)	7% (0.68)	9% (0.76)	15% (0.93)
Michigan	4,091	24% (0.57)	46% (0.67)	14% (0.46)	7% (0.35)	9% (0.38)
Ohio	4,895	26% (0.57)	47% (0.65)	11% (0.40)	7% (0.34)	9% (0.38)
Wisconsin	2,043	26% (1.08)	49% (1.22)	8% (0.66)	8% (0.67)	8% (0.67)
WEST NORTH CENTRAL	**7,678**	**26%** (0.51)	**42%** (0.57)	**8%** (0.32)	**13%** (0.39)	**11%** (0.36)
Iowa	1,187	24% (1.07)	44% (1.25)	8% (0.67)	17% (0.94)	8% (0.69)
Kansas	1,061	26% (1.09)	45% (1.24)	9% (0.70)	11% (0.79)	10% (0.74)
Minnesota	1,925	28% (1.17)	39% (1.27)	10% (0.77)	12% (0.85)	11% (0.81)
Missouri	2,263	28% (1.18)	42% (1.30)	8% (0.71)	10% (0.78)	13% (0.88)
Nebraska	682	25% (1.06)	43% (1.21)	6% (0.59)	16% (0.89)	10% (0.74)
North Dakota	268	20% (0.99)	40% (1.20)	7% (0.62)	24% (1.04)	9% (0.71)
South Dakota	292	22% (0.97)	37% (1.12)	8% (0.62)	19% (0.92)	14% (0.80)
MOUNTAIN	**5,870**	**25%** (0.48)	**40%** (0.54)	**8%** (0.29)	**11%** (0.34)	**17%** (0.42)
Arizona	1,513	27% (1.17)	35% (1.26)	8% (0.73)	11% (0.82)	19% (1.03)
Colorado	1,439	27% (1.20)	39% (1.32)	8% (0.73)	10% (0.81)	16% (1.00)
Idaho	448	20% (0.97)	43% (1.19)	6% (0.55)	14% (0.84)	18% (0.92)
Montana	351	22% (1.04)	36% (1.20)	9% (0.71)	15% (0.90)	18% (0.95)
Nevada	499	34% (1.27)	36% (1.29)	5% (0.58)	9% (0.75)	17% (1.02)
New Mexico	649	18% (0.96)	36% (1.20)	10% (0.74)	10% (0.75)	26% (1.10)
Utah	767	20% (0.97)	54% (1.22)	7% (0.62)	10% (0.74)	9% (0.70)
Wyoming	204	20% (1.19)	47% (1.48)	7% (0.78)	13% (0.99)	13% (0.99)
PACIFIC	**16,715**	**26%** (0.39)	**35%** (0.43)	**14%** (0.31)	**9%** (0.26)	**17%** (0.33)
Alaska	208	25% (1.09)	35% (1.20)	11% (0.78)	10% (0.76)	20% (1.01)
California	12,759	25% (0.46)	33% (0.50)	15% (0.38)	9% (0.30)	18% (0.41)
Hawaii	419	34% (1.35)	37% (1.38)	10% (0.87)	9% (0.83)	10% (0.85)
Oregon	1,225	27% (1.23)	42% (1.37)	9% (0.79)	8% (0.74)	14% (0.97)
Washington	2,104	29% (1.15)	38% (1.24)	11% (0.78)	11% (0.81)	11% (0.81)

Source: Three-year merged March CPS, 1989, 1990, and 1991.

TABLE A6
WHITES UNDER AGE 65: BY TYPE OF HEALTH INSURANCE COVERAGE

	Number (000s)	Employer (own)	Employer (other)	Medicaid	Other	Uninsured
UNITED STATES	178,211	34% (0.11)	35% (0.11)	7% (0.06)	10% (0.07)	14% (0.08)
NEW ENGLAND	10,363	38% (0.38)	37% (0.37)	6% (0.18)	8% (0.21)	11% (0.24)
Connecticut	2,437	42% (1.09)	38% (1.08)	4% (0.41)	7% (0.55)	9% (0.64)
Maine	1,042	33% (0.88)	36% (0.89)	9% (0.54)	10% (0.57)	11% (0.59)
Massachusetts	4,682	38% (0.50)	37% (0.49)	7% (0.26)	8% (0.28)	10% (0.31)
New Hampshire	953	36% (0.98)	36% (0.98)	3% (0.35)	10% (0.61)	16% (0.75)
Rhode Island	768	39% (1.04)	37% (1.03)	6% (0.51)	7% (0.56)	11% (0.65)
Vermont	480	36% (0.97)	35% (0.97)	7% (0.50)	10% (0.62)	11% (0.64)
MIDDLE ATLANTIC	27,103	37% (0.27)	37% (0.27)	7% (0.14)	8% (0.15)	11% (0.17)
New Jersey	5,422	41% (0.52)	37% (0.51)	4% (0.21)	8% (0.29)	10% (0.31)
New York	12,525	35% (0.41)	35% (0.41)	9% (0.25)	8% (0.23)	12% (0.28)
Pennsylvania	9,156	37% (0.48)	40% (0.48)	6% (0.23)	8% (0.27)	9% (0.29)
SOUTH ATLANTIC	26,728	37% (0.30)	33% (0.29)	4% (0.12)	10% (0.19)	15% (0.22)
Delaware	452	40% (1.09)	35% (1.06)	3% (0.36)	9% (0.65)	14% (0.77)
District of Columbia	156	48% (1.88)	14% (1.32)	5% (0.80)	15% (1.33)	18% (1.45)
Florida	8,327	34% (0.49)	30% (0.47)	4% (0.20)	12% (0.34)	21% (0.41)
Georgia	3,449	39% (1.10)	36% (1.08)	2% (0.34)	9% (0.64)	13% (0.76)
Maryland	2,788	42% (1.15)	37% (1.13)	4% (0.45)	8% (0.62)	9% (0.68)
North Carolina	4,139	41% (0.53)	32% (0.51)	4% (0.22)	11% (0.34)	12% (0.36)
South Carolina	1,968	41% (0.99)	36% (0.97)	3% (0.35)	8% (0.56)	12% (0.65)
Virginia	3,932	38% (0.91)	36% (0.90)	3% (0.32)	9% (0.55)	14% (0.65)
West Virginia	1,518	30% (0.85)	36% (0.89)	13% (0.62)	8% (0.50)	14% (0.64)
EAST SOUTH CENTRAL	10,231	33% (0.48)	35% (0.49)	7% (0.26)	10% (0.32)	15% (0.37)
Alabama	2,535	33% (1.00)	37% (1.02)	3% (0.37)	10% (0.65)	17% (0.79)
Kentucky	2,942	32% (0.88)	34% (0.90)	11% (0.60)	10% (0.57)	14% (0.65)
Mississippi	1,372	30% (1.00)	35% (1.05)	7% (0.55)	13% (0.74)	15% (0.79)
Tennessee	3,382	35% (0.93)	34% (0.92)	6% (0.48)	10% (0.58)	15% (0.69)
WEST SOUTH CENTRAL	19,337	29% (0.35)	32% (0.36)	6% (0.18)	11% (0.24)	23% (0.32)
Arkansas	1,734	29% (0.89)	34% (0.92)	5% (0.44)	12% (0.64)	19% (0.76)
Louisiana	2,539	29% (1.03)	36% (1.09)	4% (0.42)	12% (0.75)	19% (0.88)
Oklahoma	2,224	31% (0.92)	33% (0.93)	6% (0.46)	12% (0.66)	19% (0.78)
Texas	12,841	29% (0.45)	31% (0.46)	6% (0.23)	10% (0.29)	25% (0.43)

TABLE A6 (continued)
WHITES UNDER AGE 65: BY TYPE OF HEALTH INSURANCE COVERAGE

	Number (000s)	Employer (own)	Employer (other)	Medicaid	Other	Uninsured
EAST NORTH CENTRAL	**31,586**	**36%** (0.27)	**40%** (0.27)	**6%** (0.13)	**8%** (0.16)	**10%** (0.17)
Illinois	8,244	37% (0.51)	38% (0.52)	6% (0.25)	9% (0.31)	10% (0.31)
Indiana	4,281	36% (0.95)	39% (0.97)	3% (0.32)	10% (0.60)	13% (0.66)
Michigan	6,868	35% (0.49)	40% (0.50)	8% (0.28)	8% (0.27)	9% (0.30)
Ohio	8,353	35% (0.47)	41% (0.49)	7% (0.25)	8% (0.26)	9% (0.29)
Wisconsin	3,839	37% (0.86)	42% (0.88)	4% (0.36)	9% (0.51)	8% (0.49)
WEST NORTH CENTRAL	**13,981**	**33%** (0.40)	**37%** (0.41)	**5%** (0.19)	**14%** (0.30)	**11%** (0.27)
Iowa	2,319	31% (0.84)	38% (0.88)	6% (0.41)	17% (0.68)	8% (0.50)
Kansas	1,878	33% (0.88)	39% (0.92)	5% (0.42)	12% (0.61)	10% (0.56)
Minnesota	3,582	35% (0.91)	34% (0.90)	6% (0.47)	14% (0.65)	11% (0.59)
Missouri	3,866	35% (0.96)	37% (0.97)	5% (0.44)	10% (0.61)	13% (0.68)
Nebraska	1,292	31% (0.82)	37% (0.86)	5% (0.37)	16% (0.66)	12% (0.57)
North Dakota	512	26% (0.77)	36% (0.85)	4% (0.34)	26% (0.78)	9% (0.50)
South Dakota	532	28% (0.78)	34% (0.82)	4% (0.32)	20% (0.70)	14% (0.59)
MOUNTAIN	**10,982**	**31%** (0.37)	**35%** (0.39)	**6%** (0.18)	**11%** (0.25)	**18%** (0.31)
Arizona	2,888	32% (0.89)	31% (0.89)	6% (0.47)	11% (0.59)	20% (0.76)
Colorado	2,624	33% (0.94)	35% (0.96)	5% (0.45)	10% (0.60)	17% (0.76)
Idaho	871	28% (0.77)	36% (0.83)	4% (0.35)	14% (0.61)	18% (0.66)
Montana	653	28% (0.82)	33% (0.86)	6% (0.44)	17% (0.68)	17% (0.69)
Nevada	901	38% (0.97)	32% (0.93)	3% (0.32)	9% (0.57)	18% (0.78)
New Mexico	1,166	25% (0.81)	31% (0.86)	6% (0.45)	11% (0.57)	27% (0.82)
Utah	1,470	27% (0.79)	47% (0.88)	6% (0.41)	10% (0.53)	10% (0.54)
Wyoming	409	29% (0.95)	39% (1.02)	6% (0.48)	13% (0.70)	14% (0.73)
PACIFIC	**27,899**	**32%** (0.32)	**29%** (0.32)	**11%** (0.22)	**9%** (0.20)	**19%** (0.27)
Alaska	328	33% (0.95)	33% (0.95)	4% (0.41)	10% (0.62)	19% (0.80)
California	21,148	31% (0.38)	28% (0.37)	12% (0.27)	9% (0.24)	20% (0.33)
Hawaii	235	40% (1.87)	29% (1.74)	8% (1.04)	10% (1.15)	12% (1.24)
Oregon	2,334	35% (0.96)	36% (0.97)	7% (0.50)	8% (0.55)	14% (0.70)
Washington	3,854	35% (0.90)	34% (0.89)	8% (0.51)	11% (0.58)	12% (0.61)

Source: **Three-year merged March CPS, 1989, 1990, and 1991.**

TABLE A7
NONWHITES UNDER AGE 65: BY TYPE OF HEALTH INSURANCE COVERAGE

	Number (000s)	Employer (own)	Employer (other)	Medicaid	Other	Uninsured
UNITED STATES	35,368	26% (0.25)	24% (0.24)	21% (0.23)	7% (0.15)	21% (0.23)
NEW ENGLAND	794	29% (1.33)	28% (1.31)	19% (1.14)	8% (0.81)	15% (1.05)
Connecticut	324	34% (3.00)	30% (2.89)	12% (2.07)	8% (1.69)	16% (2.30)
Maine	---	--- ---	--- ---	--- ---	--- ---	--- ---
Massachusetts	379	26% (1.63)	26% (1.65)	25% (1.62)	9% (1.06)	14% (1.29)
New Hampshire	---	--- ---	--- ---	--- ---	--- ---	--- ---
Rhode Island	55	28% (3.75)	24% (3.54)	17% (3.10)	13% (2.79)	18% (3.19)
Vermont	---	--- ---	--- ---	--- ---	--- ---	--- ---
MIDDLE ATLANTIC	5,312	28% (0.59)	23% (0.55)	22% (0.55)	6% (0.32)	20% (0.52)
New Jersey	1,209	33% (1.09)	26% (1.02)	18% (0.89)	7% (0.61)	16% (0.85)
New York	2,982	27% (0.80)	23% (0.76)	23% (0.76)	6% (0.44)	22% (0.75)
Pennsylvania	1,121	28% (1.31)	21% (1.20)	27% (1.30)	5% (0.63)	20% (1.17)
SOUTH ATLANTIC	9,277	28% (0.49)	24% (0.47)	18% (0.43)	7% (0.28)	23% (0.46)
Delaware	122	32% (2.08)	26% (1.95)	16% (1.63)	4% (0.90)	23% (1.87)
District of Columbia	337	31% (1.24)	20% (1.06)	21% (1.08)	7% (0.69)	22% (1.10)
Florida	2,007	24% (0.93)	21% (0.89)	20% (0.87)	8% (0.60)	26% (0.96)
Georgia	2,026	26% (1.33)	22% (1.27)	20% (1.22)	8% (0.81)	24% (1.30)
Maryland	1,190	34% (1.75)	30% (1.69)	17% (1.40)	5% (0.79)	15% (1.31)
North Carolina	1,330	29% (0.90)	25% (0.86)	18% (0.76)	7% (0.50)	22% (0.83)
South Carolina	964	26% (1.32)	24% (1.29)	17% (1.12)	9% (0.86)	24% (1.28)
Virginia	1,234	31% (1.61)	25% (1.51)	14% (1.22)	6% (0.81)	23% (1.47)
West Virginia	68	23% (3.86)	26% (4.00)	21% (3.71)	9% (2.59)	21% (3.74)
EAST SOUTH CENTRAL	2,983	22% (0.82)	23% (0.84)	25% (0.86)	6% (0.49)	24% (0.85)
Alabama	1,034	23% (1.45)	24% (1.47)	20% (1.37)	7% (0.88)	27% (1.54)
Kentucky	181	25% (3.43)	19% (3.16)	31% (3.70)	4% (1.61)	20% (3.22)
Mississippi	913	19% (1.09)	20% (1.11)	28% (1.26)	7% (0.71)	27% (1.24)
Tennessee	855	24% (1.72)	28% (1.81)	25% (1.75)	6% (0.94)	17% (1.51)
WEST SOUTH CENTRAL	4,117	21% (0.71)	23% (0.73)	22% (0.72)	8% (0.49)	26% (0.77)
Arkansas	369	16% (1.61)	23% (1.85)	28% (1.98)	6% (1.08)	26% (1.94)
Louisiana	1,162	15% (1.24)	17% (1.32)	33% (1.64)	5% (0.77)	29% (1.58)
Oklahoma	455	16% (1.66)	22% (1.89)	22% (1.90)	9% (1.28)	32% (2.14)
Texas	2,132	27% (1.12)	25% (1.10)	14% (0.88)	10% (0.77)	24% (1.07)

	Number (000s)	Employer (own)	Employer (other)	Medicaid	Other	Uninsured
EAST NORTH CENTRAL	5,201	24% (0.61)	21% (0.59)	29% (0.65)	7% (0.37)	18% (0.55)
Illinois	1,927	23% (0.96)	18% (0.88)	31% (1.06)	7% (0.58)	20% (0.92)
Indiana	492	18% (2.33)	17% (2.28)	31% (2.81)	9% (1.78)	25% (2.66)
Michigan	1,333	25% (1.05)	24% (1.04)	29% (1.11)	7% (0.61)	15% (0.86)
Ohio	1,184	27% (1.23)	25% (1.19)	25% (1.19)	7% (0.69)	16% (1.01)
Wisconsin	265	19% (2.77)	22% (2.91)	35% (3.38)	10% (2.08)	14% (2.49)
WEST NORTH CENTRAL	1,298	24% (1.25)	28% (1.31)	23% (1.24)	7% (0.75)	18% (1.13)
Iowa	---	---	---	---	---	---
Kansas	200	27% (2.66)	28% (2.69)	23% (2.53)	6% (1.42)	15% (2.13)
Minnesota	267	19% (2.85)	25% (3.14)	34% (3.44)	4% (1.49)	17% (2.73)
Missouri	610	27% (2.33)	31% (2.45)	16% (1.95)	8% (1.40)	18% (2.03)
Nebraska	68	33% (3.78)	20% (3.21)	26% (3.51)	5% (1.81)	16% (2.95)
North Dakota	34	12% (2.32)	15% (2.55)	38% (3.50)	8% (1.96)	27% (3.19)
South Dakota	53	10% (1.72)	20% (2.28)	27% (2.54)	9% (1.64)	34% (2.70)
MOUNTAIN	730	24% (1.39)	24% (1.40)	17% (1.24)	8% (0.87)	27% (1.44)
Arizona	129	27% (4.16)	27% (4.17)	19% (3.72)	7% (2.36)	21% (3.83)
Colorado	211	25% (3.20)	29% (3.34)	14% (2.58)	8% (1.95)	24% (3.13)
Idaho	---	---	---	---	---	---
Montana	58	20% (2.54)	18% (2.47)	30% (2.93)	6% (1.53)	26% (2.81)
Nevada	110	34% (2.82)	20% (2.39)	13% (2.03)	8% (1.59)	25% (2.58)
New Mexico	136	14% (1.95)	19% (2.21)	19% (2.24)	8% (1.56)	40% (2.77)
Utah	55	29% (4.28)	29% (4.31)	17% (3.59)	6% (2.19)	19% (3.72)
Wyoming	---	---	---	---	---	---
PACIFIC	5,657	30% (0.74)	26% (0.71)	17% (0.60)	8% (0.44)	19% (0.63)
Alaska	107	17% (1.39)	22% (1.53)	20% (1.48)	7% (0.95)	33% (1.73)
California	4,440	29% (0.85)	26% (0.82)	18% (0.72)	8% (0.50)	19% (0.73)
Hawaii	615	41% (1.21)	32% (1.15)	9% (0.69)	8% (0.65)	10% (0.74)
Oregon	130	21% (3.60)	22% (3.67)	11% (2.77)	12% (2.87)	34% (4.20)
Washington	365	29% (2.87)	28% (2.85)	11% (1.98)	13% (2.13)	20% (2.54)

Source: Three-year merged March CPS, 1989, 1990, and 1991.

TABLE A8
PERSONS UNDER AGE 65 IN MARRIED-COUPLE-WITH-CHILDREN FAMILIES:
BY TYPE OF HEALTH INSURANCE COVERAGE

	Number (000s)	Employer (own)	Employer (other)	Medicaid	Other	Uninsured
UNITED STATES	106,567	25% (0.21)	51% (0.24)	5% (0.10)	7% (0.12)	12% (0.16)
NEW ENGLAND	5,482	26% (0.73)	57% (0.82)	3% (0.29)	6% (0.38)	8% (0.44)
Connecticut	1,370	28% (2.07)	58% (2.26)	2% (0.60)	4% (0.84)	8% (1.26)
Maine	554	26% (1.73)	53% (1.98)	6% (0.93)	8% (1.05)	8% (1.05)
Massachusetts	2,401	26% (0.97)	58% (1.09)	4% (0.43)	6% (0.51)	6% (0.54)
New Hampshire	516	24% (1.85)	52% (2.16)	0% (0.28)	8% (1.19)	15% (1.53)
Rhode Island	390	27% (2.05)	59% (2.27)	3% (0.75)	5% (0.97)	6% (1.13)
Vermont	250	25% (1.87)	54% (2.16)	4% (0.86)	10% (1.29)	7% (1.13)
MIDDLE ATLANTIC	16,295	27% (0.49)	54% (0.56)	5% (0.24)	6% (0.27)	9% (0.32)
New Jersey	3,346	31% (0.96)	54% (1.04)	2% (0.29)	7% (0.51)	7% (0.53)
New York	7,552	26% (0.74)	53% (0.85)	6% (0.40)	6% (0.41)	10% (0.51)
Pennsylvania	5,397	26% (0.88)	55% (0.99)	5% (0.44)	6% (0.47)	8% (0.55)
SOUTH ATLANTIC	16,496	27% (0.55)	50% (0.62)	3% (0.20)	7% (0.31)	14% (0.42)
Delaware	253	26% (2.03)	54% (2.30)	1% (0.51)	6% (1.10)	12% (1.52)
District of Columbia	107	20% (2.84)	45% (3.50)	6% (1.68)	10% (2.11)	18% (2.72)
Florida	4,477	25% (0.93)	45% (1.08)	3% (0.36)	8% (0.59)	19% (0.86)
Georgia	2,568	27% (1.78)	51% (2.01)	1% (0.38)	7% (1.05)	14% (1.42)
Maryland	1,654	29% (2.12)	60% (2.29)	1% (0.47)	3% (0.82)	6% (1.15)
North Carolina	2,587	30% (0.98)	48% (1.06)	3% (0.39)	8% (0.58)	11% (0.66)
South Carolina	1,416	30% (1.69)	50% (1.85)	2% (0.57)	6% (0.89)	11% (1.17)
Virginia	2,548	27% (1.61)	52% (1.80)	2% (0.47)	7% (0.90)	12% (1.18)
West Virginia	886	24% (1.61)	50% (1.88)	11% (1.17)	6% (0.87)	10% (1.11)
EAST SOUTH CENTRAL	6,489	25% (0.87)	49% (1.00)	5% (0.45)	7% (0.50)	14% (0.70)
Alabama	1,740	26% (1.74)	50% (1.99)	2% (0.61)	6% (0.98)	15% (1.42)
Kentucky	1,586	23% (1.70)	49% (2.01)	10% (1.18)	6% (0.96)	12% (1.30)
Mississippi	1,102	22% (1.58)	46% (1.89)	7% (0.94)	9% (1.09)	17% (1.41)
Tennessee	2,061	28% (1.73)	48% (1.93)	4% (0.78)	6% (0.92)	14% (1.33)
WEST SOUTH CENTRAL	12,331	22% (0.62)	44% (0.75)	4% (0.30)	8% (0.41)	22% (0.62)
Arkansas	1,037	23% (1.64)	48% (1.95)	4% (0.75)	8% (1.05)	17% (1.48)
Louisiana	1,871	21% (1.67)	47% (2.03)	4% (0.80)	8% (1.10)	20% (1.64)
Oklahoma	1,388	22% (1.61)	45% (1.94)	4% (0.81)	10% (1.17)	19% (1.54)
Texas	8,034	22% (0.80)	43% (0.96)	4% (0.38)	8% (0.52)	23% (0.82)

TABLE A8 (continued)
PERSONS UNDER AGE 65 IN MARRIED-COUPLE-WITH-CHILDREN FAMILIES:
BY TYPE OF HEALTH INSURANCE COVERAGE

	Number (000s)	Employer (own)	Employer (other)	Medicaid	Other	Uninsured
EAST NORTH CENTRAL	**18,448**	**26%** (0.50)	**57%** (0.56)	**4%** (0.23)	**6%** (0.28)	**7%** (0.28)
Illinois	4,936	26% (0.93)	55% (1.06)	5% (0.45)	7% (0.55)	7% (0.55)
Indiana	2,393	26% (1.81)	55% (2.05)	1% (0.47)	8% (1.14)	9% (1.21)
Michigan	3,950	25% (0.92)	57% (1.04)	6% (0.50)	5% (0.47)	6% (0.50)
Ohio	4,981	27% (0.88)	58% (0.98)	5% (0.42)	5% (0.43)	6% (0.46)
Wisconsin	2,189	26% (1.61)	58% (1.81)	3% (0.66)	7% (0.94)	5% (0.83)
WEST NORTH CENTRAL	**8,313**	**24%** (0.74)	**52%** (0.86)	**4%** (0.34)	**12%** (0.56)	**8%** (0.46)
Iowa	1,338	24% (1.58)	55% (1.83)	3% (0.58)	14% (1.27)	5% (0.78)
Kansas	1,095	25% (1.64)	56% (1.89)	4% (0.73)	9% (1.10)	6% (0.91)
Minnesota	2,061	25% (1.68)	49% (1.94)	7% (0.98)	12% (1.27)	7% (0.98)
Missouri	2,410	26% (1.72)	53% (1.97)	4% (0.75)	8% (1.08)	10% (1.18)
Nebraska	759	22% (1.50)	51% (1.80)	3% (0.59)	15% (1.28)	8% (0.99)
North Dakota	331	19% (1.33)	47% (1.71)	3% (0.59)	24% (1.46)	7% (0.88)
South Dakota	318	22% (1.43)	48% (1.73)	2% (0.47)	16% (1.26)	12% (1.13)
MOUNTAIN	**6,221**	**22%** (0.69)	**51%** (0.83)	**3%** (0.28)	**8%** (0.45)	**16%** (0.61)
Arizona	1,477	22% (1.72)	48% (2.07)	4% (0.82)	6% (1.02)	19% (1.63)
Colorado	1,419	23% (1.79)	53% (2.11)	1% (0.41)	7% (1.09)	16% (1.55)
Idaho	531	21% (1.40)	50% (1.72)	2% (0.45)	12% (1.10)	16% (1.25)
Montana	386	21% (1.51)	45% (1.84)	6% (0.85)	13% (1.25)	15% (1.32)
Nevada	449	28% (1.98)	50% (2.19)	2% (0.54)	8% (1.17)	12% (1.43)
New Mexico	725	18% (1.42)	41% (1.80)	5% (0.83)	7% (0.93)	28% (1.64)
Utah	997	22% (1.37)	60% (1.63)	2% (0.50)	8% (0.90)	8% (0.90)
Wyoming	237	22% (1.77)	54% (2.12)	5% (0.88)	11% (1.32)	9% (1.19)
PACIFIC	**16,492**	**22%** (0.58)	**44%** (0.70)	**10%** (0.42)	**7%** (0.36)	**16%** (0.51)
Alaska	228	22% (1.56)	47% (1.87)	7% (0.94)	8% (1.04)	16% (1.36)
California	12,562	21% (0.68)	42% (0.82)	11% (0.53)	7% (0.43)	18% (0.64)
Hawaii	391	29% (2.07)	51% (2.29)	6% (1.10)	6% (1.07)	8% (1.24)
Oregon	1,255	26% (1.87)	55% (2.12)	3% (0.70)	5% (0.89)	12% (1.37)
Washington	2,056	27% (1.77)	50% (2.00)	6% (0.96)	9% (1.15)	8% (1.06)

Source: Three-year merged March CPS, 1989, 1990, and 1991.

TABLE A9
PERSONS UNDER AGE 65 IN MARRIED-COUPLE-NO-CHILDREN FAMILIES:
BY TYPE OF HEALTH INSURANCE COVERAGE

	Number (000s)	Employer (own)	Employer (other)	Medicaid	Other	Uninsured
UNITED STATES	43,682	49% (0.37)	23% (0.32)	2% (0.11)	12% (0.25)	14% (0.26)
NEW ENGLAND	2,435	53% (1.24)	24% (1.06)	1% (0.30)	10% (0.74)	11% (0.77)
Connecticut	626	57% (3.35)	24% (2.88)	1% (0.61)	10% (2.00)	9% (1.91)
Maine	232	46% (3.05)	22% (2.53)	2% (0.94)	18% (2.34)	12% (1.97)
Massachusetts	1,053	53% (1.67)	26% (1.46)	2% (0.42)	9% (0.94)	11% (1.04)
New Hampshire	222	52% (3.29)	24% (2.81)	1% (0.53)	11% (2.05)	13% (2.19)
Rhode Island	208	52% (3.16)	22% (2.63)	3% (1.05)	9% (1.78)	14% (2.21)
Vermont	94	54% (3.54)	24% (3.04)	1% (0.82)	11% (2.19)	10% (2.12)
MIDDLE ATLANTIC	6,720	54% (0.87)	24% (0.74)	2% (0.24)	9% (0.50)	11% (0.55)
New Jersey	1,428	57% (1.58)	22% (1.32)	1% (0.37)	10% (0.96)	10% (0.95)
New York	2,958	52% (1.36)	24% (1.16)	3% (0.45)	9% (0.77)	13% (0.91)
Pennsylvania	2,334	54% (1.51)	25% (1.31)	1% (0.33)	9% (0.89)	10% (0.91)
SOUTH ATLANTIC	8,049	49% (0.88)	21% (0.72)	2% (0.26)	13% (0.60)	15% (0.63)
Delaware	122	53% (3.32)	24% (2.83)	1% (0.70)	10% (1.99)	12% (2.17)
District of Columbia	69	50% (4.38)	16% (3.20)	7% (2.26)	9% (2.55)	18% (3.36)
Florida	2,451	42% (1.45)	21% (1.19)	1% (0.34)	18% (1.12)	18% (1.12)
Georgia	1,136	50% (3.03)	21% (2.48)	2% (0.74)	10% (1.83)	18% (2.30)
Maryland	869	55% (3.21)	25% (2.79)	2% (0.85)	10% (1.97)	8% (1.74)
North Carolina	1,256	54% (1.52)	18% (1.17)	3% (0.55)	13% (1.02)	13% (1.01)
South Carolina	723	53% (2.58)	20% (2.05)	3% (0.87)	11% (1.63)	14% (1.78)
Virginia	1,085	50% (2.76)	21% (2.25)	2% (0.78)	12% (1.78)	15% (1.99)
West Virginia	338	43% (3.02)	25% (2.63)	5% (1.27)	11% (1.88)	17% (2.28)
EAST SOUTH CENTRAL	2,872	45% (1.50)	22% (1.25)	4% (0.60)	15% (1.07)	14% (1.06)
Alabama	803	44% (2.90)	22% (2.42)	3% (1.03)	15% (2.06)	17% (2.18)
Kentucky	731	45% (2.94)	22% (2.44)	5% (1.27)	16% (2.14)	13% (1.99)
Mississippi	415	38% (3.01)	19% (2.44)	5% (1.37)	18% (2.38)	19% (2.43)
Tennessee	923	49% (2.88)	24% (2.46)	4% (1.10)	13% (1.92)	11% (1.81)
WEST SOUTH CENTRAL	4,562	42% (1.22)	21% (1.01)	2% (0.34)	14% (0.87)	20% (0.99)
Arkansas	431	40% (2.96)	21% (2.48)	2% (0.82)	20% (2.43)	17% (2.28)
Louisiana	704	37% (3.22)	24% (2.84)	4% (1.31)	16% (2.46)	18% (2.57)
Oklahoma	602	44% (2.94)	23% (2.49)	2% (0.81)	13% (2.00)	18% (2.30)
Texas	2,825	43% (1.62)	20% (1.32)	1% (0.39)	13% (1.12)	22% (1.34)

TABLE A9 (continued)
PERSONS UNDER AGE 65 IN MARRIED-COUPLE-NO-CHILDREN FAMILIES:
BY TYPE OF HEALTH INSURANCE COVERAGE

	Number (000s)	Employer (own)	Employer (other)	Medicaid	Other	Uninsured
EAST NORTH CENTRAL	**7,651**	**51%** (0.88)	**27%** (0.78)	**1%** (0.21)	**11%** (0.54)	**10%** (0.53)
Illinois	2,028	54% (1.65)	24% (1.41)	1% (0.37)	11% (1.04)	10% (0.97)
Indiana	1,053	52% (3.10)	27% (2.76)	0% (0.40)	8% (1.71)	12% (2.01)
Michigan	1,757	49% (1.58)	29% (1.43)	2% (0.46)	10% (0.95)	9% (0.92)
Ohio	1,933	51% (1.60)	26% (1.41)	2% (0.40)	11% (0.99)	11% (0.99)
Wisconsin	879	49% (2.89)	28% (2.60)	1% (0.61)	12% (1.89)	10% (1.70)
WEST NORTH CENTRAL	**2,978**	**47%** (1.44)	**23%** (1.22)	**1%** (0.35)	**18%** (1.10)	**11%** (0.91)
Iowa	453	41% (3.11)	21% (2.58)	1% (0.68)	27% (2.81)	10% (1.91)
Kansas	430	48% (3.03)	25% (2.63)	1% (0.61)	16% (2.25)	9% (1.73)
Minnesota	701	51% (3.33)	24% (2.84)	1% (0.54)	15% (2.35)	10% (2.02)
Missouri	903	49% (3.22)	23% (2.73)	2% (0.93)	12% (2.12)	13% (2.17)
Nebraska	273	43% (2.97)	23% (2.51)	2% (0.89)	19% (2.36)	13% (2.00)
North Dakota	101	35% (2.95)	23% (2.59)	2% (0.76)	29% (2.81)	12% (2.02)
South Dakota	117	35% (2.72)	19% (2.21)	3% (0.89)	29% (2.58)	15% (2.01)
MOUNTAIN	**2,161**	**45%** (1.40)	**23%** (1.18)	**1%** (0.29)	**15%** (1.01)	**16%** (1.02)
Arizona	623	46% (3.18)	22% (2.63)	1% (0.71)	15% (2.28)	16% (2.33)
Colorado	505	48% (3.54)	25% (3.07)	1% (0.64)	14% (2.46)	12% (2.31)
Idaho	166	44% (3.05)	22% (2.54)	1% (0.53)	18% (2.35)	16% (2.26)
Montana	139	40% (3.01)	21% (2.52)	1% (0.60)	22% (2.55)	16% (2.24)
Nevada	199	50% (3.30)	20% (2.63)	1% (0.62)	11% (2.05)	18% (2.54)
New Mexico	224	35% (3.13)	23% (2.78)	2% (0.82)	16% (2.43)	24% (2.81)
Utah	220	46% (3.52)	25% (3.05)	1% (0.82)	16% (2.59)	12% (2.28)
Wyoming	86	45% (3.51)	24% (3.03)	0% (0.46)	16% (2.60)	14% (2.46)
PACIFIC	**6,255**	**47%** (1.13)	**23%** (0.95)	**3%** (0.36)	**11%** (0.72)	**16%** (0.83)
Alaska	71	45% (3.35)	20% (2.68)	1% (0.55)	12% (2.18)	23% (2.81)
California	4,566	47% (1.37)	23% (1.15)	3% (0.46)	11% (0.86)	17% (1.03)
Hawaii	218	56% (3.04)	21% (2.50)	2% (0.96)	9% (1.78)	11% (1.88)
Oregon	501	50% (3.36)	24% (2.88)	1% (0.66)	11% (2.13)	13% (2.30)
Washington	898	47% (3.01)	24% (2.57)	3% (0.94)	12% (1.97)	15% (2.14)

Source: Three-year merged March CPS, 1989, 1990, and 1991.

TABLE A10
PERSONS UNDER AGE 65 IN SINGLE-PARENT-WITH-CHILDREN FAMILIES:
BY TYPE OF HEALTH INSURANCE COVERAGE

	Number (000s)	Employer (own)	Employer (other)	Medicaid	Other	Uninsured
UNITED STATES	28,004	16% (0.34)	23% (0.39)	40% (0.46)	6% (0.22)	15% (0.34)
NEW ENGLAND	1,223	19% (1.36)	26% (1.53)	38% (1.69)	7% (0.92)	10% (1.07)
Connecticut	292	23% (4.17)	30% (4.54)	26% (4.37)	9% (2.86)	11% (3.16)
Maine	111	15% (3.17)	27% (3.92)	43% (4.38)	2% (1.18)	13% (2.95)
Massachusetts	610	17% (1.66)	24% (1.86)	43% (2.17)	7% (1.15)	9% (1.24)
New Hampshire	89	18% (3.99)	26% (4.57)	27% (4.60)	10% (3.08)	20% (4.13)
Rhode Island	73	19% (4.23)	26% (4.68)	47% (5.34)	4% (2.18)	3% (1.96)
Vermont	47	20% (3.99)	27% (4.42)	31% (4.65)	10% (2.99)	12% (3.29)
MIDDLE ATLANTIC	4,176	17% (0.82)	22% (0.92)	43% (1.09)	7% (0.55)	12% (0.71)
New Jersey	814	20% (1.69)	23% (1.78)	36% (2.02)	7% (1.10)	14% (1.47)
New York	2,218	14% (1.10)	19% (1.24)	48% (1.57)	6% (0.76)	12% (1.03)
Pennsylvania	1,144	19% (1.70)	27% (1.93)	37% (2.10)	7% (1.13)	9% (1.27)
SOUTH ATLANTIC	5,079	17% (0.84)	23% (0.93)	35% (1.06)	6% (0.53)	19% (0.87)
Delaware	82	22% (3.35)	26% (3.54)	29% (3.68)	5% (1.80)	18% (3.13)
District of Columbia	122	17% (2.48)	22% (2.75)	44% (3.27)	4% (1.37)	12% (2.16)
Florida	1,492	16% (1.39)	22% (1.57)	31% (1.74)	8% (0.99)	23% (1.57)
Georgia	834	15% (2.52)	18% (2.70)	46% (3.52)	6% (1.69)	15% (2.52)
Maryland	616	21% (3.10)	29% (3.47)	38% (3.72)	3% (1.23)	10% (2.34)
North Carolina	681	18% (1.61)	26% (1.83)	31% (1.92)	5% (0.94)	19% (1.61)
South Carolina	399	17% (2.62)	20% (2.81)	32% (3.25)	6% (1.69)	24% (2.97)
Virginia	674	19% (2.73)	25% (3.02)	28% (3.14)	6% (1.68)	23% (2.95)
West Virginia	178	13% (2.79)	19% (3.27)	47% (4.18)	7% (2.11)	15% (2.95)
EAST SOUTH CENTRAL	2,031	14% (1.24)	22% (1.49)	40% (1.76)	7% (0.89)	17% (1.36)
Alabama	537	15% (2.55)	23% (3.00)	32% (3.34)	7% (1.82)	23% (3.02)
Kentucky	385	15% (2.89)	23% (3.44)	43% (4.03)	8% (2.17)	11% (2.55)
Mississippi	437	10% (1.84)	17% (2.28)	50% (3.02)	5% (1.32)	18% (2.31)
Tennessee	671	15% (2.39)	24% (2.88)	39% (3.31)	7% (1.71)	16% (2.45)
WEST SOUTH CENTRAL	3,090	14% (1.04)	20% (1.21)	39% (1.47)	6% (0.72)	21% (1.21)
Arkansas	343	14% (2.35)	24% (2.90)	37% (3.27)	6% (1.64)	19% (2.68)
Louisiana	613	11% (2.22)	12% (2.33)	52% (3.56)	5% (1.57)	20% (2.85)
Oklahoma	312	13% (2.79)	20% (3.33)	43% (4.08)	7% (2.11)	16% (3.00)
Texas	1,822	15% (1.46)	22% (1.69)	34% (1.93)	6% (0.99)	22% (1.68)

TABLE A10 (continued)
PERSONS UNDER AGE 65 IN SINGLE-PARENT-WITH-CHILDREN FAMILIES:
BY TYPE OF HEALTH INSURANCE COVERAGE

	Number (000s)	Employer (own)	Employer (other)	Medicaid	Other	Uninsured
EAST NORTH CENTRAL	**4,991**	**16%** **(0.79)**	**24%** **(0.93)**	**43%** **(1.08)**	**6%** **(0.51)**	**12%** **(0.71)**
Illinois	1,511	14% (1.34)	19% (1.51)	48% (1.92)	5% (0.87)	13% (1.29)
Indiana	654	15% (2.84)	21% (3.23)	31% (3.64)	11% (2.42)	22% (3.25)
Michigan	1,194	14% (1.34)	25% (1.66)	47% (1.91)	5% (0.82)	8% (1.07)
Ohio	1,217	16% (1.50)	26% (1.77)	42% (1.99)	5% (0.92)	10% (1.22)
Wisconsin	416	21% (3.42)	33% (3.95)	36% (4.03)	4% (1.64)	6% (2.05)
WEST NORTH CENTRAL	**1,675**	**17%** **(1.45)**	**27%** **(1.70)**	**34%** **(1.83)**	**6%** **(0.93)**	**15%** **(1.39)**
Iowa	228	16% (3.30)	26% (3.90)	41% (4.39)	9% (2.51)	8% (2.46)
Kansas	247	18% (3.06)	30% (3.68)	36% (3.83)	5% (1.81)	11% (2.48)
Minnesota	453	18% (3.17)	25% (3.61)	35% (3.95)	6% (1.97)	16% (3.06)
Missouri	513	16% (3.17)	27% (3.78)	31% (3.97)	5% (1.79)	21% (3.49)
Nebraska	122	19% (3.54)	30% (4.12)	32% (4.19)	7% (2.29)	11% (2.78)
North Dakota	42	16% (3.47)	27% (4.24)	36% (4.60)	12% (3.14)	9% (2.80)
South Dakota	70	14% (2.55)	22% (3.07)	31% (3.40)	12% (2.35)	21% (3.02)
MOUNTAIN	**1,460**	**17%** **(1.29)**	**25%** **(1.49)**	**32%** **(1.60)**	**7%** **(0.86)**	**19%** **(1.35)**
Arizona	379	17% (3.09)	24% (3.51)	33% (3.85)	6% (1.95)	19% (3.22)
Colorado	415	17% (2.97)	25% (3.37)	33% (3.67)	6% (1.78)	20% (3.11)
Idaho	84	16% (3.15)	23% (3.65)	28% (3.88)	14% (2.96)	19% (3.38)
Montana	84	15% (2.81)	22% (3.25)	34% (3.75)	11% (2.47)	18% (3.05)
Nevada	140	21% (3.20)	31% (3.65)	19% (3.08)	8% (2.09)	21% (3.23)
New Mexico	163	16% (2.86)	23% (3.25)	30% (3.54)	6% (1.84)	24% (3.28)
Utah	151	13% (2.91)	31% (3.94)	42% (4.20)	5% (1.86)	9% (2.42)
Wyoming	43	17% (3.79)	23% (4.22)	30% (4.59)	7% (2.61)	22% (4.14)
PACIFIC	**4,279**	**16%** **(0.99)**	**21%** **(1.12)**	**44%** **(1.36)**	**5%** **(0.59)**	**15%** **(0.98)**
Alaska	55	15% (2.72)	19% (2.98)	34% (3.61)	5% (1.71)	26% (3.34)
California	3,359	15% (1.14)	20% (1.27)	46% (1.60)	5% (0.67)	15% (1.16)
Hawaii	88	20% (3.85)	22% (4.00)	43% (4.79)	6% (2.36)	9% (2.74)
Oregon	286	12% (2.94)	22% (3.67)	39% (4.35)	7% (2.32)	20% (3.53)
Washington	491	22% (3.39)	32% (3.80)	34% (3.87)	5% (1.81)	7% (2.09)

Source: Three-year merged March CPS, 1989, 1990, and 1991.

TABLE A11
PERSONS UNDER AGE 65 IN SINGLE-PERSON-WITHOUT-CHILDREN FAMILIES:
BY TYPE OF HEALTH INSURANCE COVERAGE

	Number (000s)	Employer (own)	Employer (other)	Medicaid	Other	Uninsured
UNITED STATES	35,327	52% (0.42)	1% (0.07)	6% (0.19)	14% (0.29)	27% (0.37)
NEW ENGLAND	2,018	62% (1.32)	0% (0.16)	5% (0.58)	14% (0.94)	19% (1.08)
Connecticut	473	69% (3.60)	0% (0.52)	4% (1.53)	11% (2.46)	15% (2.80)
Maine	157	52% (3.72)	1% (0.70)	9% (2.16)	15% (2.69)	22% (3.09)
Massachusetts	998	61% (1.67)	0% (0.16)	5% (0.74)	15% (1.21)	19% (1.36)
New Hampshire	145	62% (3.95)	*** ***	1% (0.79)	12% (2.66)	25% (3.52)
Rhode Island	152	57% (3.67)	1% (0.61)	4% (1.42)	17% (2.77)	22% (3.07)
Vermont	93	58% (3.51)	0% (0.48)	6% (1.71)	12% (2.34)	23% (3.00)
MIDDLE ATLANTIC	5,224	56% (0.98)	0% (0.12)	7% (0.52)	12% (0.65)	24% (0.84)
New Jersey	1,043	61% (1.83)	0% (0.19)	5% (0.81)	12% (1.21)	22% (1.56)
New York	2,779	52% (1.40)	0% (0.16)	9% (0.81)	12% (0.91)	26% (1.24)
Pennsylvania	1,403	60% (1.92)	1% (0.28)	6% (0.91)	14% (1.35)	20% (1.57)
SOUTH ATLANTIC	6,382	52% (0.99)	1% (0.17)	6% (0.47)	14% (0.68)	27% (0.88)
Delaware	117	58% (3.35)	0% (0.26)	3% (1.09)	14% (2.35)	25% (2.94)
District of Columbia	194	53% (2.61)	1% (0.45)	6% (1.22)	12% (1.73)	28% (2.35)
Florida	1,914	49% (1.66)	1% (0.30)	5% (0.71)	14% (1.16)	31% (1.54)
Georgia	937	54% (3.32)	1% (0.66)	7% (1.71)	11% (2.11)	27% (2.95)
Maryland	838	57% (3.26)	0% (0.42)	6% (1.53)	14% (2.25)	24% (2.79)
North Carolina	945	52% (1.76)	1% (0.30)	7% (0.89)	15% (1.25)	26% (1.54)
South Carolina	394	48% (3.50)	1% (0.69)	9% (1.99)	15% (2.52)	27% (3.12)
Virginia	859	58% (3.07)	1% (0.58)	5% (1.39)	12% (2.01)	24% (2.65)
West Virginia	184	46% (4.11)	*** ***	8% (2.18)	16% (3.00)	31% (3.81)
EAST SOUTH CENTRAL	1,822	44% (1.88)	1% (0.38)	9% (1.06)	15% (1.35)	31% (1.75)
Alabama	489	40% (3.67)	0% (0.33)	9% (2.14)	14% (2.62)	37% (3.61)
Kentucky	420	51% (3.90)	2% (0.99)	7% (1.94)	14% (2.74)	26% (3.43)
Mississippi	332	38% (3.37)	1% (0.75)	11% (2.19)	14% (2.41)	35% (3.30)
Tennessee	581	47% (3.63)	1% (0.77)	8% (2.01)	16% (2.67)	27% (3.24)
WEST SOUTH CENTRAL	3,472	43% (1.41)	1% (0.22)	5% (0.62)	16% (1.04)	35% (1.35)
Arkansas	292	38% (3.58)	0% (0.49)	9% (2.09)	16% (2.73)	36% (3.54)
Louisiana	512	38% (3.77)	1% (0.66)	10% (2.38)	16% (2.85)	35% (3.73)
Oklahoma	376	40% (3.67)	1% (0.65)	4% (1.51)	20% (3.02)	35% (3.57)
Texas	2,291	46% (1.81)	1% (0.27)	3% (0.66)	15% (1.31)	35% (1.73)

PERSONS UNDER AGE 65 IN SINGLE-PERSON-WITHOUT-CHILDREN FAMILIES: BY TYPE OF HEALTH INSURANCE COVERAGE

	Number (000s)	Employer (own)	Employer (other)	Medicaid	Other	Uninsured
EAST NORTH CENTRAL	**5,696**	**55%** (1.02)	**1%** (0.18)	**5%** (0.46)	**14%** (0.70)	**25%** (0.89)
Illinois	1,696	55% (1.80)	1% (0.34)	5% (0.76)	14% (1.24)	26% (1.59)
Indiana	673	52% (3.88)	1% (0.79)	3% (1.41)	17% (2.94)	26% (3.40)
Michigan	1,301	54% (1.83)	1% (0.31)	8% (0.99)	13% (1.22)	25% (1.58)
Ohio	1,406	54% (1.87)	1% (0.31)	6% (0.87)	13% (1.28)	26% (1.65)
Wisconsin	620	61% (3.35)	1% (0.61)	4% (1.34)	14% (2.35)	21% (2.78)
WEST NORTH CENTRAL	**2,313**	**53%** (1.63)	**0%** (0.20)	**4%** (0.62)	**19%** (1.28)	**24%** (1.39)
Iowa	367	54% (3.51)	1% (0.61)	4% (1.31)	20% (2.82)	22% (2.91)
Kansas	305	50% (3.60)	0% (0.47)	3% (1.31)	18% (2.78)	28% (3.25)
Minnesota	635	54% (3.49)	0% (0.44)	3% (1.21)	19% (2.74)	24% (2.97)
Missouri	650	57% (3.77)	*** ***	4% (1.48)	16% (2.81)	23% (3.20)
Nebraska	206	51% (3.45)	0% (0.39)	5% (1.47)	19% (2.72)	24% (2.97)
North Dakota	72	43% (3.63)	*** ***	7% (1.90)	29% (3.34)	20% (2.96)
South Dakota	79	43% (3.44)	2% (0.88)	4% (1.30)	26% (3.06)	25% (3.02)
MOUNTAIN	**1,870**	**49%** (1.51)	**0%** (0.19)	**3%** (0.52)	**18%** (1.16)	**29%** (1.38)
Arizona	537	51% (3.43)	*** ***	3% (1.20)	19% (2.70)	27% (3.05)
Colorado	497	53% (3.57)	1% (0.58)	3% (1.19)	17% (2.68)	27% (3.17)
Idaho	116	41% (3.62)	1% (0.63)	5% (1.55)	22% (3.06)	31% (3.40)
Montana	101	42% (3.56)	1% (0.74)	5% (1.55)	22% (2.98)	30% (3.31)
Nevada	222	55% (3.10)	0% (0.16)	2% (0.81)	10% (1.86)	33% (2.94)
New Mexico	190	40% (3.49)	0% (0.42)	4% (1.43)	20% (2.87)	36% (3.42)
Utah	157	51% (4.18)	1% (0.77)	2% (1.27)	17% (3.13)	29% (3.78)
Wyoming	49	41% (4.63)	1% (0.78)	*** ***	22% (3.89)	36% (4.51)
PACIFIC	**6,530**	**50%** (1.11)	**1%** (0.18)	**5%** (0.50)	**14%** (0.78)	**30%** (1.02)
Alaska	81	44% (3.11)	1% (0.45)	2% (0.76)	14% (2.15)	40% (3.08)
California	5,101	49% (1.30)	1% (0.22)	6% (0.60)	13% (0.89)	31% (1.21)
Hawaii	153	63% (3.55)	0% (0.50)	4% (1.42)	15% (2.58)	18% (2.84)
Oregon	422	54% (3.65)	*** ***	5% (1.54)	16% (2.71)	25% (3.17)
Washington	773	50% (3.26)	1% (0.46)	4% (1.34)	18% (2.49)	27% (2.90)

Source: Three-year merged March CPS, 1989, 1990, and 1991.

TABLE A12
TOTAL POPULATION UNDER AGE 65 WITH INCOME BELOW 100 PERCENT OF POVERTY:
BY TYPE OF HEALTH INSURANCE COVERAGE

	Number (000s)	Employer (own)	Employer (other)	Medicaid	Other	Uninsured
UNITED STATES	30,630	5% (0.27)	9% (0.36)	49% (0.62)	8% (0.34)	29% (0.56)
NEW ENGLAND	916	6% (1.33)	8% (1.53)	57% (2.78)	9% (1.64)	20% (2.25)
Connecticut	127	9% (6.00)	5% (4.33)	54% (10.41)	12% (6.80)	20% (8.39)
Maine	131	4% (2.33)	10% (3.34)	58% (5.60)	9% (3.32)	18% (4.40)
Massachusetts	476	5% (1.49)	8% (1.83)	61% (3.37)	9% (1.93)	18% (2.66)
New Hampshire	64	6% (4.04)	7% (4.35)	39% (8.31)	8% (4.73)	40% (8.34)
Rhode Island	73	9% (4.28)	13% (4.99)	50% (7.44)	10% (4.38)	18% (5.75)
Vermont	44	8% (3.83)	13% (4.82)	48% (7.20)	12% (4.65)	20% (5.75)
MIDDLE ATLANTIC	3,978	5% (0.66)	9% (0.92)	58% (1.54)	6% (0.76)	21% (1.28)
New Jersey	577	5% (1.59)	9% (2.01)	56% (3.46)	7% (1.77)	22% (2.90)
New York	2,231	4% (0.83)	7% (1.11)	61% (2.12)	6% (1.03)	22% (1.80)
Pennsylvania	1,170	6% (1.37)	14% (2.09)	54% (2.97)	7% (1.47)	19% (2.35)
SOUTH ATLANTIC	5,157	6% (0.70)	10% (0.91)	45% (1.52)	8% (0.85)	31% (1.42)
Delaware	54	8% (3.73)	14% (4.78)	49% (6.95)	6% (3.19)	24% (5.97)
District of Columbia	97	5% (2.23)	6% (2.43)	61% (5.04)	5% (2.29)	23% (4.34)
Florida	1,563	5% (1.17)	10% (1.51)	38% (2.48)	10% (1.56)	36% (2.46)
Georgia	926	5% (1.96)	10% (2.76)	47% (4.66)	6% (2.20)	32% (4.37)
Maryland	404	4% (2.56)	8% (3.50)	63% (6.35)	7% (3.35)	18% (5.07)
North Carolina	740	7% (1.41)	12% (1.80)	45% (2.76)	10% (1.64)	26% (2.43)
South Carolina	478	6% (2.13)	10% (2.63)	39% (4.31)	8% (2.40)	37% (4.28)
Virginia	599	6% (2.49)	10% (3.10)	42% (5.11)	7% (2.70)	34% (4.91)
West Virginia	296	5% (1.98)	10% (2.70)	54% (4.51)	8% (2.43)	24% (3.85)
EAST SOUTH CENTRAL	2,695	6% (1.00)	10% (1.31)	45% (2.16)	8% (1.19)	31% (2.00)
Alabama	748	6% (1.99)	10% (2.57)	33% (3.97)	9% (2.47)	41% (4.15)
Kentucky	531	5% (2.05)	8% (2.57)	55% (4.79)	7% (2.39)	26% (4.21)
Mississippi	617	6% (1.63)	11% (2.24)	48% (3.53)	7% (1.81)	28% (3.16)
Tennessee	798	6% (2.05)	10% (2.64)	47% (4.31)	9% (2.48)	28% (3.86)
WEST SOUTH CENTRAL	4,531	4% (0.69)	8% (0.94)	38% (1.67)	8% (0.91)	43% (1.71)
Arkansas	424	4% (1.75)	10% (2.49)	41% (4.18)	10% (2.50)	36% (4.07)
Louisiana	914	5% (1.73)	7% (2.08)	48% (4.06)	6% (1.94)	34% (3.85)
Oklahoma	440	4% (1.86)	5% (2.17)	43% (4.77)	11% (2.98)	37% (4.67)
Texas	2,753	4% (0.90)	9% (1.29)	33% (2.17)	7% (1.19)	47% (2.30)

TOTAL POPULATION UNDER AGE 65 WITH INCOME BELOW 100 PERCENT OF POVERTY:
BY TYPE OF HEALTH INSURANCE COVERAGE

	Population (000s)	Employer (own)	Employer (other)	Medicaid	Other	Uninsured
EAST NORTH CENTRAL	**4,974**	**5%** **(0.64)**	**10%** **(0.92)**	**57%** **(1.51)**	**7%** **(0.80)**	**21%** **(1.24)**
Illinois	1,443	4% (1.08)	7% (1.43)	63% (2.64)	6% (1.28)	20% (2.19)
Indiana	678	6% (2.53)	15% (3.80)	34% (5.10)	10% (3.29)	35% (5.13)
Michigan	1,261	4% (1.05)	10% (1.56)	61% (2.53)	5% (1.12)	20% (2.07)
Ohio	1,228	5% (1.25)	11% (1.75)	59% (2.75)	8% (1.54)	17% (2.09)
Wisconsin	365	4% (2.53)	10% (3.74)	55% (6.22)	13% (4.24)	18% (4.78)
WEST NORTH CENTRAL	**1,917**	**6%** **(1.19)**	**11%** **(1.56)**	**46%** **(2.49)**	**14%** **(1.75)**	**23%** **(2.11)**
Iowa	269	4% (2.31)	10% (3.48)	46% (5.70)	18% (4.44)	21% (4.66)
Kansas	240	4% (2.27)	11% (3.61)	47% (5.64)	8% (3.08)	29% (5.15)
Minnesota	514	5% (2.30)	11% (3.34)	53% (5.41)	16% (4.01)	16% (3.93)
Missouri	566	8% (3.15)	12% (3.68)	44% (5.63)	9% (3.26)	26% (4.99)
Nebraska	161	8% (2.91)	9% (3.12)	41% (5.34)	16% (3.95)	26% (4.78)
North Dakota	78	4% (1.91)	9% (2.80)	34% (4.65)	35% (4.68)	17% (3.72)
South Dakota	90	7% (2.32)	10% (2.77)	32% (4.22)	17% (3.39)	34% (4.29)
MOUNTAIN	**1,726**	**6%** **(1.04)**	**10%** **(1.33)**	**37%** **(2.12)**	**10%** **(1.32)**	**37%** **(2.11)**
Arizona	484	7% (2.58)	9% (2.90)	40% (4.94)	9% (2.92)	34% (4.77)
Colorado	401	5% (2.37)	11% (3.45)	38% (5.38)	8% (2.96)	38% (5.38)
Idaho	121	7% (2.59)	9% (2.91)	27% (4.47)	18% (3.85)	38% (4.85)
Montana	121	6% (2.20)	12% (2.98)	36% (4.40)	17% (3.41)	30% (4.19)
Nevada	115	10% (3.59)	11% (3.73)	30% (5.52)	8% (3.32)	42% (5.95)
New Mexico	287	5% (1.74)	9% (2.28)	30% (3.71)	8% (2.23)	48% (4.04)
Utah	145	5% (2.54)	15% (4.37)	51% (6.06)	9% (3.53)	19% (4.78)
Wyoming	51	4% (2.36)	7% (3.30)	39% (6.23)	14% (4.39)	37% (6.16)
PACIFIC	**4,737**	**4%** **(0.73)**	**7%** **(0.94)**	**54%** **(1.80)**	**6%** **(0.88)**	**28%** **(1.62)**
Alaska	67	4% (1.82)	6% (2.21)	45% (4.76)	6% (2.21)	40% (4.70)
California	3,809	4% (0.78)	7% (1.07)	55% (2.07)	5% (0.95)	28% (1.88)
Hawaii	119	10% (3.40)	12% (3.76)	48% (5.77)	11% (3.65)	19% (4.58)
Oregon	320	8% (3.20)	10% (3.49)	42% (5.78)	11% (3.74)	29% (5.31)
Washington	422	6% (2.90)	6% (2.80)	56% (6.08)	8% (3.31)	24% (5.26)

Source: Three-year merged March CPS, 1989, 1990, and 1991.

TABLE A13
TOTAL POPULATION UNDER AGE 65 WITH INCOME BETWEEN 100 AND 199 PERCENT OF POVERTY:
BY TYPE OF HEALTH INSURANCE COVERAGE

	Number (000s)	Employer (own)	Employer (other)	Medicaid	Other	Uninsured
UNITED STATES	36,463	20% (0.45)	30% (0.52)	9% (0.32)	12% (0.38)	29% (0.52)
NEW ENGLAND	1,259	22% (1.97)	32% (2.23)	14% (1.67)	12% (1.54)	21% (1.95)
Connecticut	241	22% (6.32)	36% (7.28)	15% (5.38)	9% (4.36)	18% (5.81)
Maine	191	23% (3.93)	35% (4.48)	10% (2.79)	13% (3.13)	20% (3.76)
Massachusetts	539	21% (2.62)	28% (2.91)	18% (2.51)	12% (2.11)	21% (2.64)
New Hampshire	94	19% (5.47)	33% (6.63)	2% (1.96)	13% (4.73)	33% (6.62)
Rhode Island	122	25% (4.99)	37% (5.54)	10% (3.50)	11% (3.66)	16% (4.25)
Vermont	71	23% (4.75)	22% (4.69)	14% (3.92)	15% (4.10)	26% (4.98)
MIDDLE ATLANTIC	4,641	21% (1.18)	35% (1.38)	12% (0.93)	10% (0.87)	23% (1.21)
New Jersey	598	23% (2.88)	31% (3.17)	10% (2.10)	10% (2.09)	25% (2.99)
New York	2,345	19% (1.67)	32% (1.98)	15% (1.52)	9% (1.22)	24% (1.80)
Pennsylvania	1,698	23% (2.08)	39% (2.41)	7% (1.30)	11% (1.56)	20% (1.98)
SOUTH ATLANTIC	6,308	22% (1.14)	28% (1.24)	6% (0.63)	12% (0.91)	33% (1.30)
Delaware	79	24% (4.93)	29% (5.21)	5% (2.56)	12% (3.78)	30% (5.25)
District of Columbia	81	23% (4.77)	20% (4.49)	14% (3.89)	9% (3.30)	34% (5.37)
Florida	1,971	19% (1.77)	24% (1.94)	5% (0.95)	13% (1.51)	41% (2.24)
Georgia	996	23% (3.76)	29% (4.10)	3% (1.57)	14% (3.10)	31% (4.17)
Maryland	476	21% (4.97)	33% (5.71)	10% (3.72)	10% (3.63)	25% (5.28)
North Carolina	1,013	25% (2.04)	29% (2.15)	6% (1.09)	12% (1.53)	28% (2.13)
South Carolina	541	24% (3.57)	32% (3.88)	4% (1.68)	12% (2.69)	27% (3.71)
Virginia	781	21% (3.70)	28% (4.06)	5% (1.98)	13% (3.05)	33% (4.26)
West Virginia	369	23% (3.41)	34% (3.84)	11% (2.58)	9% (2.35)	22% (3.36)
EAST SOUTH CENTRAL	2,850	21% (1.72)	31% (1.95)	6% (1.00)	13% (1.42)	29% (1.90)
Alabama	777	22% (3.41)	32% (3.87)	4% (1.61)	14% (2.85)	28% (3.73)
Kentucky	724	21% (3.36)	31% (3.83)	8% (2.26)	13% (2.78)	27% (3.66)
Mississippi	511	20% (3.08)	26% (3.41)	7% (2.04)	14% (2.73)	32% (3.63)
Tennessee	838	22% (3.50)	33% (3.96)	5% (1.87)	12% (2.71)	28% (3.79)
WEST SOUTH CENTRAL	4,771	18% (1.31)	27% (1.49)	4% (0.69)	12% (1.11)	38% (1.63)
Arkansas	541	19% (2.96)	34% (3.57)	4% (1.52)	14% (2.64)	28% (3.38)
Louisiana	702	19% (3.65)	26% (4.08)	4% (1.75)	14% (3.17)	37% (4.48)
Oklahoma	579	16% (3.06)	27% (3.74)	5% (1.91)	16% (3.09)	36% (4.03)
Texas	2,949	19% (1.74)	25% (1.94)	4% (0.91)	11% (1.39)	41% (2.19)

TOTAL POPULATION UNDER AGE 65 WITH INCOME BETWEEN 100 AND 199 PERCENT OF POVERTY: BY TYPE OF HEALTH INSURANCE COVERAGE

	Number (000s)	Employer (own)	Employer (other)	Medicaid	Other	Uninsured
EAST NORTH CENTRAL	**5,544**	**22%** (1.19)	**35%** (1.38)	**8%** (0.77)	**12%** (0.95)	**23%** (1.22)
Illinois	1,426	20% (2.22)	32% (2.57)	8% (1.53)	13% (1.84)	26% (2.41)
Indiana	839	22% (4.00)	35% (4.60)	3% (1.68)	16% (3.56)	24% (4.14)
Michigan	1,150	22% (2.24)	36% (2.60)	12% (1.73)	10% (1.65)	21% (2.19)
Ohio	1,547	22% (2.08)	39% (2.43)	7% (1.25)	10% (1.47)	23% (2.08)
Wisconsin	581	24% (4.23)	30% (4.53)	8% (2.75)	16% (3.64)	21% (4.06)
WEST NORTH CENTRAL	**2,834**	**19%** (1.63)	**32%** (1.93)	**4%** (0.85)	**20%** (1.65)	**24%** (1.75)
Iowa	452	21% (3.57)	32% (4.12)	4% (1.66)	27% (3.92)	16% (3.25)
Kansas	360	22% (3.82)	36% (4.44)	7% (2.36)	15% (3.28)	20% (3.68)
Minnesota	604	17% (3.72)	30% (4.58)	5% (2.25)	23% (4.23)	25% (4.31)
Missouri	919	20% (3.56)	33% (4.17)	4% (1.78)	14% (3.07)	29% (4.05)
Nebraska	257	20% (3.44)	39% (4.19)	2% (1.32)	19% (3.40)	20% (3.41)
North Dakota	110	15% (2.98)	25% (3.56)	4% (1.52)	36% (3.95)	21% (3.34)
South Dakota	133	19% (2.92)	28% (3.34)	3% (1.35)	27% (3.30)	23% (3.14)
MOUNTAIN	**2,375**	**18%** (1.43)	**34%** (1.77)	**3%** (0.66)	**14%** (1.30)	**31%** (1.74)
Arizona	554	17% (3.56)	30% (4.32)	2% (1.38)	12% (3.10)	38% (4.56)
Colorado	487	19% (3.92)	28% (4.51)	2% (1.54)	14% (3.44)	37% (4.86)
Idaho	248	18% (2.67)	39% (3.40)	2% (1.03)	17% (2.61)	25% (3.00)
Montana	153	17% (3.04)	27% (3.61)	8% (2.26)	21% (3.32)	27% (3.63)
Nevada	161	23% (4.29)	33% (4.78)	2% (1.39)	13% (3.39)	30% (4.67)
New Mexico	308	18% (2.99)	29% (3.55)	4% (1.45)	11% (2.44)	38% (3.79)
Utah	389	16% (2.72)	50% (3.70)	4% (1.45)	14% (2.56)	16% (2.72)
Wyoming	74	18% (4.05)	29% (4.79)	5% (2.32)	20% (4.24)	29% (4.80)
PACIFIC	**5,882**	**15%** (1.16)	**21%** (1.32)	**19%** (1.29)	**10%** (0.97)	**35%** (1.55)
Alaska	78	17% (3.36)	22% (3.66)	7% (2.24)	16% (3.24)	39% (4.33)
California	4,639	14% (1.30)	18% (1.47)	22% (1.57)	9% (1.08)	37% (1.82)
Hawaii	141	28% (4.76)	37% (5.14)	8% (2.82)	8% (2.94)	19% (4.14)
Oregon	418	18% (3.91)	31% (4.74)	7% (2.61)	11% (3.20)	33% (4.84)
Washington	606	18% (3.93)	30% (4.67)	13% (3.42)	15% (3.65)	25% (4.41)

Source: Three-year merged March CPS, 1989, 1990, and 1991.

TABLE A14
TOTAL POPULATION UNDER AGE 65 WITH INCOME AT OR ABOVE 200 PERCENT OF POVERTY:
BY TYPE OF HEALTH INSURANCE COVERAGE

	Number (000s)	Employer (own)	Employer (other)	Medicaid	Other	Uninsured
UNITED STATES	146,487	42% (0.28)	39% (0.28)	1% (0.05)	9% (0.16)	9% (0.17)
NEW ENGLAND	8,982	43% (0.89)	40% (0.88)	1% (0.16)	8% (0.48)	9% (0.50)
Connecticut	2,393	45% (2.40)	39% (2.35)	1% (0.45)	6% (1.17)	9% (1.34)
Maine	733	41% (2.36)	41% (2.35)	1% (0.43)	10% (1.43)	8% (1.28)
Massachusetts	4,046	43% (1.17)	40% (1.16)	1% (0.21)	8% (0.63)	8% (0.64)
New Hampshire	814	40% (2.35)	38% (2.32)	0% (0.23)	9% (1.39)	12% (1.57)
Rhode Island	628	44% (2.52)	39% (2.47)	1% (0.54)	7% (1.29)	9% (1.46)
Vermont	369	42% (2.46)	41% (2.44)	0% (0.28)	9% (1.45)	7% (1.31)
MIDDLE ATLANTIC	23,796	44% (0.64)	39% (0.62)	1% (0.12)	8% (0.34)	9% (0.36)
New Jersey	5,456	45% (1.13)	38% (1.10)	1% (0.20)	8% (0.62)	8% (0.62)
New York	10,931	43% (0.97)	38% (0.95)	1% (0.21)	8% (0.52)	10% (0.59)
Pennsylvania	7,409	44% (1.18)	41% (1.17)	1% (0.19)	7% (0.62)	7% (0.59)
SOUTH ATLANTIC	24,540	45% (0.70)	36% (0.67)	0% (0.10)	9% (0.40)	10% (0.42)
Delaware	441	44% (2.42)	36% (2.33)	0% (0.23)	8% (1.32)	12% (1.59)
District of Columbia	316	50% (2.86)	21% (2.33)	2% (0.80)	11% (1.78)	16% (2.11)
Florida	6,799	42% (1.21)	33% (1.16)	1% (0.18)	11% (0.78)	13% (0.82)
Georgia	3,553	45% (2.37)	37% (2.30)	1% (0.37)	8% (1.26)	9% (1.39)
Maryland	3,097	47% (2.37)	39% (2.32)	0% (0.23)	6% (1.16)	8% (1.28)
North Carolina	3,716	47% (1.23)	34% (1.17)	0% (0.17)	9% (0.72)	9% (0.70)
South Carolina	1,913	47% (2.21)	38% (2.14)	1% (0.33)	8% (1.19)	7% (1.14)
Virginia	3,786	44% (2.04)	38% (2.00)	0% (0.16)	8% (1.11)	10% (1.23)
West Virginia	920	40% (2.51)	44% (2.55)	1% (0.49)	8% (1.36)	8% (1.39)
EAST SOUTH CENTRAL	7,669	42% (1.27)	40% (1.26)	1% (0.23)	9% (0.72)	8% (0.69)
Alabama	2,045	42% (2.52)	41% (2.51)	0% (0.23)	8% (1.36)	9% (1.43)
Kentucky	1,867	43% (2.54)	41% (2.53)	2% (0.63)	9% (1.49)	6% (1.19)
Mississippi	1,157	38% (2.51)	39% (2.52)	1% (0.53)	11% (1.61)	10% (1.56)
Tennessee	2,600	44% (2.38)	39% (2.34)	1% (0.39)	8% (1.30)	7% (1.26)
WEST SOUTH CENTRAL	14,153	39% (0.95)	39% (0.95)	0% (0.12)	10% (0.60)	12% (0.63)
Arkansas	1,137	39% (2.53)	39% (2.54)	0% (0.25)	10% (1.59)	11% (1.61)
Louisiana	2,085	36% (2.57)	42% (2.65)	1% (0.40)	11% (1.67)	11% (1.71)
Oklahoma	1,660	39% (2.42)	39% (2.42)	0% (0.29)	11% (1.53)	11% (1.58)
Texas	9,271	39% (1.23)	38% (1.22)	0% (0.14)	10% (0.76)	12% (0.83)

TABLE A14 (continued)
TOTAL POPULATION UNDER AGE 65 WITH INCOME AT OR ABOVE 200 PERCENT OF POVERTY: BY TYPE OF HEALTH INSURANCE COVERAGE

	Number (000s)	Employer (own)	Employer (other)	Medicaid	Other	Uninsured
EAST NORTH CENTRAL	**26,269**	**43%** (0.66)	**43%** (0.66)	**0%** (0.09)	**8%** (0.35)	**6%** (0.32)
Illinois	7,302	44% (1.21)	40% (1.19)	1% (0.18)	9% (0.68)	7% (0.63)
Indiana	3,256	43% (2.43)	41% (2.42)	0% (0.17)	8% (1.35)	7% (1.26)
Michigan	5,791	42% (1.19)	44% (1.20)	1% (0.21)	7% (0.63)	6% (0.57)
Ohio	6,762	42% (1.18)	44% (1.18)	0% (0.16)	7% (0.60)	6% (0.58)
Wisconsin	3,158	42% (2.09)	46% (2.11)	0% (0.23)	7% (1.08)	5% (0.95)
WEST NORTH CENTRAL	**10,529**	**40%** (1.05)	**41%** (1.05)	**0%** (0.14)	**11%** (0.68)	**6%** (0.52)
Iowa	1,665	38% (2.23)	43% (2.28)	0% (0.26)	14% (1.58)	5% (0.97)
Kansas	1,479	40% (2.23)	43% (2.26)	1% (0.32)	11% (1.45)	5% (1.01)
Minnesota	2,732	43% (2.32)	39% (2.29)	1% (0.38)	10% (1.41)	8% (1.25)
Missouri	2,991	43% (2.44)	42% (2.43)	0% (0.26)	9% (1.39)	7% (1.22)
Nebraska	942	38% (2.17)	40% (2.20)	0% (0.31)	15% (1.59)	7% (1.17)
North Dakota	358	32% (2.13)	44% (2.27)	0% (0.30)	19% (1.79)	5% (1.00)
South Dakota	363	34% (2.13)	40% (2.21)	0% (0.15)	17% (1.71)	8% (1.24)
MOUNTAIN	**7,611**	**39%** (1.02)	**40%** (1.02)	**0%** (0.09)	**10%** (0.63)	**10%** (0.64)
Arizona	1,978	42% (2.45)	37% (2.40)	0% (0.21)	10% (1.50)	11% (1.57)
Colorado	1,947	41% (2.47)	41% (2.47)	0% (0.20)	9% (1.46)	9% (1.40)
Idaho	527	37% (2.31)	40% (2.35)	0% (0.20)	12% (1.58)	11% (1.47)
Montana	436	36% (2.33)	39% (2.36)	0% (0.18)	14% (1.67)	11% (1.51)
Nevada	735	45% (2.38)	33% (2.25)	0% (0.23)	8% (1.30)	13% (1.62)
New Mexico	707	35% (2.45)	39% (2.51)	0% (0.31)	11% (1.62)	15% (1.86)
Utah	992	35% (2.21)	49% (2.31)	0% (0.25)	8% (1.27)	7% (1.21)
Wyoming	290	36% (2.57)	46% (2.67)	0% (0.21)	11% (1.66)	7% (1.34)
PACIFIC	**22,937**	**41%** (0.81)	**35%** (0.79)	**1%** (0.19)	**9%** (0.48)	**13%** (0.54)
Alaska	290	38% (2.24)	38% (2.24)	0% (0.25)	9% (1.31)	14% (1.61)
California	17,141	41% (0.97)	34% (0.93)	1% (0.24)	10% (0.58)	14% (0.68)
Hawaii	589	50% (2.60)	34% (2.46)	1% (0.51)	8% (1.39)	7% (1.31)
Oregon	1,726	43% (2.50)	41% (2.48)	0% (0.34)	7% (1.29)	8% (1.39)
Washington	3,191	42% (2.20)	38% (2.16)	1% (0.47)	11% (1.37)	9% (1.27)

Source: Three-year merged March CPS, 1989, 1990, and 1991.

TABLE A15

ALL PERSONS IN FAMILY UNDER AGE 65 BY WORK STATUS OF SPOUSE AND HEAD,
AT LEAST ONE FULL-TIME WORKER: BY TYPE OF HEALTH INSURANCE COVERAGE

	Number (000s)	Employer (own)	Employer (other)	Medicaid	Other	Uninsured
UNITED STATES	174,084	37%	38%	3%	8%	14%
		(0.13)	(0.13)	(0.05)	(0.07)	(0.09)
NEW ENGLAND	9,278	41%	41%	2%	7%	9%
		(0.45)	(0.45)	(0.13)	(0.23)	(0.27)
Connecticut	2,366	44%	41%	1%	5%	9%
		(1.25)	(1.23)	(0.29)	(0.57)	(0.71)
Maine	864	37%	41%	3%	9%	10%
		(1.10)	(1.12)	(0.39)	(0.65)	(0.69)
Massachusetts	4,094	41%	42%	2%	7%	9%
		(0.60)	(0.60)	(0.18)	(0.30)	(0.34)
New Hampshire	865	38%	38%	1%	8%	15%
		(1.17)	(1.17)	(0.20)	(0.67)	(0.85)
Rhode Island	676	40%	41%	3%	5%	10%
		(1.24)	(1.25)	(0.42)	(0.57)	(0.77)
Vermont	412	39%	40%	3%	9%	9%
		(1.19)	(1.20)	(0.40)	(0.69)	(0.70)
MIDDLE ATLANTIC	25,722	39%	41%	3%	7%	11%
		(0.31)	(0.31)	(0.10)	(0.16)	(0.20)
New Jersey	5,574	42%	39%	2%	7%	9%
		(0.58)	(0.57)	(0.17)	(0.30)	(0.34)
New York	11,599	38%	40%	3%	7%	12%
		(0.48)	(0.48)	(0.17)	(0.25)	(0.32)
Pennsylvania	8,549	39%	43%	3%	6%	9%
		(0.56)	(0.57)	(0.20)	(0.28)	(0.33)
SOUTH ATLANTIC	29,482	39%	36%	3%	8%	15%
		(0.32)	(0.32)	(0.11)	(0.18)	(0.24)
Delaware	482	40%	36%	2%	7%	15%
		(1.18)	(1.16)	(0.33)	(0.62)	(0.86)
District of Columbia	362	43%	23%	6%	9%	19%
		(1.37)	(1.16)	(0.67)	(0.78)	(1.09)
Florida	8,357	36%	32%	3%	9%	20%
		(0.55)	(0.53)	(0.19)	(0.33)	(0.46)
Georgia	4,402	39%	36%	2%	7%	15%
		(1.08)	(1.07)	(0.34)	(0.58)	(0.78)
Maryland	3,306	44%	40%	2%	5%	9%
		(1.18)	(1.17)	(0.32)	(0.52)	(0.69)
North Carolina	4,604	42%	34%	3%	8%	13%
		(0.57)	(0.54)	(0.19)	(0.32)	(0.39)
South Carolina	2,471	40%	36%	3%	8%	13%
		(0.99)	(0.97)	(0.35)	(0.54)	(0.67)
Virginia	4,293	39%	38%	1%	7%	14%
		(0.98)	(0.97)	(0.23)	(0.52)	(0.69)
West Virginia	1,206	34%	43%	6%	6%	12%
		(1.10)	(1.15)	(0.53)	(0.55)	(0.75)
EAST SOUTH CENTRAL	10,411	36%	38%	4%	8%	14%
		(0.55)	(0.56)	(0.22)	(0.30)	(0.40)
Alabama	2,758	35%	39%	2%	8%	16%
		(1.09)	(1.11)	(0.32)	(0.60)	(0.83)
Kentucky	2,456	36%	39%	5%	8%	11%
		(1.12)	(1.14)	(0.53)	(0.62)	(0.74)
Mississippi	1,757	31%	36%	7%	9%	17%
		(1.00)	(1.04)	(0.56)	(0.63)	(0.82)
Tennessee	3,440	38%	38%	3%	6%	14%
		(1.05)	(1.05)	(0.37)	(0.53)	(0.75)
WEST SOUTH CENTRAL	19,074	32%	35%	3%	9%	21%
		(0.41)	(0.42)	(0.16)	(0.24)	(0.35)
Arkansas	1,683	32%	38%	4%	9%	17%
		(1.03)	(1.07)	(0.43)	(0.63)	(0.83)
Louisiana	2,748	30%	38%	4%	8%	19%
		(1.11)	(1.18)	(0.49)	(0.67)	(0.96)
Oklahoma	2,199	32%	36%	4%	9%	19%
		(1.05)	(1.07)	(0.42)	(0.65)	(0.87)
Texas	12,444	32%	34%	3%	9%	22%
		(0.53)	(0.53)	(0.19)	(0.31)	(0.47)

ALL PERSONS IN FAMILY UNDER AGE 65 BY WORK STATUS OF SPOUSE AND HEAD,
AT LEAST ONE FULL-TIME WORKER: BY TYPE OF HEALTH INSURANCE COVERAGE

	Number (000s)	Employer (own)	Employer (other)	Medicaid	Other	Uninsured
EAST NORTH CENTRAL	**30,180**	**38%** (0.31)	**43%** (0.32)	**3%** (0.11)	**7%** (0.16)	**9%** (0.18)
Illinois	8,290	39% (0.58)	40% (0.58)	3% (0.21)	7% (0.31)	10% (0.35)
Indiana	4,039	38% (1.11)	41% (1.12)	2% (0.29)	8% (0.63)	11% (0.72)
Michigan	6,458	38% (0.58)	44% (0.59)	4% (0.23)	6% (0.28)	8% (0.32)
Ohio	7,843	38% (0.56)	45% (0.57)	3% (0.21)	6% (0.27)	8% (0.31)
Wisconsin	3,550	38% (1.01)	45% (1.03)	3% (0.35)	7% (0.54)	7% (0.54)
WEST NORTH CENTRAL	**13,054**	**35%** (0.47)	**40%** (0.49)	**3%** (0.17)	**12%** (0.32)	**10%** (0.29)
Iowa	2,031	34% (1.02)	42% (1.06)	2% (0.31)	15% (0.78)	7% (0.53)
Kansas	1,809	35% (1.02)	43% (1.05)	3% (0.38)	10% (0.65)	8% (0.59)
Minnesota	3,236	37% (1.08)	38% (1.09)	3% (0.40)	12% (0.71)	10% (0.67)
Missouri	3,801	37% (1.09)	40% (1.11)	3% (0.38)	8% (0.63)	12% (0.72)
Nebraska	1,210	33% (0.96)	40% (1.00)	3% (0.35)	14% (0.72)	10% (0.62)
North Dakota	461	27% (0.93)	40% (1.02)	2% (0.29)	22% (0.87)	9% (0.58)
South Dakota	506	29% (0.90)	36% (0.95)	3% (0.35)	18% (0.76)	13% (0.67)
MOUNTAIN	**9,791**	**33%** (0.45)	**39%** (0.47)	**2%** (0.14)	**9%** (0.27)	**16%** (0.35)
Arizona	2,479	35% (1.10)	35% (1.10)	3% (0.38)	8% (0.64)	18% (0.89)
Colorado	2,376	36% (1.13)	39% (1.15)	1% (0.25)	9% (0.66)	15% (0.84)
Idaho	781	29% (0.93)	39% (1.00)	2% (0.29)	13% (0.68)	16% (0.76)
Montana	585	30% (0.99)	35% (1.03)	4% (0.40)	15% (0.78)	16% (0.80)
Nevada	861	41% (1.12)	34% (1.08)	1% (0.27)	8% (0.61)	16% (0.84)
New Mexico	1,032	27% (0.98)	35% (1.05)	4% (0.43)	8% (0.59)	26% (0.96)
Utah	1,319	29% (0.95)	51% (1.04)	3% (0.33)	8% (0.56)	9% (0.60)
Wyoming	357	31% (1.15)	42% (1.24)	3% (0.42)	11% (0.79)	13% (0.83)
PACIFIC	**27,093**	**36%** (0.38)	**34%** (0.37)	**5%** (0.18)	**8%** (0.21)	**17%** (0.30)
Alaska	356	32% (1.01)	34% (1.02)	4% (0.41)	9% (0.63)	21% (0.87)
California	20,517	35% (0.45)	32% (0.44)	6% (0.22)	8% (0.25)	19% (0.37)
Hawaii	684	45% (1.24)	36% (1.20)	4% (0.46)	6% (0.61)	9% (0.71)
Oregon	2,002	38% (1.18)	40% (1.19)	3% (0.43)	6% (0.56)	13% (0.82)
Washington	3,533	38% (1.07)	37% (1.06)	4% (0.43)	9% (0.64)	11% (0.69)

Source: Three-year merged March CPS, 1989, 1990, and 1991.

42

TABLE A16
ALL PERSONS IN FAMILY UNDER AGE 65 BY WORK STATUS OF SPOUSE AND HEAD,
AT LEAST ONE PART-TIME WORKER AND NO FULL-TIME WORKERS:
BY TYPE OF HEALTH INSURANCE COVERAGE

	Number (000s)	Employer (own)	Employer (other)	Medicaid	Other	Uninsured
UNITED STATES	17,101	20% (0.35)	15% (0.31)	18% (0.33)	17% (0.33)	29% (0.39)
NEW ENGLAND	951	28% (1.29)	19% (1.13)	16% (1.04)	17% (1.08)	19% (1.12)
Connecticut	249	29% (3.51)	25% (3.36)	13% (2.59)	16% (2.85)	17% (2.91)
Maine	90	19% (2.78)	17% (2.69)	26% (3.11)	18% (2.72)	20% (2.82)
Massachusetts	447	29% (1.68)	18% (1.40)	18% (1.42)	17% (1.39)	18% (1.41)
New Hampshire	56	20% (3.75)	18% (3.58)	9% (2.62)	21% (3.85)	33% (4.41)
Rhode Island	73	40% (3.77)	20% (3.10)	7% (2.03)	17% (2.88)	15% (2.77)
Vermont	36	25% (3.54)	7% (2.08)	13% (2.75)	24% (3.52)	32% (3.82)
MIDDLE ATLANTIC	2,790	31% (0.90)	23% (0.81)	14% (0.68)	12% (0.64)	20% (0.78)
New Jersey	488	35% (1.88)	20% (1.57)	10% (1.16)	15% (1.41)	20% (1.57)
New York	1,678	32% (1.21)	24% (1.11)	14% (0.91)	9% (0.76)	21% (1.06)
Pennsylvania	623	25% (1.85)	22% (1.74)	17% (1.58)	19% (1.66)	17% (1.61)
SOUTH ATLANTIC	2,708	19% (0.86)	13% (0.75)	15% (0.78)	18% (0.84)	35% (1.04)
Delaware	40	33% (3.90)	22% (3.43)	16% (3.04)	11% (2.61)	19% (3.26)
District of Columbia	44	28% (3.57)	6% (1.91)	22% (3.30)	16% (2.94)	27% (3.53)
Florida	850	18% (1.38)	12% (1.18)	12% (1.15)	22% (1.48)	36% (1.73)
Georgia	443	17% (2.62)	13% (2.32)	13% (2.32)	13% (2.38)	44% (3.47)
Maryland	280	21% (3.36)	15% (2.96)	18% (3.13)	20% (3.28)	25% (3.57)
North Carolina	373	21% (1.63)	13% (1.36)	16% (1.48)	20% (1.62)	30% (1.86)
South Carolina	188	13% (2.48)	12% (2.41)	20% (2.95)	12% (2.39)	42% (3.60)
Virginia	368	23% (2.86)	15% (2.41)	13% (2.29)	17% (2.60)	33% (3.21)
West Virginia	122	19% (2.89)	18% (2.81)	31% (3.36)	9% (2.07)	23% (3.07)
EAST SOUTH CENTRAL	1,067	15% (1.26)	13% (1.20)	23% (1.49)	18% (1.38)	32% (1.66)
Alabama	301	19% (2.67)	13% (2.33)	16% (2.52)	14% (2.42)	38% (3.34)
Kentucky	254	19% (2.84)	14% (2.51)	15% (2.55)	21% (2.95)	31% (3.34)
Mississippi	209	8% (1.74)	9% (1.82)	31% (2.91)	16% (2.30)	35% (3.00)
Tennessee	302	11% (2.28)	14% (2.54)	30% (3.32)	21% (2.98)	24% (3.09)
WEST SOUTH CENTRAL	2,014	12% (0.86)	11% (0.83)	18% (1.03)	17% (1.01)	43% (1.33)
Arkansas	182	9% (1.95)	7% (1.77)	19% (2.63)	22% (2.80)	42% (3.32)
Louisiana	313	11% (2.28)	8% (1.96)	16% (2.61)	20% (2.86)	45% (3.58)
Oklahoma	242	10% (2.03)	9% (1.96)	24% (2.87)	22% (2.78)	35% (3.22)
Texas	1,278	12% (1.15)	12% (1.13)	18% (1.33)	15% (1.24)	44% (1.74)

TABLE A16 (continued)
ALL PERSONS IN FAMILY UNDER AGE 65 BY WORK STATUS OF SPOUSE AND HEAD,
AT LEAST ONE PART-TIME WORKER AND NO FULL-TIME WORKERS:
BY TYPE OF HEALTH INSURANCE COVERAGE

	Number (000s)	Employer (own)	Employer (other)	Medicaid	Other	Uninsured
EAST NORTH CENTRAL	**2,630**	**20%** (0.86)	**15%** (0.78)	**21%** (0.89)	**17%** (0.82)	**26%** (0.96)
Illinois	710	21% (1.65)	15% (1.45)	23% (1.69)	18% (1.54)	23% (1.70)
Indiana	299	12% (2.73)	9% (2.43)	12% (2.77)	18% (3.23)	48% (4.20)
Michigan	649	19% (1.47)	17% (1.42)	24% (1.59)	18% (1.43)	22% (1.55)
Ohio	667	21% (1.59)	17% (1.48)	22% (1.63)	14% (1.37)	26% (1.72)
Wisconsin	305	22% (2.94)	14% (2.45)	20% (2.85)	21% (2.88)	23% (2.97)
WEST NORTH CENTRAL	**1,220**	**18%** (1.24)	**14%** (1.13)	**16%** (1.20)	**25%** (1.41)	**27%** (1.44)
Iowa	202	19% (2.70)	13% (2.29)	17% (2.57)	28% (3.09)	22% (2.85)
Kansas	145	15% (2.72)	8% (2.05)	16% (2.77)	25% (3.27)	35% (3.59)
Minnesota	359	18% (2.57)	13% (2.29)	20% (2.70)	26% (2.93)	23% (2.82)
Missouri	341	19% (2.99)	21% (3.09)	13% (2.53)	17% (2.84)	30% (3.45)
Nebraska	77	17% (3.09)	8% (2.23)	12% (2.61)	35% (3.89)	28% (3.65)
North Dakota	48	15% (2.28)	8% (1.74)	18% (2.45)	41% (3.17)	19% (2.52)
South Dakota	49	11% (2.00)	9% (1.86)	16% (2.34)	30% (2.91)	34% (3.01)
MOUNTAIN	**982**	**15%** (1.08)	**14%** (1.06)	**17%** (1.12)	**20%** (1.21)	**33%** (1.42)
Arizona	248	17% (2.75)	18% (2.79)	13% (2.46)	18% (2.78)	34% (3.46)
Colorado	233	14% (2.65)	13% (2.53)	19% (2.96)	19% (2.95)	34% (3.57)
Idaho	77	14% (2.27)	13% (2.22)	19% (2.53)	21% (2.64)	33% (3.05)
Montana	73	16% (2.26)	17% (2.30)	18% (2.34)	17% (2.32)	31% (2.83)
Nevada	70	20% (3.23)	16% (2.90)	6% (1.97)	15% (2.83)	43% (3.96)
New Mexico	137	12% (1.95)	11% (1.88)	12% (1.97)	24% (2.59)	42% (2.99)
Utah	110	12% (2.35)	13% (2.39)	28% (3.24)	28% (3.22)	19% (2.83)
Wyoming	32	19% (3.26)	15% (2.94)	19% (3.23)	23% (3.48)	25% (3.57)
PACIFIC	**2,740**	**20%** (0.99)	**12%** (0.80)	**21%** (1.01)	**17%** (0.93)	**30%** (1.13)
Alaska	45	16% (2.24)	16% (2.23)	28% (2.74)	9% (1.72)	31% (2.81)
California	1,999	19% (1.17)	11% (0.93)	21% (1.23)	17% (1.13)	32% (1.40)
Hawaii	73	31% (3.54)	14% (2.69)	15% (2.72)	12% (2.51)	27% (3.40)
Oregon	261	20% (2.71)	16% (2.45)	15% (2.42)	20% (2.70)	28% (3.03)
Washington	362	24% (2.93)	14% (2.36)	25% (2.95)	17% (2.59)	21% (2.77)

Source: Three-year merged March CPS, 1989, 1990, and 1991.

TABLE A17
ALL PERSONS IN FAMILY UNDER AGE 65 BY WORK STATUS OF SPOUSE AND HEAD,
NO FULL-TIME OR PART-TIME WORKERS: BY TYPE OF HEALTH INSURANCE COVERAGE

	Number (000s)	Employer (own)	Employer (other)	Medicaid	Other	Uninsured
UNITED STATES	22,394	12% (0.25)	7% (0.19)	46% (0.38)	14% (0.27)	20% (0.30)
NEW ENGLAND	928	17% (1.08)	6% (0.67)	47% (1.44)	14% (1.01)	17% (1.07)
Connecticut	146	24% (4.34)	5% (2.24)	41% (4.98)	13% (3.40)	16% (3.70)
Maine	101	14% (2.28)	7% (1.66)	50% (3.34)	15% (2.41)	14% (2.33)
Massachusetts	520	16% (1.24)	6% (0.80)	49% (1.71)	13% (1.15)	17% (1.27)
New Hampshire	51	16% (3.65)	6% (2.34)	35% (4.74)	17% (3.73)	26% (4.33)
Rhode Island	74	15% (2.75)	5% (1.70)	44% (3.80)	21% (3.14)	15% (2.71)
Vermont	36	19% (3.23)	5% (1.83)	44% (4.10)	15% (2.91)	17% (3.07)
MIDDLE ATLANTIC	3,903	15% (0.58)	6% (0.38)	51% (0.82)	12% (0.53)	17% (0.62)
New Jersey	569	16% (1.34)	6% (0.86)	47% (1.82)	13% (1.22)	19% (1.42)
New York	2,230	12% (0.72)	5% (0.47)	57% (1.12)	10% (0.67)	17% (0.85)
Pennsylvania	1,105	20% (1.27)	8% (0.85)	40% (1.56)	15% (1.14)	17% (1.19)
SOUTH ATLANTIC	3,815	14% (0.64)	7% (0.48)	42% (0.91)	16% (0.68)	21% (0.75)
Delaware	51	26% (3.23)	6% (1.73)	31% (3.41)	18% (2.85)	20% (2.95)
District of Columbia	87	15% (2.02)	3% (0.97)	51% (2.82)	9% (1.58)	23% (2.36)
Florida	1,127	13% (1.04)	9% (0.91)	34% (1.47)	21% (1.27)	23% (1.31)
Georgia	630	11% (1.85)	6% (1.40)	53% (2.93)	13% (1.96)	17% (2.21)
Maryland	391	15% (2.49)	4% (1.38)	52% (3.47)	13% (2.31)	16% (2.57)
North Carolina	492	14% (1.22)	7% (0.89)	44% (1.74)	17% (1.34)	18% (1.35)
South Carolina	273	16% (2.21)	6% (1.46)	38% (2.94)	15% (2.14)	26% (2.65)
Virginia	506	16% (2.14)	8% (1.59)	39% (2.84)	14% (2.02)	23% (2.47)
West Virginia	257	12% (1.65)	8% (1.39)	41% (2.47)	18% (1.91)	21% (2.05)
EAST SOUTH CENTRAL	1,736	9% (0.80)	6% (0.68)	45% (1.39)	16% (1.03)	23% (1.18)
Alabama	510	10% (1.62)	9% (1.50)	35% (2.53)	16% (1.95)	29% (2.41)
Kentucky	413	10% (1.67)	8% (1.50)	51% (2.83)	13% (1.92)	19% (2.21)
Mississippi	319	7% (1.29)	4% (1.05)	49% (2.54)	15% (1.83)	24% (2.17)
Tennessee	494	8% (1.54)	4% (1.13)	49% (2.84)	20% (2.25)	20% (2.26)
WEST SOUTH CENTRAL	2,367	9% (0.72)	7% (0.63)	40% (1.22)	17% (0.94)	26% (1.08)
Arkansas	238	7% (1.49)	6% (1.39)	42% (2.90)	20% (2.35)	26% (2.56)
Louisiana	640	9% (1.42)	7% (1.27)	49% (2.51)	14% (1.74)	22% (2.08)
Oklahoma	238	8% (1.86)	7% (1.71)	36% (3.26)	23% (2.88)	26% (2.96)
Texas	1,250	10% (1.08)	7% (0.92)	37% (1.71)	18% (1.35)	28% (1.59)

ALL PERSONS IN FAMILY UNDER AGE 65 BY WORK STATUS OF SPOUSE AND HEAD, NO FULL-TIME OR PART-TIME WORKERS: BY TYPE OF HEALTH INSURANCE COVERAGE

	Number (000s)	Employer (own)	Employer (other)	Medicaid	Other	Uninsured
EAST NORTH CENTRAL	**3,977**	**14%** **(0.62)**	**8%** **(0.47)**	**46%** **(0.88)**	**13%** **(0.60)**	**18%** **(0.68)**
Illinois	1,172	11% (0.97)	5% (0.68)	53% (1.57)	12% (1.02)	19% (1.24)
Indiana	436	15% (2.50)	10% (2.13)	36% (3.34)	20% (2.76)	18% (2.70)
Michigan	1,094	16% (1.04)	9% (0.83)	49% (1.44)	10% (0.85)	17% (1.08)
Ohio	1,026	15% (1.12)	8% (0.86)	43% (1.57)	15% (1.14)	19% (1.24)
Wisconsin	249	24% (3.34)	10% (2.34)	37% (3.78)	16% (2.84)	13% (2.67)
WEST NORTH CENTRAL	**1,006**	**11%** **(1.12)**	**7%** **(0.90)**	**47%** **(1.79)**	**17%** **(1.36)**	**18%** **(1.38)**
Iowa	153	8% (2.19)	8% (2.14)	45% (3.90)	19% (3.09)	20% (3.13)
Kansas	125	11% (2.51)	11% (2.58)	49% (4.06)	14% (2.81)	15% (2.87)
Minnesota	254	15% (2.83)	6% (1.89)	55% (3.97)	13% (2.71)	11% (2.50)
Missouri	334	11% (2.38)	5% (1.72)	43% (3.78)	18% (2.95)	23% (3.20)
Nebraska	74	9% (2.41)	4% (1.66)	43% (4.12)	19% (3.26)	25% (3.58)
North Dakota	36	8% (1.97)	5% (1.67)	41% (3.67)	31% (3.44)	15% (2.67)
South Dakota	30	5% (1.81)	11% (2.54)	30% (3.68)	28% (3.63)	26% (3.52)
MOUNTAIN	**939**	**13%** **(1.03)**	**8%** **(0.84)**	**36%** **(1.48)**	**18%** **(1.18)**	**25%** **(1.34)**
Arizona	290	12% (2.23)	8% (1.79)	38% (3.26)	21% (2.74)	21% (2.76)
Colorado	226	10% (2.32)	5% (1.67)	43% (3.78)	14% (2.64)	28% (3.44)
Idaho	39	12% (3.02)	9% (2.61)	25% (3.96)	32% (4.28)	23% (3.84)
Montana	52	13% (2.46)	10% (2.12)	44% (3.59)	18% (2.78)	16% (2.63)
Nevada	79	18% (2.89)	8% (2.06)	28% (3.40)	15% (2.67)	31% (3.50)
New Mexico	133	11% (1.91)	7% (1.60)	33% (2.88)	17% (2.32)	32% (2.87)
Utah	96	18% (2.98)	15% (2.79)	29% (3.50)	14% (2.69)	23% (3.24)
Wyoming	25	13% (3.17)	10% (2.87)	29% (4.28)	24% (4.03)	23% (3.97)
PACIFIC	**3,724**	**9%** **(0.62)**	**7%** **(0.54)**	**52%** **(1.06)**	**12%** **(0.69)**	**19%** **(0.84)**
Alaska	34	14% (2.43)	8% (1.91)	31% (3.23)	14% (2.40)	33% (3.30)
California	3,072	8% (0.67)	6% (0.59)	56% (1.20)	10% (0.74)	19% (0.95)
Hawaii	93	20% (2.73)	9% (1.96)	41% (3.34)	20% (2.70)	10% (1.99)
Oregon	201	18% (2.97)	10% (2.32)	34% (3.62)	19% (2.98)	19% (3.03)
Washington	324	11% (2.30)	10% (2.19)	36% (3.49)	20% (2.90)	22% (3.00)

Source: Three-year merged March CPS, 1989, 1990, and 1991.

Notes for tables A1–A17

A1   Categorization by type of health insurance coverage is hierarchial. Individuals reporting more than one type of coverage are categorized in the following order: own-employer group, employer group from another source, Medicaid, other government insurance (includes CHAMPUS), and other private insurance. An individual is categorized as uninsured if none of the above types are reported.

A2–A3   The category "Employer" includes individuals covered by employer group health insurance from their own employer or as a dependent.

A2–A17   The category "Other" includes individuals covered by non-Medicaid government insurance and nonemployer-sponsored private insurance.

A11   Three asterisks (***) indicate that there are no observations available in the three-year merged March CPS for that cell.

A12–A17   These tables include all persons under age 65 by the work status of the head or spouse. Single individuals are included as a family. The work status of other adults in the family is not considered. For example, a man who is working and living with his brother and brother's wife who are both not working would be included in table A17.

A15   This table includes all persons in families where either the head or the spouse or both is a full-time worker. Full-time workers are defined as individuals who reported that their usual number of hours of work per week in the previous year was more than 35 hours.

A16   This table includes all persons in families where neither the spouse nor the head is a full-time worker and at least one of them is a part-time worker. Part-time workers are defined as individuals who reported that their usual number of hours of work per week in the previous year was 35 or less.

A17   This table includes all persons in families where neither the head nor the spouse is working. Nonworkers are defined as individuals who reported that their usual number of hours of work per week in the previous year was zero.

     Individuals in nonworker families may have employer group insurance for several reasons. These include individuals covered by the Consolidated Budget Reconciliation Act of 1986 (COBRA), early retirees, children covered by an adult not living in the household, and coverage by individuals who are not the head or spouse, but are working.

SECTION B

Health Insurance Coverage of Workers

This section provides more information about insurance coverage of workers. Since many policy proposals to expand health insurance access focus on the workplace, it is important to understand the job characteristics of workers with and without employment-based insurance.

The first two tables in this section (tables B1 and B2) show insurance coverage for persons working full-time (more than 35 hours a week) and persons working part-time, respectively. The number of hours usually worked per week is important because many employers only insure full-time workers. Many policies seeking to expand the employment-based insurance system would also exclude part-time workers. Thus, the percentage of full-time workers without health insurance from their own employer indicates the proportion of workers in a state who could be affected by a policy that expanded employment-based coverage to all full-time workers using a definition of more than 35 hours a week.

In the entire United States 14 percent of full-time workers have no source of health insurance (table B1). The rate of uninsurance for this group varies from 8 percent in states such as Iowa, Hawaii, and Wisconsin to 20 percent and higher in states such as Texas, Alaska, and New Mexico. States with low rates of uninsurance for full-time workers tend to have higher incidences of employer group insurance, higher rates of other types of private health insurance, or both. For example, in Wisconsin 83 percent of full-time workers have employer group insurance either through their own employer or their spouse's employer, compared to the national average of 77 percent.

Insurance status for part-time workers (table B2) indicates that relatively few (20 percent) have insurance through their own employment. Part-time workers are more likely to be covered as dependents on other workers' policies (37 percent) or to be covered through other private and government policies (17 percent). This group also has a high rate of uninsurance—more than one-in-five part-time workers has no health insurance coverage. Insurance coverage for part-time workers also varies across the states. For example, only 15 percent or fewer of part-time workers have insurance through their employment in many of the southern and western states (for example, Texas, Arkansas, Tennessee, and the Dakotas). In contrast, the proportion of part-time workers insured through their employer is more than 20 percent in many of the New England and Middle Atlantic states.

EMPLOYMENT CHARACTERISTICS

Focusing on the employment characteristics of persons who are working (full-time or part-time), we show the incidence of employer group coverage and uninsurance by firm size (tables B3 and B4), by sector of employment (tables B5 and B6), and by industry (tables B7 and B8). These tables show important coverage differences across employers' characteristics that generally hold across all states. Note that these data indicate how many are *enrolled* in their own employer's plan, not the number *offered* health insurance. Persons not enrolled may have chosen not to enroll, for example, because they are insured through a spouse's plan, or they may not have access to employer-group health insurance.

Firms with fewer than 25 workers are less likely to provide health insurance, whereas those with 100 or more workers are more likely to provide insurance. States that have lower-than-average or higher-than-average rates of own-employer group health insurance across all firm size categories stand out, however. For example, employer group insurance is less common in all West South Central states (Arkansas, Louisiana, Oklahoma, and Texas) than it is across the entire United States. Thus, mandates requiring all employers to provide health insurance will have a greater impact on employers in these states than in states in the New England and Middle Atlantic regions that already have higher-than-average rates of employer group insurance coverage.

Statistics presented for workers without any source of health insurance (table B4) show the reverse of the employer group insurance picture.

Workers in small firms (less than 25 workers) are much more likely to lack insurance than are other workers. Although this holds true across the country, workers in some states have generally higher rates of uninsurance than in others. In general, states mentioned earlier that have lower-than-average employer group coverage rates have higher rates of uninsurance (for example, workers in all firm-size categories in the West South Central region).

The table showing employer group insurance by employment sector (table B5) highlights the high enrollment rates in employer group insurance plans among workers in the government sector. Nationwide, 71 percent of government employees are insured through their own employer, compared to 56 percent of private-sector workers. Only 27 percent of those who are self-employed report having health insurance through their own employment-based plans. Not surprisingly, self-employed workers have the highest rate of uninsurance (20 percent) among the three employment sectors (table B6). There is wide variation in the incidence of uninsurance among self-employed workers across the country, however. For example, the percentage of self-employed workers without health insurance is 14 percent in the West North Central region compared to 27 percent in the West South Central region.

The last two tables in this section (tables B7 and B8) show the percent of private-sector workers with employer group insurance and without insurance by industry. Workers in manufacturing are much more likely to have insurance through their employer than are other workers. Insurance coverage among the manufacturing industry is relatively high across all states, but there are some important differences across the states. For example, 82 percent of workers in manufacturing in Michigan and Ohio have employer group insurance, compared to 63 percent in New Mexico and 65 percent in Alaska (table B7). This reflects the high concentration of large manufacturing firms in the East North Central, many of which provide generous insurance coverage established through union bargaining agreements.

The rates of uninsurance among private-sector workers (table B8) also indicate some important variations across the states. Nationwide, 17 percent of workers in service industries are uninsured. However, 22 percent of service sector employees in California and 30 percent in New Mexico have no health insurance. Workers in the wholesale and retail industry have the highest rates of uninsurance. In the Mountain and Pacific regions, for example, one-quarter of workers in this industry group lack insurance.

TABLE B1
FULL-TIME WORKERS AGES 18-64: BY TYPE OF HEALTH INSURANCE COVERAGE

	Population (000s)	Employer (own)	Employer (other)	Medicaid	Other	Uninsured
UNITED STATES	95,625	66% (0.17)	11% (0.12)	1% (0.04)	8% (0.10)	14% (0.13)
NEW ENGLAND	5,340	69% (0.56)	13% (0.41)	1% (0.12)	7% (0.30)	10% (0.36)
Connecticut	1,362	73% (1.47)	12% (1.08)	1% (0.28)	5% (0.73)	9% (0.96)
Maine	474	65% (1.48)	14% (1.08)	1% (0.33)	8% (0.86)	12% (0.99)
Massachusetts	2,404	69% (0.74)	14% (0.54)	1% (0.16)	7% (0.41)	10% (0.47)
New Hampshire	483	65% (1.53)	14% (1.11)	1% (0.26)	9% (0.92)	11% (1.02)
Rhode Island	377	68% (1.58)	13% (1.13)	1% (0.36)	5% (0.72)	13% (1.14)
Vermont	240	65% (1.53)	15% (1.15)	1% (0.39)	8% (0.86)	11% (0.98)
MIDDLE ATLANTIC	14,080	70% (0.40)	11% (0.27)	1% (0.09)	6% (0.21)	12% (0.28)
New Jersey	3,176	72% (0.69)	11% (0.48)	1% (0.14)	6% (0.38)	10% (0.46)
New York	6,334	68% (0.63)	11% (0.41)	1% (0.12)	7% (0.34)	14% (0.46)
Pennsylvania	4,570	72% (0.70)	11% (0.50)	1% (0.18)	6% (0.37)	9% (0.45)
SOUTH ATLANTIC	17,255	66% (0.41)	11% (0.27)	1% (0.09)	8% (0.23)	14% (0.30)
Delaware	286	67% (1.48)	10% (0.96)	1% (0.30)	8% (0.83)	15% (1.10)
District of Columbia	252	65% (1.58)	5% (0.75)	2% (0.50)	9% (0.94)	18% (1.28)
Florida	4,852	61% (0.73)	10% (0.45)	1% (0.17)	9% (0.43)	19% (0.59)
Georgia	2,550	66% (1.38)	12% (0.93)	1% (0.32)	7% (0.72)	14% (1.02)
Maryland	2,020	70% (1.39)	13% (1.02)	1% (0.30)	6% (0.72)	10% (0.92)
North Carolina	2,752	68% (0.69)	10% (0.44)	1% (0.17)	8% (0.40)	13% (0.49)
South Carolina	1,412	69% (1.24)	12% (0.85)	1% (0.28)	7% (0.69)	11% (0.85)
Virginia	2,513	67% (1.23)	12% (0.84)	1% (0.19)	7% (0.67)	13% (0.89)
West Virginia	620	65% (1.54)	13% (1.09)	3% (0.58)	6% (0.74)	13% (1.09)
EAST SOUTH CENTRAL	5,583	65% (0.74)	12% (0.51)	1% (0.18)	7% (0.49)	14% (0.54)
Alabama	1,464	64% (1.50)	13% (1.04)	0% (0.19)	7% (0.79)	16% (1.15)
Kentucky	1,295	67% (1.51)	12% (1.04)	3% (0.52)	8% (0.85)	11% (0.99)
Mississippi	924	57% (1.48)	13% (1.00)	2% (0.44)	9% (0.86)	19% (1.16)
Tennessee	1,900	68% (1.35)	12% (0.95)	1% (0.26)	6% (0.69)	13% (0.97)
WEST SOUTH CENTRAL	10,042	59% (0.59)	11% (0.38)	1% (0.14)	8% (0.33)	20% (0.48)
Arkansas	893	58% (1.50)	14% (1.05)	2% (0.39)	9% (0.87)	17% (1.15)
Louisiana	1,397	58% (1.68)	14% (1.19)	2% (0.47)	7% (0.88)	19% (1.33)
Oklahoma	1,190	58% (1.50)	13% (1.02)	1% (0.35)	9% (0.85)	19% (1.20)
Texas	6,562	60% (0.76)	10% (0.46)	1% (0.17)	8% (0.43)	20% (0.62)

FULL-TIME WORKERS AGES 18-64: BY TYPE OF HEALTH INSURANCE COVERAGE

	Population (000s)	Employer (own)	Employer (other)	Medicaid	Other	Uninsured
EAST NORTH CENTRAL	**16,308**	**70%** (0.40)	**13%** (0.29)	**2%** (0.11)	**7%** (0.22)	**10%** (0.26)
Illinois	4,549	70% (0.73)	11% (0.50)	1% (0.19)	7% (0.41)	10% (0.48)
Indiana	2,222	67% (1.45)	14% (1.07)	1% (0.28)	7% (0.80)	11% (0.96)
Michigan	3,418	71% (0.74)	12% (0.53)	2% (0.23)	6% (0.39)	9% (0.47)
Ohio	4,164	70% (0.72)	13% (0.53)	2% (0.20)	6% (0.37)	9% (0.45)
Wisconsin	1,955	69% (1.30)	14% (0.97)	2% (0.37)	7% (0.72)	8% (0.77)
WEST NORTH CENTRAL	**6,999**	**64%** (0.65)	**13%** (0.45)	**2%** (0.17)	**12%** (0.44)	**10%** (0.41)
Iowa	1,078	62% (1.44)	14% (1.01)	1% (0.31)	15% (1.05)	8% (0.82)
Kansas	977	64% (1.39)	14% (1.00)	2% (0.38)	11% (0.90)	10% (0.85)
Minnesota	1,764	65% (1.44)	11% (0.94)	2% (0.45)	11% (0.95)	10% (0.92)
Missouri	2,055	67% (1.45)	12% (1.00)	2% (0.38)	8% (0.85)	11% (0.98)
Nebraska	634	61% (1.38)	14% (0.97)	1% (0.30)	13% (0.96)	11% (0.89)
North Dakota	228	53% (1.48)	15% (1.05)	1% (0.22)	22% (1.22)	10% (0.90)
South Dakota	263	53% (1.37)	14% (0.95)	1% (0.30)	19% (1.07)	13% (0.92)
MOUNTAIN	**5,069**	**62%** (0.64)	**12%** (0.43)	**1%** (0.13)	**9%** (0.38)	**16%** (0.48)
Arizona	1,349	63% (1.51)	12% (1.01)	1% (0.30)	8% (0.87)	16% (1.13)
Colorado	1,287	64% (1.54)	13% (1.09)	1% (0.27)	9% (0.90)	13% (1.09)
Idaho	380	57% (1.45)	12% (0.93)	1% (0.28)	13% (0.97)	18% (1.12)
Montana	301	55% (1.50)	12% (0.97)	2% (0.40)	16% (1.10)	16% (1.11)
Nevada	506	67% (1.40)	9% (0.85)	0% (0.19)	7% (0.74)	17% (1.12)
New Mexico	512	54% (1.56)	11% (0.99)	2% (0.39)	8% (0.86)	25% (1.36)
Utah	557	67% (1.51)	13% (1.09)	1% (0.38)	8% (0.89)	10% (0.98)
Wyoming	177	59% (1.74)	14% (1.22)	1% (0.40)	11% (1.11)	15% (1.25)
PACIFIC	**14,948**	**62%** (0.51)	**10%** (0.31)	**3%** (0.17)	**8%** (0.29)	**17%** (0.40)
Alaska	194	56% (1.45)	11% (0.90)	1% (0.33)	9% (0.85)	23% (1.22)
California	11,346	61% (0.61)	9% (0.36)	3% (0.21)	8% (0.34)	19% (0.49)
Hawaii	426	71% (1.43)	13% (1.06)	2% (0.43)	6% (0.77)	8% (0.84)
Oregon	1,077	67% (1.56)	12% (1.07)	2% (0.45)	7% (0.82)	13% (1.11)
Washington	1,905	66% (1.41)	10% (0.91)	1% (0.36)	9% (0.87)	13% (0.99)

Source: Three-year merged March CPS, 1989, 1990, and 1991.

TABLE B2
PART-TIME WORKERS AGES 18-64: BY TYPE OF HEALTH INSURANCE COVERAGE

	Number (000s)	Employer (own)	Employer (other)	Medicaid	Other	Uninsured
UNITEED STATES	27,145	20% (0.28)	37% (0.33)	4% (0.14)	17% (0.26)	21% (0.28)
NEW ENGLAND	1,663	26% (0.94)	43% (1.07)	4% (0.43)	15% (0.77)	13% (0.72)
Connecticut	421	30% (2.73)	42% (2.94)	4% (1.22)	12% (1.96)	11% (1.86)
Maine	149	21% (2.25)	40% (2.71)	6% (1.35)	17% (2.05)	15% (1.99)
Massachusetts	761	24% (1.20)	44% (1.40)	4% (0.57)	16% (1.03)	12% (0.92)
New Hampshire	131	21% (2.52)	44% (3.06)	2% (0.95)	14% (2.15)	18% (2.37)
Rhode Island	129	36% (2.79)	35% (2.77)	2% (0.90)	14% (2.00)	13% (1.93)
Vermont	72	20% (2.35)	42% (2.87)	3% (1.02)	19% (2.27)	16% (2.13)
MIDDLE ATLANTIC	4,364	30% (0.71)	37% (0.75)	3% (0.27)	14% (0.54)	15% (0.56)
New Jersey	851	32% (1.39)	37% (1.43)	2% (0.44)	15% (1.06)	14% (1.03)
New York	2,194	34% (1.07)	33% (1.07)	3% (0.41)	14% (0.78)	17% (0.85)
Pennsylvania	1,319	22% (1.21)	46% (1.45)	4% (0.54)	14% (1.02)	14% (1.01)
SOUTH ATLANTIC	4,146	20% (0.71)	33% (0.83)	4% (0.33)	17% (0.67)	27% (0.78)
Delaware	71	27% (2.78)	37% (3.04)	3% (1.09)	15% (2.24)	19% (2.44)
District of Columbia	50	23% (3.11)	14% (2.55)	6% (1.81)	20% (2.97)	37% (3.57)
Florida	1,270	20% (1.16)	29% (1.33)	3% (0.49)	21% (1.19)	28% (1.31)
Georgia	618	19% (2.31)	29% (2.69)	4% (1.09)	14% (2.03)	35% (2.82)
Maryland	493	20% (2.48)	43% (3.06)	3% (1.08)	15% (2.21)	18% (2.39)
North Carolina	602	21% (1.29)	33% (1.50)	4% (0.61)	18% (1.21)	25% (1.37)
South Carolina	286	19% (2.35)	28% (2.67)	4% (1.22)	17% (2.24)	30% (2.73)
Virginia	589	20% (2.15)	37% (2.61)	3% (0.94)	16% (1.98)	24% (2.32)
West Virginia	168	20% (2.49)	36% (2.99)	11% (1.92)	13% (2.07)	21% (2.52)
EAST SOUTH CENTRAL	1,514	16% (1.11)	35% (1.43)	6% (0.69)	18% (1.16)	25% (1.30)
Alabama	388	21% (2.48)	31% (2.80)	4% (1.16)	15% (2.19)	29% (2.75)
Kentucky	427	17% (2.11)	37% (2.69)	6% (1.34)	18% (2.15)	21% (2.29)
Mississippi	240	13% (2.00)	26% (2.57)	8% (1.57)	19% (2.31)	34% (2.77)
Tennessee	459	13% (1.99)	41% (2.90)	6% (1.35)	20% (2.35)	20% (2.37)
WEST SOUTH CENTRAL	2,725	15% (0.82)	32% (1.07)	5% (0.48)	19% (0.90)	30% (1.06)
Arkansas	247	15% (2.07)	30% (2.65)	5% (1.30)	20% (2.31)	29% (2.62)
Louisiana	430	13% (2.07)	34% (2.90)	3% (1.03)	23% (2.56)	28% (2.75)
Oklahoma	331	13% (1.95)	33% (2.72)	6% (1.35)	21% (2.36)	26% (2.54)
Texas	1,716	15% (1.09)	31% (1.40)	5% (0.63)	17% (1.15)	32% (1.41)

	Number (000s)	Employer (own)	Employer (other)	Medicaid	Other	Uninsured
EAST NORTH CENTRAL	**4,887**	**17%** (0.60)	**45%** (0.79)	**5%** (0.34)	**16%** (0.58)	**17%** (0.60)
Illinois	1,276	19% (1.19)	43% (1.49)	4% (0.61)	17% (1.13)	16% (1.11)
Indiana	626	15% (2.04)	44% (2.88)	2% (0.89)	18% (2.24)	20% (2.34)
Michigan	1,137	16% (1.05)	46% (1.41)	7% (0.70)	16% (1.04)	15% (1.00)
Ohio	1,234	17% (1.08)	46% (1.44)	5% (0.61)	14% (1.00)	18% (1.12)
Wisconsin	614	15% (1.76)	48% (2.49)	5% (1.07)	16% (1.84)	16% (1.84)
WEST NORTH CENTRAL	**2,237**	**16%** (0.87)	**41%** (1.18)	**4%** (0.47)	**23%** (1.01)	**17%** (0.90)
Iowa	378	15% (1.80)	39% (2.44)	4% (0.98)	28% (2.23)	14% (1.73)
Kansas	292	12% (1.74)	44% (2.63)	4% (1.03)	23% (2.23)	17% (1.99)
Minnesota	630	17% (1.92)	38% (2.46)	5% (1.15)	21% (2.08)	17% (1.92)
Missouri	578	17% (2.21)	44% (2.88)	3% (0.96)	16% (2.12)	20% (2.31)
Nebraska	177	13% (1.82)	40% (2.63)	2% (0.75)	30% (2.45)	15% (1.94)
North Dakota	94	13% (1.54)	36% (2.22)	4% (0.92)	34% (2.20)	12% (1.52)
South Dakota	87	14% (1.64)	34% (2.25)	4% (0.97)	28% (2.14)	20% (1.90)
MOUNTAIN	**1,516**	**17%** (0.91)	**33%** (1.14)	**4%** (0.50)	**20%** (0.97)	**25%** (1.06)
Arizona	346	19% (2.41)	26% (2.72)	4% (1.18)	22% (2.56)	29% (2.80)
Colorado	364	17% (2.25)	34% (2.85)	5% (1.34)	19% (2.38)	25% (2.60)
Idaho	128	17% (1.90)	36% (2.42)	3% (0.90)	20% (2.02)	24% (2.15)
Montana	112	17% (1.85)	33% (2.32)	5% (1.09)	20% (1.96)	25% (2.14)
Nevada	110	24% (2.73)	31% (2.96)	1% (0.64)	14% (2.24)	29% (2.90)
New Mexico	181	13% (1.80)	30% (2.40)	4% (1.01)	20% (2.12)	33% (2.48)
Utah	209	15% (1.88)	45% (2.60)	6% (1.21)	19% (2.06)	15% (1.87)
Wyoming	65	16% (2.14)	41% (2.88)	6% (1.43)	18% (2.26)	19% (2.28)
PACIFIC	**4,094**	**22%** (0.84)	**31%** (0.93)	**6%** (0.48)	**16%** (0.75)	**25%** (0.87)
Alaska	55	23% (2.31)	25% (2.38)	6% (1.31)	14% (1.94)	32% (2.57)
California	2,974	21% (1.00)	30% (1.13)	6% (0.59)	16% (0.91)	26% (1.08)
Hawaii	88	33% (3.27)	30% (3.18)	4% (1.42)	14% (2.44)	19% (2.71)
Oregon	362	25% (2.48)	33% (2.68)	4% (1.16)	15% (2.04)	23% (2.39)
Washington	615	26% (2.29)	33% (2.48)	6% (1.28)	17% (1.97)	18% (2.01)

Source: Three-year merged March CPS, 1989, 1990, and 1991.

TABLE B3

ALL WORKERS AGES 18-64: PERCENTAGE IN FIRM SIZE WITH OWN-EMPLOYER GROUP INSURANCE

	<25		25-99		100+	
	Number (000s)	Percent Insured	Number (000s)	Percent Insured	Number (000s)	Percent Insured
UNITED STATES	35,961	29% (0.27)	16,209	55% (0.44)	70,599	69% (0.20)
NEW ENGLAND	2,002	33% (0.93)	978	56% (1.40)	4,023	72% (0.63)
Connecticut	486	35% (2.65)	249	59% (3.81)	1,048	76% (1.60)
Maine	208	30% (2.13)	97	54% (3.40)	317	70% (1.72)
Massachusetts	843	33% (1.27)	429	55% (1.87)	1,893	69% (0.83)
New Hampshire	195	31% (2.35)	84	51% (3.86)	336	71% (1.75)
Rhode Island	144	37% (2.65)	77	62% (3.66)	285	71% (1.76)
Vermont	126	31% (2.04)	42	60% (3.77)	144	73% (1.83)
MIDDLE ATLANTIC	5,028	35% (0.69)	2,611	60% (0.98)	10,806	73% (0.44)
New Jersey	1,082	37% (1.27)	578	62% (1.75)	2,367	76% (0.76)
New York	2,395	33% (1.02)	1,193	59% (1.52)	4,940	72% (0.68)
Pennsylvania	1,551	36% (1.29)	840	61% (1.78)	3,498	72% (0.81)
SOUTH ATLANTIC	6,017	29% (0.67)	2,553	55% (1.12)	12,831	70% (0.46)
Delaware	88	31% (2.61)	38	61% (4.19)	230	69% (1.61)
District of Columbia	65	33% (3.07)	36	59% (4.33)	201	66% (1.76)
Florida	2,027	27% (1.03)	788	54% (1.86)	3,307	67% (0.85)
Georgia	842	31% (2.35)	353	58% (3.86)	1,973	68% (1.55)
Maryland	635	34% (2.58)	306	53% (3.91)	1,572	73% (1.54)
North Carolina	877	30% (1.20)	398	54% (1.95)	2,080	73% (0.76)
South Carolina	434	28% (2.15)	201	57% (3.50)	1,063	74% (1.34)
Virginia	800	30% (2.12)	330	54% (3.60)	1,972	71% (1.34)
West Virginia	250	29% (2.32)	105	60% (3.85)	432	70% (1.78)
EAST SOUTH CENTRAL	1,967	26% (1.15)	807	54% (2.04)	4,322	68% (0.83)
Alabama	506	26% (2.33)	214	50% (4.08)	1,132	69% (1.64)
Kentucky	526	26% (2.20)	186	60% (4.13)	1,010	68% (1.69)
Mississippi	342	26% (2.16)	126	46% (4.04)	696	60% (1.69)
Tennessee	593	25% (2.24)	281	58% (3.72)	1,485	70% (1.50)
WEST SOUTH CENTRAL	3,997	23% (0.80)	1,507	47% (1.55)	7,263	65% (0.67)
Arkansas	375	22% (1.93)	138	53% (3.86)	628	64% (1.74)
Louisiana	577	23% (2.22)	244	53% (4.06)	1,006	60% (1.96)
Oklahoma	485	23% (2.01)	201	42% (3.65)	836	64% (1.74)
Texas	2,560	23% (1.05)	925	45% (2.05)	4,794	67% (0.85)

ALL WORKERS AGES 18-64: PERCENTAGE IN FIRM SIZE WITH OWN-EMPLOYER GROUP INSURANCE

	<25		25-99		100+	
	Number (000s)	Percent Insured	Number (000s)	Percent Insured	Number (000s)	Percent Insured
EAST NORTH CENTRAL	**5,551**	**31%** **(0.69)**	**2,964**	**57%** **(1.01)**	**12,679**	**69%** **(0.46)**
Illinois	1,492	32% (1.30)	832	57% (1.84)	3,500	71% (0.83)
Indiana	732	26% (2.37)	407	57% (3.56)	1,709	67% (1.65)
Michigan	1,257	29% (1.22)	601	58% (1.92)	2,698	70% (0.84)
Ohio	1,335	32% (1.30)	731	55% (1.87)	3,333	69% (0.81)
Wisconsin	734	31% (2.10)	395	58% (3.07)	1,439	68% (1.52)
WEST NORTH CENTRAL	**2,983**	**26%** **(0.91)**	**1,319**	**53%** **(1.56)**	**4,934**	**68%** **(0.76)**
Iowa	475	21% (1.82)	212	51% (3.34)	769	67% (1.64)
Kansas	413	27% (1.98)	191	55% (3.26)	665	67% (1.66)
Minnesota	779	28% (2.04)	354	51% (3.38)	1,262	69% (1.66)
Missouri	744	30% (2.34)	346	56% (3.73)	1,544	69% (1.65)
Nebraska	282	24% (1.81)	114	52% (3.33)	414	68% (1.64)
North Dakota	141	20% (1.50)	47	47% (3.28)	135	62% (1.88)
South Dakota	149	22% (1.50)	55	53% (3.00)	146	62% (1.79)
MOUNTAIN	**2,186**	**27%** **(0.89)**	**790**	**50%** **(1.68)**	**3,609**	**67%** **(0.74)**
Arizona	536	29% (2.24)	224	48% (3.83)	935	70% (1.71)
Colorado	500	28% (2.31)	164	52% (4.48)	987	67% (1.72)
Idaho	196	23% (1.72)	70	49% (3.41)	242	66% (1.74)
Montana	188	24% (1.63)	56	53% (3.51)	170	64% (1.93)
Nevada	166	32% (2.44)	84	53% (3.66)	367	73% (1.55)
New Mexico	266	22% (1.81)	85	44% (3.83)	342	60% (1.88)
Utah	238	26% (2.15)	80	48% (4.22)	449	67% (1.67)
Wyoming	97	24% (2.06)	28	56% (4.46)	118	65% (2.07)
PACIFIC	**6,230**	**28%** **(0.73)**	**2,681**	**55%** **(1.24)**	**10,131**	**69%** **(0.59)**
Alaska	90	22% (1.79)	28	52% (3.83)	130	67% (1.68)
California	4,721	27% (0.87)	2,061	54% (1.47)	7,538	68% (0.72)
Hawaii	141	47% (2.74)	74	67% (3.57)	299	73% (1.68)
Oregon	485	30% (2.26)	183	59% (3.95)	771	72% (1.76)
Washington	793	28% (2.07)	334	58% (3.52)	1,393	72% (1.56)

Source: Three-year merged March CPS, 1989, 1990, and 1991.

TABLE B4
ALL WORKERS AGES 18-64: PERCENTAGE IN FIRM SIZE THAT ARE UNINSURED

	<25		25-99		100+	
	Number (000s)	Percent Uninsured	Number (000s)	Percent Uninsured	Number (000s)	Percent Uninsured
UNITED STATES	35,961	26% (0.26)	16,209	18% (0.34)	70,599	10% (0.13)
NEW ENGLAND	2,002	19% (0.77)	978	12% (0.93)	4,023	6% (0.34)
Connecticut	486	18% (2.11)	249	11% (2.43)	1,048	6% (0.86)
Maine	208	19% (1.84)	97	18% (2.64)	317	6% (0.91)
Massachusetts	843	18% (1.02)	429	11% (1.18)	1,893	7% (0.45)
New Hampshire	195	24% (2.15)	84	12% (2.53)	336	7% (0.96)
Rhode Island	144	22% (2.27)	77	16% (2.78)	285	7% (1.02)
Vermont	126	19% (1.74)	42	11% (2.40)	144	5% (0.94)
MIDDLE ATLANTIC	5,028	21% (0.59)	2,611	15% (0.71)	10,806	8% (0.26)
New Jersey	1,082	19% (1.03)	578	13% (1.22)	2,367	7% (0.45)
New York	2,395	25% (0.95)	1,193	18% (1.19)	4,940	9% (0.43)
Pennsylvania	1,551	16% (1.00)	840	11% (1.16)	3,498	7% (0.46)
SOUTH ATLANTIC	6,017	28% (0.66)	2,553	20% (0.90)	12,831	11% (0.31)
Delaware	88	30% (2.58)	38	14% (2.95)	230	10% (1.05)
District of Columbia	65	33% (3.05)	36	22% (3.66)	201	18% (1.41)
Florida	2,027	33% (1.10)	788	22% (1.56)	3,307	12% (0.60)
Georgia	842	30% (2.33)	353	20% (3.11)	1,973	13% (1.10)
Maryland	635	19% (2.13)	306	19% (3.06)	1,572	7% (0.90)
North Carolina	877	24% (1.13)	398	19% (1.55)	2,080	10% (0.51)
South Carolina	434	28% (2.15)	201	19% (2.75)	1,063	8% (0.85)
Virginia	800	27% (2.06)	330	16% (2.67)	1,972	10% (0.90)
West Virginia	250	25% (2.20)	105	18% (2.99)	432	8% (1.06)
EAST SOUTH CENTRAL	1,967	29% (1.20)	807	17% (1.54)	4,322	10% (0.54)
Alabama	506	33% (2.49)	214	23% (3.41)	1,132	12% (1.14)
Kentucky	526	24% (2.16)	186	10% (2.57)	1,010	8% (1.00)
Mississippi	342	32% (2.29)	126	26% (3.55)	696	16% (1.26)
Tennessee	593	29% (2.35)	281	13% (2.53)	1,485	9% (0.92)
WEST SOUTH CENTRAL	3,997	34% (0.90)	1,507	27% (1.37)	7,263	14% (0.50)
Arkansas	375	30% (2.14)	138	21% (3.17)	628	13% (1.24)
Louisiana	577	30% (2.42)	244	21% (3.34)	1,006	16% (1.46)
Oklahoma	485	32% (2.23)	201	26% (3.26)	836	13% (1.21)
Texas	2,560	36% (1.19)	925	29% (1.86)	4,794	14% (0.64)

	<25		25-99		100+	
	Number (000s)	**Percent Uninsured**	**Number (000s)**	**Percent Uninsured**	**Number (000s)**	**Percent Uninsured**
EAST NORTH CENTRAL	**5,551**	**19% (0.58)**	**2,964**	**13% (0.69)**	**12,679**	**7% (0.26)**
Illinois	1,492	19% (1.08)	832	13% (1.27)	3,500	8% (0.49)
Indiana	732	23% (2.24)	407	15% (2.55)	1,709	9% (0.98)
Michigan	1,257	17% (1.02)	601	14% (1.35)	2,698	7% (0.45)
Ohio	1,335	19% (1.09)	731	14% (1.28)	3,333	7% (0.46)
Wisconsin	734	16% (1.69)	395	10% (1.90)	1,439	7% (0.82)
WEST NORTH CENTRAL	**2,983**	**18% (0.80)**	**1,319**	**14% (1.07)**	**4,934**	**8% (0.44)**
Iowa	475	13% (1.51)	212	13% (2.25)	769	7% (0.88)
Kansas	413	16% (1.64)	191	14% (2.25)	665	7% (0.93)
Minnesota	779	20% (1.82)	354	12% (2.17)	1,262	8% (0.95)
Missouri	744	22% (2.11)	346	16% (2.78)	1,544	9% (0.99)
Nebraska	282	17% (1.60)	114	13% (2.26)	414	8% (0.97)
North Dakota	141	13% (1.28)	47	13% (2.22)	135	8% (1.02)
South Dakota	149	18% (1.40)	55	13% (2.03)	146	12% (1.19)
MOUNTAIN	**2,186**	**27% (0.90)**	**790**	**24% (1.43)**	**3,609**	**11% (0.49)**
Arizona	536	27% (2.20)	224	25% (3.32)	935	12% (1.21)
Colorado	500	26% (2.24)	164	20% (3.59)	987	10% (1.10)
Idaho	196	25% (1.77)	70	27% (3.03)	242	12% (1.20)
Montana	188	25% (1.66)	56	19% (2.74)	170	11% (1.28)
Nevada	166	32% (2.44)	84	27% (3.24)	367	12% (1.12)
New Mexico	266	39% (2.11)	85	34% (3.65)	342	16% (1.42)
Utah	238	21% (1.99)	80	14% (2.90)	449	7% (0.88)
Wyoming	97	23% (2.03)	28	20% (3.57)	118	9% (1.22)
PACIFIC	**6,230**	**31% (0.76)**	**2,681**	**22% (1.03)**	**10,131**	**11% (0.40)**
Alaska	90	37% (2.07)	28	26% (3.38)	130	16% (1.30)
California	4,721	33% (0.92)	2,061	24% (1.26)	7,538	11% (0.49)
Hawaii	141	15% (1.98)	74	9% (2.14)	299	7% (0.96)
Oregon	485	26% (2.17)	183	14% (2.79)	771	9% (1.11)
Washington	793	23% (1.96)	334	15% (2.57)	1,393	8% (0.95)

Source: Three-Year merged March CPS, 1989, 1990, and 1991.

58

TABLE B5
WORKERS AGES 18-64: PERCENTAGE WITH OWN-EMPLOYER GROUP INSURANCE BY SECTOR

	Private Workers (000s)	Percent with Own-Employer Group Insurance	Government Workers (000s)	Percent with Own-Employer Group Insurance	Self-Employed Workers (000s)	Percent with Own-Employer Group Insurance
UNITED STATES	91,950	56% (0.18)	18,545	71% (0.38)	12,274	27% (0.45)
NEW ENGLAND	5,416	59% (0.59)	920	73% (1.29)	668	32% (1.59)
Connecticut	1,403	63% (1.57)	226	78% (3.38)	154	34% (4.66)
Maine	445	56% (1.58)	92	70% (3.21)	85	25% (3.16)
Massachusetts	2,463	58% (0.77)	432	70% (1.72)	269	34% (2.25)
New Hampshire	482	58% (1.59)	63	72% (4.01)	70	27% (3.78)
Rhode Island	401	60% (1.61)	61	76% (3.58)	44	37% (4.81)
Vermont	221	56% (1.65)	46	74% (3.21)	45	29% (3.34)
MIDDLE ATLANTIC	14,039	60% (0.42)	2,774	78% (0.81)	1,631	33% (1.19)
New Jersey	3,097	64% (0.75)	563	81% (1.44)	367	33% (2.13)
New York	6,264	58% (0.66)	1,485	77% (1.16)	780	33% (1.80)
Pennsylvania	4,678	61% (0.75)	726	76% (1.67)	485	32% (2.24)
SOUTH ATLANTIC	15,852	57% (0.45)	3,582	74% (0.84)	1,967	28% (1.15)
Delaware	277	59% (1.56)	50	70% (3.43)	30	34% (4.57)
District of Columbia	185	53% (1.93)	97	72% (2.40)	---	---
Florida	4,495	52% (0.78)	907	76% (1.49)	719	25% (1.69)
Georgia	2,462	57% (1.47)	468	71% (3.09)	238	30% (4.37)
Maryland	1,757	59% (1.61)	555	72% (2.60)	200	38% (4.71)
North Carolina	2,578	61% (0.75)	485	74% (1.55)	291	24% (1.95)
South Carolina	1,300	61% (1.36)	261	78% (2.55)	137	24% (3.63)
Virginia	2,204	58% (1.38)	635	73% (2.32)	263	28% (3.64)
West Virginia	594	56% (1.64)	124	68% (3.39)	69	30% (4.43)
EAST SOUTH CENTRAL	5,323	55% (0.79)	1,108	71% (1.58)	665	24% (1.93)
Alabama	1,363	54% (1.61)	319	75% (2.89)	170	27% (4.07)
Kentucky	1,301	55% (1.59)	248	69% (3.37)	174	26% (3.85)
Mississippi	861	49% (1.55)	190	62% (3.20)	113	20% (3.40)
Tennessee	1,798	58% (1.47)	353	74% (2.95)	208	21% (3.59)
WEST SOUTH CENTRAL	9,434	50% (0.62)	1,971	68% (1.26)	1,362	25% (1.41)
Arkansas	834	50% (1.57)	165	65% (3.37)	141	22% (3.18)
Louisiana	1,341	47% (1.73)	300	61% (3.58)	185	29% (4.25)
Oklahoma	1,050	48% (1.62)	279	66% (2.97)	193	22% (3.11)
Texas	6,209	50% (0.79)	1,227	71% (1.62)	843	25% (1.87)

WORKERS AGES 18-64: PERCENTAGE WITH OWN-EMPLOYER GROUP INSURANCE BY SECTOR

	Private Workers (000s)	Percent with Own-Employer Group Insurance	Government Workers (000s)	Percent with Own-Employer Group Insurance	Self-Employed Workers (000s)	Percent with Own-Employer Group Insurance
EAST NORTH CENTRAL	**16,468**	**59%** **(0.43)**	**2,932**	**67%** **(0.96)**	**1,794**	**29%** **(1.19)**
Illinois	4,566	60% (0.78)	777	70% (1.77)	482	30% (2.25)
Indiana	2,296	57% (1.50)	348	63% (3.76)	204	21% (4.15)
Michigan	3,520	58% (0.79)	636	67% (1.78)	400	32% (2.23)
Ohio	4,169	59% (0.77)	781	69% (1.68)	449	31% (2.21)
Wisconsin	1,919	58% (1.39)	389	65% (3.00)	260	24% (3.26)
WEST NORTH CENTRAL	**6,723**	**55%** **(0.69)**	**1,362**	**65%** **(1.46)**	**1,152**	**19%** **(1.32)**
Iowa	1,024	53% (1.51)	229	70% (2.95)	203	12% (2.22)
Kansas	906	55% (1.50)	207	63% (3.04)	156	20% (2.90)
Minnesota	1,795	57% (1.49)	310	61% (3.52)	290	19% (2.91)
Missouri	2,024	57% (1.54)	352	69% (3.46)	257	29% (3.94)
Nebraska	554	53% (1.51)	136	69% (2.85)	122	17% (2.42)
North Dakota	200	44% (1.57)	66	57% (2.74)	57	14% (2.05)
South Dakota	221	45% (1.49)	62	64% (2.70)	67	17% (2.05)
MOUNTAIN	**4,690**	**53%** **(0.69)**	**1,098**	**66%** **(1.35)**	**797**	**24%** **(1.44)**
Arizona	1,279	55% (1.59)	219	67% (3.65)	197	33% (3.85)
Colorado	1,181	57% (1.66)	283	62% (3.31)	187	20% (3.38)
Idaho	356	47% (1.51)	82	66% (2.99)	70	23% (2.88)
Montana	259	45% (1.62)	85	63% (2.74)	69	17% (2.39)
Nevada	491	59% (1.49)	75	82% (2.97)	51	27% (4.17)
New Mexico	440	42% (1.67)	154	61% (2.78)	99	21% (2.92)
Utah	530	52% (1.64)	146	71% (2.84)	90	24% (3.39)
Wyoming	153	46% (1.90)	54	70% (2.95)	35	22% (3.28)
PACIFIC	**14,005**	**54%** **(0.55)**	**2,798**	**72%** **(1.09)**	**2,239**	**25%** **(1.18)**
Alaska	146	48% (1.68)	70	64% (2.34)	32	21% (2.92)
California	10,663	53% (0.65)	1,982	72% (1.35)	1,675	24% (1.40)
Hawaii	358	68% (1.61)	107	69% (2.94)	49	36% (4.46)
Oregon	1,036	57% (1.67)	218	74% (3.23)	186	30% (3.64)
Washington	1,801	57% (1.52)	421	76% (2.73)	297	25% (3.27)

Source: Three-year merged March CPS, 1989, 1990, and 1991.

TABLE B6
WORKERS AGES 18-64: PERCENTAGE UNINSURED BY SECTOR

	Private Workers (000s)	Percent Uninsured	Government Workers (000s)	Percent Uninsured	Self-Employed Workers (000s)	Percent Uninsured
UNITED STATES	91,950	16% (0.14)	18,545	7% (0.21)	12,274	20% (0.41)
NEW ENGLAND	5,416	11% (0.37)	920	5% (0.62)	668	18% (1.30)
Connecticut	1,403	9% (0.95)	226	3% (1.32)	154	21% (4.00)
Maine	445	13% (1.06)	92	5% (1.50)	85	20% (2.93)
Massachusetts	2,463	11% (0.49)	432	6% (0.90)	269	13% (1.60)
New Hampshire	482	13% (1.07)	63	1% (1.07)	70	24% (3.63)
Rhode Island	401	13% (1.11)	61	7% (2.22)	44	19% (3.93)
Vermont	221	13% (1.10)	46	3% (1.33)	45	16% (2.73)
MIDDLE ATLANTIC	14,039	13% (0.29)	2,774	6% (0.47)	1,631	17% (0.95)
New Jersey	3,097	11% (0.49)	563	6% (0.88)	367	15% (1.63)
New York	6,264	16% (0.50)	1,485	6% (0.68)	780	18% (1.48)
Pennsylvania	4,678	10% (0.47)	726	6% (0.90)	485	16% (1.77)
SOUTH ATLANTIC	15,852	18% (0.35)	3,582	7% (0.50)	1,967	23% (1.07)
Delaware	277	16% (1.16)	50	7% (1.95)	30	23% (4.06)
District of Columbia	185	26% (1.70)	97	13% (1.77)	---	---
Florida	4,495	23% (0.65)	907	6% (0.84)	719	27% (1.73)
Georgia	2,462	19% (1.17)	468	10% (2.01)	238	23% (4.03)
Maryland	1,757	13% (1.09)	555	7% (1.49)	200	14% (3.38)
North Carolina	2,578	15% (0.55)	485	8% (0.96)	291	21% (1.88)
South Carolina	1,300	15% (1.00)	261	7% (1.62)	137	23% (3.59)
Virginia	2,204	17% (1.06)	635	6% (1.25)	263	20% (3.25)
West Virginia	594	16% (1.22)	124	6% (1.77)	69	16% (3.54)
EAST SOUTH CENTRAL	5,323	18% (0.61)	1,108	7% (0.90)	665	21% (1.84)
Alabama	1,363	22% (1.34)	319	6% (1.53)	170	18% (3.52)
Kentucky	1,301	14% (1.12)	248	6% (1.78)	174	17% (3.27)
Mississippi	861	23% (1.30)	190	13% (2.22)	113	28% (3.84)
Tennessee	1,798	15% (1.06)	353	6% (1.58)	208	23% (3.67)
WEST SOUTH CENTRAL	9,434	24% (0.53)	1,971	10% (0.89)	1,362	27% (1.45)
Arkansas	834	20% (1.25)	165	14% (2.48)	141	26% (3.36)
Louisiana	1,341	23% (1.46)	300	12% (2.41)	185	19% (3.66)
Oklahoma	1,050	23% (1.36)	279	8% (1.73)	193	27% (3.37)
Texas	6,209	25% (0.69)	1,227	9% (1.00)	843	29% (1.95)

	Private Workers (000s)	Percent Uninsured	Government Workers (000s)	Percent Uninsured	Self-Employed Workers (000s)	Percent Uninsured
EAST NORTH CENTRAL	**16,468**	**12% (0.28)**	**2,932**	**6% (0.50)**	**1,794**	**16% (0.95)**
Illinois	4,566	12% (0.51)	777	6% (0.93)	482	16% (1.81)
Indiana	2,296	13% (1.03)	348	7% (2.03)	204	18% (3.93)
Michigan	3,520	11% (0.51)	636	5% (0.80)	400	14% (1.65)
Ohio	4,169	11% (0.50)	781	8% (0.98)	449	16% (1.74)
Wisconsin	1,919	10% (0.86)	389	6% (1.44)	260	15% (2.72)
WEST NORTH CENTRAL	**6,723**	**13% (0.47)**	**1,362**	**6% (0.72)**	**1,152**	**14% (1.15)**
Iowa	1,024	11% (0.95)	229	4% (1.30)	203	10% (2.07)
Kansas	906	13% (1.01)	207	5% (1.34)	156	11% (2.25)
Minnesota	1,795	13% (1.00)	310	6% (1.76)	290	16% (2.73)
Missouri	2,024	14% (1.08)	352	6% (1.78)	257	16% (3.20)
Nebraska	554	14% (1.04)	136	5% (1.40)	122	13% (2.15)
North Dakota	200	12% (1.05)	66	7% (1.42)	57	10% (1.76)
South Dakota	221	16% (1.10)	62	10% (1.66)	67	15% (1.94)
MOUNTAIN	**4,690**	**20% (0.55)**	**1,098**	**9% (0.81)**	**797**	**20% (1.34)**
Arizona	1,279	20% (1.29)	219	9% (2.27)	197	15% (2.91)
Colorado	1,181	17% (1.26)	283	9% (1.93)	187	17% (3.19)
Idaho	356	22% (1.24)	82	8% (1.69)	70	21% (2.76)
Montana	259	21% (1.32)	85	12% (1.83)	69	19% (2.46)
Nevada	491	20% (1.22)	75	8% (2.09)	51	26% (4.13)
New Mexico	440	30% (1.56)	154	13% (1.94)	99	34% (3.37)
Utah	530	12% (1.08)	146	5% (1.33)	90	19% (3.11)
Wyoming	153	19% (1.50)	54	4% (1.32)	35	19% (3.11)
PACIFIC	**14,005**	**20% (0.44)**	**2,798**	**7% (0.64)**	**2,239**	**25% (1.18)**
Alaska	146	27% (1.49)	70	17% (1.83)	32	31% (3.34)
California	10,663	22% (0.54)	1,982	7% (0.79)	1,675	25% (1.43)
Hawaii	358	9% (1.00)	107	7% (1.62)	49	16% (3.41)
Oregon	1,036	15% (1.22)	218	7% (1.89)	186	26% (3.48)
Washington	1,801	14% (1.07)	421	6% (1.51)	297	23% (3.18)

Source: Three-year merged March CPS, 1989, 1990, and 1991.

TABLE B7
PRIVATE-SECTOR WORKERS AGES 18-64:
PERCENTAGE IN INDUSTRY WITH OWN-EMPLOYER GROUP INSURANCE

	Private Sector	Manufacturing	Services	Wholesale/ Retail	Other
UNITED STATES	56%	76%	49%	42%	61%
	(0.18)	(0.33)	(0.35)	(0.37)	(0.37)
NEW ENGLAND	59%	77%	52%	45%	62%
	(0.59)	(0.97)	(1.10)	(1.29)	(1.22)
Connecticut	63%	81%	55%	46%	65%
	(1.57)	(2.36)	(3.06)	(3.73)	(3.19)
Maine	56%	77%	49%	41%	62%
	(1.58)	(2.69)	(3.06)	(3.09)	(3.31)
Massachusetts	58%	75%	51%	46%	61%
	(0.77)	(1.37)	(1.38)	(1.70)	(1.62)
New Hampshire	58%	75%	46%	44%	60%
	(1.59)	(2.49)	(3.33)	(3.33)	(3.32)
Rhode Island	60%	76%	55%	46%	61%
	(1.61)	(2.61)	(3.17)	(3.37)	(3.49)
Vermont	56%	80%	50%	45%	52%
	(1.65)	(2.91)	(2.96)	(3.52)	(3.31)
MIDDLE ATLANTIC	60%	77%	55%	44%	68%
	(0.42)	(0.77)	(0.79)	(0.90)	(0.82)
New Jersey	64%	77%	59%	47%	72%
	(0.75)	(1.34)	(1.43)	(1.66)	(1.38)
New York	58%	74%	53%	42%	65%
	(0.66)	(1.31)	(1.20)	(1.37)	(1.28)
Pennsylvania	61%	80%	54%	43%	68%
	(0.75)	(1.23)	(1.43)	(1.62)	(1.49)
SOUTH ATLANTIC	57%	75%	50%	45%	60%
	(0.45)	(0.83)	(0.87)	(0.90)	(0.88)
Delaware	59%	83%	52%	39%	60%
	(1.56)	(2.36)	(3.04)	(3.39)	(3.03)
District of Columbia	53%	***	58%	31%	55%
	(1.93)	***	(2.62)	(4.06)	(4.05)
Florida	52%	69%	49%	43%	55%
	(0.78)	(1.94)	(1.43)	(1.46)	(1.45)
Georgia	57%	71%	48%	46%	64%
	(1.47)	(2.76)	(2.98)	(2.86)	(2.86)
Maryland	59%	83%	53%	47%	64%
	(1.61)	(3.10)	(2.74)	(3.42)	(3.05)
North Carolina	61%	77%	50%	47%	59%
	(0.75)	(1.08)	(1.69)	(1.62)	(1.63)
South Carolina	61%	80%	47%	43%	60%
	(1.36)	(1.86)	(2.92)	(3.05)	(2.91)
Virginia	58%	77%	51%	48%	59%
	(1.38)	(2.54)	(2.66)	(2.81)	(2.69)
West Virginia	56%	74%	51%	37%	66%
	(1.64)	(3.33)	(3.38)	(3.06)	(2.88)
EAST SOUTH CENTRAL	55%	76%	45%	36%	58%
	(0.79)	(1.24)	(1.68)	(1.55)	(1.66)
Alabama	54%	75%	45%	38%	50%
	(1.61)	(2.51)	(3.43)	(3.10)	(3.50)
Kentucky	55%	78%	43%	34%	65%
	(1.59)	(2.56)	(3.31)	(2.97)	(3.10)
Mississippi	49%	66%	41%	32%	51%
	(1.55)	(2.65)	(3.32)	(2.88)	(3.22)
Tennessee	58%	79%	47%	36%	61%
	(1.47)	(2.11)	(3.10)	(3.08)	(3.11)
WEST SOUTH CENTRAL	50%	71%	39%	38%	56%
	(0.62)	(1.27)	(1.15)	(1.19)	(1.18)
Arkansas	50%	72%	36%	34%	54%
	(1.57)	(2.66)	(3.24)	(2.89)	(3.23)
Louisiana	47%	73%	40%	32%	57%
	(1.73)	(4.26)	(3.10)	(3.10)	(3.16)
Oklahoma	48%	70%	34%	35%	57%
	(1.62)	(3.28)	(2.94)	(3.16)	(3.00)
Texas	50%	71%	40%	40%	55%
	(0.79)	(1.63)	(1.47)	(1.54)	(1.52)

TABLE B7 (continued)
PRIVATE-SECTOR WORKERS AGES 18-64:
PERCENTAGE IN INDUSTRY WITH OWN-EMPLOYER GROUP INSURANCE

	Private Sector	Manufacturing	Services	Wholesale/ Retail	Other
EAST NORTH CENTRAL	**59%**	**80%**	**48%**	**41%**	**63%**
	(0.43)	**(0.64)**	**(0.86)**	**(0.86)**	**(0.91)**
Illinois	60%	78%	51%	44%	69%
	(0.78)	(1.35)	(1.53)	(1.58)	(1.50)
Indiana	57%	79%	47%	38%	58%
	(1.50)	(2.20)	(3.12)	(2.99)	(3.28)
Michigan	58%	82%	46%	40%	61%
	(0.79)	(1.11)	(1.60)	(1.57)	(1.82)
Ohio	59%	82%	47%	42%	61%
	(0.77)	(1.12)	(1.53)	(1.58)	(1.70)
Wisconsin	58%	82%	45%	37%	61%
	(1.39)	(1.88)	(2.83)	(2.83)	(3.10)
WEST NORTH CENTRAL	**55%**	**76%**	**46%**	**42%**	**61%**
	(0.69)	**(1.26)**	**(1.31)**	**(1.33)**	**(1.39)**
Iowa	53%	78%	40%	40%	58%
	(1.51)	(2.60)	(2.88)	(2.84)	(3.17)
Kansas	55%	83%	45%	41%	56%
	(1.50)	(2.35)	(2.87)	(2.91)	(3.07)
Minnesota	57%	76%	46%	46%	63%
	(1.49)	(2.66)	(2.77)	(2.99)	(3.04)
Missouri	57%	72%	52%	42%	66%
	(1.54)	(2.93)	(2.99)	(2.98)	(2.99)
Nebraska	53%	77%	44%	39%	62%
	(1.51)	(2.84)	(2.83)	(2.83)	(2.99)
North Dakota	44%	65%	41%	31%	51%
	(1.57)	(4.89)	(2.80)	(2.68)	(2.94)
South Dakota	45%	67%	41%	33%	49%
	(1.49)	(3.43)	(2.68)	(2.65)	(3.00)
MOUNTAIN	**53%**	**74%**	**48%**	**41%**	**58%**
	(0.69)	**(1.53)**	**(1.27)**	**(1.31)**	**(1.28)**
Arizona	55%	75%	47%	46%	61%
	(1.59)	(3.32)	(2.97)	(3.06)	(3.05)
Colorado	57%	81%	49%	42%	62%
	(1.66)	(3.17)	(3.21)	(3.29)	(2.94)
Idaho	47%	73%	42%	38%	44%
	(1.51)	(3.02)	(2.99)	(2.75)	(2.90)
Montana	45%	66%	42%	37%	51%
	(1.62)	(5.14)	(2.96)	(2.71)	(3.06)
Nevada	59%	69%	65%	45%	59%
	(1.49)	(5.16)	(2.19)	(3.16)	(2.89)
New Mexico	42%	63%	40%	28%	50%
	(1.67)	(4.44)	(3.19)	(2.76)	(3.12)
Utah	52%	69%	43%	41%	62%
	(1.64)	(3.34)	(2.96)	(3.19)	(3.25)
Wyoming	46%	***	35%	31%	59%
	(1.90)	***	(3.82)	(3.34)	(2.87)
PACIFIC	**54%**	**73%**	**48%**	**43%**	**56%**
	(0.55)	**(1.03)**	**(1.03)**	**(1.08)**	**(1.09)**
Alaska	48%	65%	41%	41%	54%
	(1.68)	(5.59)	(2.99)	(3.28)	(2.82)
California	53%	72%	48%	42%	55%
	(0.65)	(1.24)	(1.23)	(1.28)	(1.29)
Hawaii	68%	***	64%	61%	74%
	(1.61)	***	(2.88)	(3.15)	(2.71)
Oregon	57%	76%	47%	45%	63%
	(1.67)	(2.81)	(3.15)	(3.36)	(3.65)
Washington	57%	80%	49%	45%	59%
	(1.52)	(2.62)	(2.90)	(2.98)	(3.13)

Source: Three-year merged March CPS, 1989, 1990, and 1991.

TABLE B8
PRIVATE-SECTOR WORKERS AGES 18-64:
PERCENTAGE IN INDUSTRY THAT ARE UNINSURED

	Private Sector	Manufacturing	Services	Wholesale/ Retail	Other
UNITED STATES	16%	10%	17%	21%	17%
	(0.14)	(0.23)	(0.27)	(0.31)	(0.29)
NEW ENGLAND	11%	8%	10%	14%	13%
	(0.37)	(0.61)	(0.67)	(0.90)	(0.84)
Connecticut	9%	7%	11%	11%	10%
	(0.95)	(1.51)	(1.90)	(2.37)	(2.00)
Maine	13%	9%	11%	17%	14%
	(1.06)	(1.77)	(1.91)	(2.38)	(2.35)
Massachusetts	11%	8%	9%	14%	13%
	(0.49)	(0.85)	(0.80)	(1.18)	(1.12)
New Hampshire	13%	7%	13%	17%	15%
	(1.07)	(1.50)	(2.25)	(2.51)	(2.45)
Rhode Island	13%	11%	11%	16%	15%
	(1.11)	(1.90)	(1.97)	(2.51)	(2.59)
Vermont	13%	4%	12%	17%	16%
	(1.10)	(1.46)	(1.95)	(2.64)	(2.43)
MIDDLE ATLANTIC	13%	9%	13%	18%	12%
	(0.29)	(0.52)	(0.54)	(0.69)	(0.58)
New Jersey	11%	9%	11%	16%	10%
	(0.49)	(0.90)	(0.89)	(1.22)	(0.92)
New York	16%	13%	16%	21%	15%
	(0.50)	(0.99)	(0.89)	(1.13)	(0.96)
Pennsylvania	10%	6%	11%	14%	11%
	(0.47)	(0.71)	(0.89)	(1.15)	(0.99)
SOUTH ATLANTIC	18%	12%	18%	22%	20%
	(0.35)	(0.63)	(0.66)	(0.75)	(0.71)
Delaware	16%	6%	18%	24%	17%
	(1.16)	(1.45)	(2.35)	(2.96)	(2.33)
District of Columbia	26%	***	21%	42%	26%
	(1.70)	***	(2.18)	(4.32)	(3.57)
Florida	23%	16%	22%	26%	23%
	(0.65)	(1.54)	(1.19)	(1.30)	(1.22)
Georgia	19%	16%	20%	25%	16%
	(1.17)	(2.23)	(2.38)	(2.47)	(2.19)
Maryland	13%	6%	12%	13%	18%
	(1.09)	(1.95)	(1.78)	(2.28)	(2.46)
North Carolina	15%	11%	14%	19%	20%
	(0.55)	(0.80)	(1.19)	(1.29)	(1.32)
South Carolina	15%	7%	16%	21%	21%
	(1.00)	(1.23)	(2.16)	(2.52)	(2.40)
Virginia	17%	14%	16%	20%	19%
	(1.06)	(2.08)	(1.96)	(2.27)	(2.14)
West Virginia	16%	12%	15%	20%	17%
	(1.22)	(2.46)	(2.40)	(2.52)	(2.27)
EAST SOUTH CENTRAL	18%	12%	17%	25%	19%
	(0.61)	(0.92)	(1.28)	(1.40)	(1.32)
Alabama	22%	13%	22%	30%	25%
	(1.34)	(1.96)	(2.84)	(2.92)	(3.05)
Kentucky	14%	9%	15%	20%	13%
	(1.12)	(1.77)	(2.41)	(2.50)	(2.18)
Mississippi	23%	17%	21%	31%	23%
	(1.30)	(2.11)	(2.73)	(2.84)	(2.72)
Tennessee	15%	10%	14%	21%	17%
	(1.06)	(1.52)	(2.18)	(2.63)	(2.39)
WEST SOUTH CENTRAL	24%	15%	25%	28%	25%
	(0.53)	(1.02)	(1.02)	(1.10)	(1.03)
Arkansas	20%	13%	20%	24%	23%
	(1.25)	(1.98)	(2.72)	(2.61)	(2.71)
Louisiana	23%	18%	22%	28%	22%
	(1.46)	(3.71)	(2.61)	(3.01)	(2.63)
Oklahoma	23%	18%	26%	24%	23%
	(1.36)	(2.74)	(2.71)	(2.81)	(2.56)
Texas	25%	15%	26%	30%	27%
	(0.69)	(1.29)	(1.31)	(1.44)	(1.35)

	Private Sector	Manufacturing	Services	Wholesale/ Retail	Other
EAST NORTH CENTRAL	**12%**	**6%**	**13%**	**16%**	**12%**
	(0.28)	**(0.39)**	**(0.58)**	**(0.65)**	**(0.61)**
Illinois	12%	8%	12%	16%	10%
	(0.51)	(0.90)	(1.01)	(1.17)	(0.99)
Indiana	13%	7%	17%	18%	15%
	(1.03)	(1.37)	(2.32)	(2.34)	(2.35)
Michigan	11%	6%	14%	15%	12%
	(0.51)	(0.68)	(1.10)	(1.14)	(1.20)
Ohio	11%	5%	13%	16%	12%
	(0.50)	(0.61)	(1.04)	(1.18)	(1.14)
Wisconsin	10%	5%	10%	18%	12%
	(0.86)	(1.05)	(1.69)	(2.23)	(2.06)
WEST NORTH CENTRAL	**13%**	**9%**	**14%**	**17%**	**11%**
	(0.47)	**(0.86)**	**(0.91)**	**(1.01)**	**(0.90)**
Iowa	11%	9%	13%	12%	10%
	(0.95)	(1.81)	(1.98)	(1.85)	(1.90)
Kansas	13%	7%	15%	15%	13%
	(1.01)	(1.62)	(2.05)	(2.12)	(2.10)
Minnesota	13%	8%	15%	16%	11%
	(1.00)	(1.73)	(1.96)	(2.20)	(1.93)
Missouri	14%	11%	14%	21%	11%
	(1.08)	(2.03)	(2.06)	(2.44)	(1.96)
Nebraska	14%	10%	13%	20%	11%
	(1.04)	(1.99)	(1.93)	(2.30)	(1.90)
North Dakota	12%	11%	10%	16%	12%
	(1.05)	(3.19)	(1.71)	(2.09)	(1.94)
South Dakota	16%	12%	15%	18%	18%
	(1.10)	(2.39)	(1.95)	(2.16)	(2.29)
MOUNTAIN	**20%**	**11%**	**20%**	**24%**	**21%**
	(0.55)	**(1.07)**	**(1.01)**	**(1.15)**	**(1.05)**
Arizona	20%	10%	24%	23%	20%
	(1.29)	(2.34)	(2.54)	(2.61)	(2.50)
Colorado	17%	9%	16%	23%	19%
	(1.26)	(2.30)	(2.32)	(2.82)	(2.36)
Idaho	22%	12%	19%	28%	25%
	(1.24)	(2.18)	(2.38)	(2.54)	(2.53)
Montana	21%	19%	22%	22%	19%
	(1.32)	(4.23)	(2.48)	(2.34)	(2.41)
Nevada	20%	12%	16%	26%	24%
	(1.22)	(3.62)	(1.70)	(2.78)	(2.52)
New Mexico	30%	18%	30%	37%	30%
	(1.56)	(3.49)	(2.98)	(2.98)	(2.86)
Utah	12%	7%	14%	14%	14%
	(1.08)	(1.83)	(2.05)	(2.26)	(2.30)
Wyoming	19%	***	18%	25%	16%
	(1.50)	***	(3.07)	(3.15)	(2.16)
PACIFIC	**20%**	**14%**	**21%**	**24%**	**22%**
	(0.44)	**(0.80)**	**(0.83)**	**(0.93)**	**(0.91)**
Alaska	27%	15%	24%	32%	28%
	(1.49)	(4.25)	(2.60)	(3.10)	(2.55)
California	22%	15%	22%	26%	24%
	(0.54)	(0.99)	(1.02)	(1.14)	(1.10)
Hawaii	9%	***	9%	10%	10%
	(1.00)	***	(1.68)	(1.93)	(1.89)
Oregon	15%	9%	18%	19%	17%
	(1.22)	(1.84)	(2.40)	(2.64)	(2.82)
Washington	14%	8%	14%	18%	17%
	(1.07)	(1.74)	(2.00)	(2.29)	(2.38)

Source: Three-year merged March CPS, 1989, 1990, and 1991.

Notes for tables B1–B8

B1–B3, B5, B7	Employer group health insurance includes only own-employer coverage.
B1–B8	Workers are defined as individuals who reported a positive number of usual hours of work per week in the previous year.
B1	Full-time workers are defined as individuals who reported that their usual number of hours of work per week in the previous year was more than 35.
B2	Part-time workers are defined as individuals who reported that their usual number of hours of work per week in the previous year was 35 or less.
B5–B6	Sector is based upon the longest job held in the previous year.
B7–B8	This table includes only private-sector workers. Industry is based upon the longest job held in the previous year. The category "Other" includes agriculture, forestry, fisheries, mining, construction, transportation, communication, other public utilities, finance, insurance, and real estate.

Three asterisks (***) indicate that there were no observations available in the three-year merged March CPS for that cell.

SECTION C

Characteristics of the Uninsured

This section highlights characteristics of persons without health insurance. Statistics already presented indicate the relative incidence of uninsurance for various subpopulations. Here we show the demographic, income, and work characteristics of the uninsured population alone. These data can help states to estimate the number of uninsured persons who could be targeted through various types of health insurance expansion strategies.

It is important to use these statistics in conjunction with other data showing the relative sizes of the various subpopulations (see sections A and G) because they reflect the relative size of the population subgroup in the state as well as the degree to which that subgroup may be uninsured. For example, some states have larger percentages of low-income persons or persons working in small firms than other states. Because these characteristics are also associated with higher rates of uninsurance, those states will have large concentrations of their uninsured populations with these characteristics. The numbers in this section can be used with those presented earlier to gain a more complete picture of the uninsured population in a state.

Demographic Characteristics

The first tables (C1–C3) show the percentage of the uninsured population by race and sex, by age, and by family type. The percentage of the uninsured population that is nonwhite varies widely across the states, in part because some states have higher concentrations of nonwhites and because nonwhites have characteristics that are associated with higher rates of uninsurance (low income, higher unemployment rates, and so on). Women are somewhat less likely to be uninsured than men across the country—46 percent for women compared to 54 percent for men. This probably reflects the higher rates of Medicaid coverage for women than men (see tables A4 and A5). Medicaid covers low-income pregnant women and mothers eligible for Aid to Families with Dependent Children.

Table C2 indicates that the uninsured tend to be young adults (aged 18–34). In fact, young adults comprise about one-half of the uninsured population in some states (Michigan, Wisconsin, Massachusetts, and Rhode Island). This category includes persons who are still in school; persons in entry-level jobs that do not provide health insurance; and, because young adults have a relatively high unemployment rate, persons without jobs.

Table C3 categorizes uninsured persons by the type of family in which they live. It shows, for example, that 40 percent of uninsured persons live in two-parent families with children. In some states (for example, Texas and New Mexico) half of uninsured persons fall into this family status category. A large share of the uninsured also live alone—29 percent across the country. As noted earlier, single adults have low rates of employer group insurance coverage and high rates of uninsurance. In addition, public health plan coverage is not typically available to single persons unless they have severe disabilities.

The focus on uninsured persons by the work status of the head and spouse of the family reveals some surprising statistics (table C4). Despite the fact that persons in families with a full-time worker have relatively low rates of uninsurance (14 percent, as shown in table A15), they comprise a large share of the uninsured population because *most* families have a full-time worker. Thus, 71 percent of the uninsured population live in a family in which either the head or the spouse works more than 35 hours a week. This statistic has led many to conclude that expanding the employer-group health insurance system could go far toward reducing the number of uninsured Americans. It is important to notice the variation in the percentage of the uninsured in full-time worker families across the states. In some states (New Hampshire and Delaware, for example) as many as 80 percent of the uninsured live in a family with a full-time worker. In Michigan, however, only 60 percent of the uninsured have this characteristic, and 22 percent live in families without a worker. Thus, expansion of the employment-based insurance system would have a relatively larger effect on the uninsurance rate in states like New Hampshire and Delaware than it would in Michigan.

INCOME CHARACTERISTICS

Table C5 provides some indication of whether some of the uninsured may be able to pay for a share of their insurance coverage. Forty-one percent of the uninsured live in families with incomes more than twice the poverty line. There is wide variation in this statistic across states and regions, however, reflecting widely different economic circumstances across the states. Policymakers need to assess the ability to pay for insurance within their own state environment. In the Middle Atlantic region, for example, more than half of the uninsured live in families with incomes above 200 percent of poverty, compared to about one-quarter of families in the East South Central region. However, some families in a state with high insurance costs like New York, for example, may find it difficult to afford insurance even when their incomes exceed two times the poverty level. On the other hand, families with incomes between 150 percent and 200 percent of the poverty line living in lower-cost areas may be able to pay a reasonable share of their health insurance costs.

WORKER CHARACTERISTICS

The distribution of uninsured adults (table C6) by own-work status indicates that the majority of uninsured adults work part-time (53 percent), about one-quarter are full-time workers, and approximately another quarter are not working. Thus, policies focused on employment-based insurance will not encompass a large share of workers unless they include part-time workers (defined as working 35 or fewer hours a week). In addition, a residual insurance program would be required to cover adults who are not working. This may seem at odds with the statistic shown earlier that a large share of *all* uninsured persons live in families with at least one full-time worker. This simply indicates that many full-time working adults have dependents who would qualify for coverage under their group policy. Thus, expansion of the employment-based insurance system to all full-time workers and their dependents would reduce the number of uninsured persons significantly. But many adults who work part-time or do not have jobs would remain without coverage unless a broader coverage expansion policy were implemented.

Table C7 shows that nearly one-half of all uninsured workers are in firms with fewer than 25 workers. Variations across the states in the distribution of uninsured workers by firm size indicate variations in employment patterns across the states more than they indicate different propensities for firms of a given size to provide health insurance. For example, 58 percent or more of uninsured workers are in small firms in New Hampshire, Wyoming, and Montana. These states have higher-than-average concentrations of their employment base in small firms (table G11). There are important exceptions to this generalization, however, and each state's employment base must be reviewed separately.

Data for uninsured workers by sector of employment (table C8) show that such individuals work in the private sector (80 percent). The high rate of employment-based coverage in the government sector discussed earlier means that relatively few uninsured workers are in the government sector. Nationwide, 7 percent of the uninsured work in the government sector, despite the fact that they comprise 15 percent of all employment (shown later in table G12). In contrast, 12 percent of the uninsured are in the self-employed sector which comprises 10 percent of all workers (table G12).

The last table in this section (table C9) shows the distribution of the uninsured by industry. Not surprisingly, the uninsured are more likely to work in the service or wholesale and retail industries than in manufacturing. This holds true across the country, although the differences across industry groups are not as sharp in some states as they are in others. For example, among uninsured workers in Georgia, 20 percent are employed in manufacturing, 25 percent are in the service industry, and 34 percent are in the wholesale and retail group. And in Ohio, 12 percent of the uninsured work in manufacturing, 31 percent work in services, and 35 percent work in wholesale and retail industries. As noted earlier, the extent of employment-based coverage in the manufacturing industry differs across the states. States with very large manufacturing firms and long-established benefit plans have above-average rates of employer-group coverage, and states with small manufacturers have lower-than-average rates of employer-group coverage. In addition, the concentration of workers by industry affects these results (see table G13 and others in that section to review differences in employers' characteristics across states).

TABLE C1
UNINSURED UNDER AGE 65: BY RACE AND SEX

	Number (000s)	White	Nonwhite	Male	Female
UNITED STATES	33,202	77% (0.23)	23% (0.24)	54% (0.28)	46% (0.28)
NEW ENGLAND	1,211	90% (0.68)	10% (0.71)	56% (1.13)	44% (1.13)
Connecticut	272	81% (2.59)	19% (2.69)	57% (3.28)	43% (3.28)
Maine	118	100% (0.39)	0% (0.40)	54% (2.76)	46% (2.76)
Massachusetts	517	90% (0.93)	10% (0.97)	55% (1.53)	45% (1.53)
New Hampshire	157	95% (1.05)	5% (1.09)	51% (2.52)	49% (2.52)
Rhode Island	91	89% (1.92)	11% (2.00)	62% (3.00)	38% (3.00)
Vermont	55	99% (0.52)	1% (0.55)	55% (2.98)	45% (2.98)
MIDDLE ATLANTIC	3,935	73% (0.65)	27% (0.68)	54% (0.73)	46% (0.73)
New Jersey	723	74% (1.28)	26% (1.33)	55% (1.44)	45% (1.44)
New York	2,148	70% (0.95)	30% (0.98)	54% (1.03)	46% (1.03)
Pennsylvania	1,064	79% (1.18)	21% (1.22)	54% (1.45)	46% (1.45)
SOUTH ATLANTIC	6,146	65% (0.62)	35% (0.64)	54% (0.65)	46% (0.65)
Delaware	90	69% (2.30)	31% (2.39)	49% (2.50)	51% (2.50)
District of Columbia	101	28% (2.10)	72% (2.18)	56% (2.32)	44% (2.32)
Florida	2,239	76% (0.84)	24% (0.88)	55% (0.98)	45% (0.98)
Georgia	947	48% (2.14)	52% (2.23)	54% (2.13)	46% (2.13)
Maryland	437	60% (2.88)	40% (3.00)	53% (2.94)	47% (2.94)
North Carolina	808	64% (1.18)	36% (1.23)	53% (1.23)	47% (1.23)
South Carolina	463	50% (2.09)	50% (2.17)	56% (2.07)	44% (2.07)
Virginia	836	65% (1.93)	35% (2.01)	53% (2.03)	47% (2.03)
West Virginia	225	94% (1.18)	6% (1.23)	52% (2.41)	48% (2.41)
EAST SOUTH CENTRAL	2,243	68% (1.02)	32% (1.07)	54% (1.10)	46% (1.10)
Alabama	701	60% (1.98)	40% (2.06)	54% (2.02)	46% (2.02)
Kentucky	436	92% (1.38)	8% (1.43)	56% (2.45)	44% (2.45)
Mississippi	455	46% (1.90)	54% (1.98)	55% (1.90)	45% (1.90)
Tennessee	651	78% (1.84)	22% (1.91)	53% (2.21)	47% (2.21)
WEST SOUTH CENTRAL	5,444	80% (0.58)	20% (0.61)	54% (0.73)	46% (0.73)
Arkansas	426	77% (1.65)	23% (1.72)	56% (1.96)	44% (1.96)
Louisiana	811	58% (1.97)	42% (2.05)	51% (2.00)	49% (2.00)
Oklahoma	560	74% (1.74)	26% (1.81)	55% (1.97)	45% (1.97)
Texas	3,648	86% (0.64)	14% (0.66)	54% (0.93)	46% (0.93)

	Number (000s)	White	Nonwhite	Male	Female
EAST NORTH CENTRAL	**4,017**	**76%** (0.67)	**24%** (0.69)	**55%** (0.78)	**45%** (0.78)
Illinois	1,182	67% (1.32)	33% (1.37)	59% (1.38)	41% (1.38)
Indiana	670	81% (1.96)	19% (2.04)	47% (2.50)	53% (2.50)
Michigan	828	76% (1.26)	24% (1.31)	56% (1.47)	44% (1.47)
Ohio	980	81% (1.15)	19% (1.19)	54% (1.45)	46% (1.45)
Wisconsin	358	89% (1.81)	11% (1.88)	53% (2.92)	47% (2.92)
WEST NORTH CENTRAL	**1,785**	**87%** (0.82)	**13%** (0.85)	**53%** (1.20)	**47%** (1.20)
Iowa	208	94% (1.45)	6% (1.50)	54% (3.01)	46% (3.01)
Kansas	218	86% (1.90)	14% (1.97)	53% (2.75)	47% (2.75)
Minnesota	437	90% (1.67)	10% (1.74)	51% (2.73)	49% (2.73)
Missouri	616	82% (1.93)	18% (2.01)	53% (2.52)	47% (2.52)
Nebraska	161	93% (1.27)	7% (1.32)	57% (2.49)	43% (2.49)
North Dakota	54	83% (2.03)	17% (2.12)	54% (2.72)	46% (2.72)
South Dakota	91	81% (1.66)	19% (1.72)	56% (2.07)	44% (2.07)
MOUNTAIN	**2,168**	**91%** (0.52)	**9%** (0.54)	**53%** (0.91)	**47%** (0.91)
Arizona	598	96% (0.87)	4% (0.90)	53% (2.10)	47% (2.10)
Colorado	502	90% (1.38)	10% (1.43)	53% (2.29)	47% (2.29)
Idaho	162	95% (0.91)	5% (0.95)	52% (2.00)	48% (2.00)
Montana	125	88% (1.36)	12% (1.42)	51% (2.09)	49% (2.09)
Nevada	194	86% (1.50)	14% (1.56)	55% (2.14)	45% (2.14)
New Mexico	363	85% (1.19)	15% (1.24)	53% (1.66)	47% (1.66)
Utah	164	94% (1.29)	6% (1.34)	58% (2.60)	42% (2.60)
Wyoming	59	97% (0.89)	3% (0.92)	56% (2.73)	44% (2.73)
PACIFIC	**6,254**	**83%** (0.55)	**17%** (0.57)	**56%** (0.73)	**44%** (0.73)
Alaska	99	65% (1.76)	35% (1.83)	58% (1.81)	42% (1.81)
California	5,154	84% (0.62)	16% (0.64)	56% (0.83)	44% (0.83)
Hawaii	90	31% (2.85)	69% (2.97)	54% (3.07)	46% (3.07)
Oregon	376	88% (1.62)	12% (1.69)	54% (2.50)	46% (2.50)
Washington	535	86% (1.73)	14% (1.80)	55% (2.51)	45% (2.51)

Source: Three-year merged March CPS, 1989, 1990, and 1991.

TABLE C2
UNINSURED UNDER AGE 65: BY AGE

	Number (000s)	Ages <18	Ages 18-34	Ages 35-53	Ages 54-64
UNITED STATES	33,202	26% (0.38)	43% (0.43)	22% (0.36)	9% (0.24)
NEW ENGLAND	1,211	22% (1.46)	46% (1.75)	23% (1.47)	9% (1.00)
Connecticut	272	24% (4.38)	42% (5.07)	27% (4.56)	7% (2.66)
Maine	118	20% (3.45)	42% (4.22)	26% (3.78)	12% (2.75)
Massachusetts	517	20% (1.91)	51% (2.38)	21% (1.93)	9% (1.33)
New Hampshire	157	35% (3.72)	34% (3.71)	21% (3.19)	10% (2.35)
Rhode Island	91	15% (3.41)	59% (4.72)	15% (3.46)	11% (3.00)
Vermont	55	20% (3.73)	46% (4.62)	27% (4.09)	7% (2.39)
MIDDLE ATLANTIC	3,935	20% (0.90)	46% (1.13)	24% (0.97)	10% (0.67)
New Jersey	723	21% (1.83)	48% (2.24)	22% (1.86)	8% (1.24)
New York	2,148	18% (1.22)	48% (1.59)	25% (1.38)	9% (0.92)
Pennsylvania	1,064	23% (1.89)	42% (2.22)	24% (1.91)	12% (1.45)
SOUTH ATLANTIC	6,146	27% (0.89)	40% (0.99)	23% (0.85)	10% (0.60)
Delaware	90	26% (3.41)	43% (3.83)	22% (3.21)	9% (2.19)
District of Columbia	101	18% (2.78)	45% (3.61)	27% (3.22)	11% (2.23)
Florida	2,239	27% (1.37)	40% (1.50)	22% (1.27)	10% (0.93)
Georgia	947	25% (2.88)	41% (3.27)	24% (2.82)	10% (1.95)
Maryland	437	19% (3.59)	44% (4.52)	26% (4.01)	11% (2.80)
North Carolina	808	26% (1.67)	42% (1.88)	23% (1.60)	9% (1.10)
South Carolina	463	30% (2.97)	37% (3.12)	22% (2.66)	11% (2.04)
Virginia	836	32% (2.93)	35% (3.01)	25% (2.71)	9% (1.76)
West Virginia	225	22% (3.11)	40% (3.66)	27% (3.30)	10% (2.28)
EAST SOUTH CENTRAL	2,243	28% (1.54)	41% (1.68)	22% (1.40)	9% (1.00)
Alabama	701	30% (2.88)	41% (3.08)	20% (2.51)	9% (1.77)
Kentucky	436	25% (3.33)	44% (3.80)	20% (3.09)	10% (2.28)
Mississippi	455	27% (2.62)	42% (2.92)	22% (2.45)	9% (1.70)
Tennessee	651	29% (3.12)	37% (3.32)	23% (2.91)	10% (2.08)
WEST SOUTH CENTRAL	5,444	32% (1.05)	39% (1.10)	22% (0.93)	8% (0.60)
Arkansas	426	33% (2.87)	36% (2.93)	22% (2.53)	9% (1.71)
Louisiana	811	31% (2.86)	37% (2.99)	24% (2.65)	8% (1.68)
Oklahoma	560	28% (2.75)	37% (2.97)	25% (2.67)	10% (1.83)
Texas	3,648	32% (1.34)	40% (1.41)	21% (1.16)	7% (0.74)

	Number (000s)	Ages <18	Ages 18-34	Ages 35-53	Ages 54-64
EAST NORTH CENTRAL	**4,017**	**21%** **(1.00)**	**46%** **(1.21)**	**22%** **(1.01)**	**10%** **(0.74)**
Illinois	1,182	20% (1.75)	47% (2.17)	22% (1.79)	10% (1.33)
Indiana	670	29% (3.52)	39% (3.80)	22% (3.24)	10% (2.28)
Michigan	828	20% (1.83)	50% (2.30)	20% (1.85)	10% (1.36)
Ohio	980	20% (1.80)	44% (2.23)	24% (1.92)	12% (1.45)
Wisconsin	358	18% (3.52)	50% (4.53)	23% (3.81)	8% (2.49)
WEST NORTH CENTRAL	**1,785**	**27%** **(1.66)**	**43%** **(1.85)**	**21%** **(1.53)**	**8%** **(1.04)**
Iowa	208	20% (3.76)	42% (4.61)	29% (4.25)	8% (2.59)
Kansas	218	23% (3.60)	48% (4.26)	20% (3.42)	9% (2.42)
Minnesota	437	27% (3.75)	43% (4.18)	21% (3.46)	9% (2.38)
Missouri	616	30% (3.59)	43% (3.87)	20% (3.09)	7% (1.98)
Nebraska	161	26% (3.43)	42% (3.86)	19% (3.06)	12% (2.57)
North Dakota	54	26% (3.71)	44% (4.19)	23% (3.56)	7% (2.17)
South Dakota	91	33% (3.05)	36% (3.11)	20% (2.61)	10% (1.97)
MOUNTAIN	**2,168**	**32%** **(1.31)**	**40%** **(1.38)**	**21%** **(1.14)**	**7%** **(0.72)**
Arizona	598	34% (3.09)	39% (3.18)	19% (2.55)	7% (1.71)
Colorado	502	33% (3.36)	40% (3.48)	21% (2.92)	5% (1.61)
Idaho	162	31% (2.88)	40% (3.04)	22% (2.58)	7% (1.59)
Montana	125	30% (2.98)	39% (3.16)	23% (2.73)	8% (1.78)
Nevada	194	25% (2.87)	44% (3.31)	23% (2.83)	8% (1.85)
New Mexico	363	33% (2.43)	38% (2.51)	22% (2.13)	7% (1.32)
Utah	164	31% (3.79)	43% (4.05)	19% (3.18)	7% (2.09)
Wyoming	59	25% (3.69)	42% (4.19)	21% (3.48)	12% (2.78)
PACIFIC	**6,254**	**26%** **(0.99)**	**44%** **(1.13)**	**22%** **(0.95)**	**8%** **(0.61)**
Alaska	99	24% (2.44)	41% (2.80)	26% (2.51)	8% (1.53)
California	5,154	26% (1.14)	44% (1.29)	22% (1.07)	7% (0.67)
Hawaii	90	27% (4.23)	42% (4.71)	20% (3.78)	11% (2.99)
Oregon	376	29% (3.51)	37% (3.76)	25% (3.34)	10% (2.30)
Washington	535	20% (3.13)	44% (3.88)	25% (3.40)	11% (2.41)

Source: Three-year merged March CPS, 1989, 1990, and 1991.

76

TABLE C3
UNINSURED UNDER AGE 65: BY FAMILY TYPE

	Number (000s)	Married	Married with Children	Single with Children	Single
UNITED STATES	33,202	18% (0.33)	40% (0.42)	13% (0.29)	29% (0.39)
NEW ENGLAND	1,211	22% (1.45)	35% (1.68)	10% (1.08)	32% (1.64)
Connecticut	272	20% (4.10)	41% (5.06)	12% (3.38)	27% (4.53)
Maine	118	23% (3.60)	36% (4.11)	12% (2.79)	29% (3.90)
Massachusetts	517	22% (1.97)	30% (2.18)	10% (1.45)	38% (2.30)
New Hampshire	157	18% (3.00)	48% (3.91)	11% (2.46)	23% (3.28)
Rhode Island	91	33% (4.50)	28% (4.28)	3% (1.58)	37% (4.63)
Vermont	55	17% (3.47)	33% (4.36)	11% (2.85)	40% (4.53)
MIDDLE ATLANTIC	3,935	19% (0.89)	37% (1.09)	12% (0.75)	32% (1.06)
New Jersey	723	20% (1.78)	32% (2.10)	16% (1.64)	32% (2.10)
New York	2,148	18% (1.22)	36% (1.53)	13% (1.06)	34% (1.51)
Pennsylvania	1,064	22% (1.87)	41% (2.21)	10% (1.36)	27% (1.99)
SOUTH ATLANTIC	6,146	20% (0.80)	36% (0.97)	16% (0.73)	28% (0.91)
Delaware	90	16% (2.87)	35% (3.68)	17% (2.88)	32% (3.62)
District of Columbia	101	12% (2.38)	19% (2.87)	15% (2.58)	53% (3.62)
Florida	2,239	20% (1.22)	39% (1.49)	15% (1.10)	27% (1.36)
Georgia	947	21% (2.70)	39% (3.24)	13% (2.24)	26% (2.93)
Maryland	437	16% (3.31)	24% (3.92)	15% (3.21)	45% (4.53)
North Carolina	808	20% (1.51)	35% (1.81)	16% (1.38)	30% (1.75)
South Carolina	463	21% (2.65)	35% (3.07)	21% (2.61)	23% (2.73)
Virginia	836	20% (2.51)	37% (3.04)	19% (2.45)	25% (2.72)
West Virginia	225	25% (3.24)	38% (3.62)	12% (2.38)	25% (3.24)
EAST SOUTH CENTRAL	2,243	18% (1.32)	41% (1.68)	16% (1.24)	25% (1.48)
Alabama	701	19% (2.46)	38% (3.03)	18% (2.40)	26% (2.73)
Kentucky	436	22% (3.16)	43% (3.79)	10% (2.27)	25% (3.33)
Mississippi	455	17% (2.24)	40% (2.89)	17% (2.23)	26% (2.58)
Tennessee	651	16% (2.50)	44% (3.41)	16% (2.52)	24% (2.95)
WEST SOUTH CENTRAL	5,444	17% (0.85)	49% (1.13)	12% (0.73)	22% (0.94)
Arkansas	426	17% (2.31)	42% (3.01)	16% (2.21)	25% (2.63)
Louisiana	811	16% (2.26)	47% (3.09)	15% (2.22)	22% (2.58)
Oklahoma	560	20% (2.45)	48% (3.07)	9% (1.74)	23% (2.60)
Texas	3,648	17% (1.07)	51% (1.44)	11% (0.90)	22% (1.19)

	Number (000s)	Married	Married with Children	Single with Children	Single
EAST NORTH CENTRAL	**4,017**	**19%** **(0.96)**	**30%** **(1.12)**	**15%** **(0.86)**	**36%** **(1.17)**
Illinois	1,182	16% (1.60)	30% (1.99)	17% (1.61)	37% (2.10)
Indiana	670	19% (3.04)	34% (3.68)	21% (3.18)	26% (3.42)
Michigan	828	20% (1.83)	29% (2.09)	12% (1.50)	39% (2.24)
Ohio	980	21% (1.83)	29% (2.04)	13% (1.50)	37% (2.17)
Wisconsin	358	24% (3.85)	33% (4.28)	7% (2.38)	36% (4.34)
WEST NORTH CENTRAL	**1,785**	**19%** **(1.46)**	**36%** **(1.79)**	**15%** **(1.31)**	**31%** **(1.72)**
Iowa	208	22% (3.86)	30% (4.29)	9% (2.68)	39% (4.55)
Kansas	218	18% (3.24)	30% (3.92)	12% (2.79)	40% (4.17)
Minnesota	437	16% (3.13)	33% (3.96)	17% (3.16)	34% (4.01)
Missouri	616	19% (3.07)	39% (3.81)	18% (2.97)	24% (3.35)
Nebraska	161	22% (3.20)	39% (3.81)	8% (2.14)	31% (3.61)
North Dakota	54	23% (3.53)	43% (4.18)	7% (2.20)	27% (3.76)
South Dakota	91	19% (2.54)	42% (3.20)	17% (2.41)	22% (2.69)
MOUNTAIN	**2,168**	**16%** **(1.02)**	**46%** **(1.40)**	**13%** **(0.94)**	**25%** **(1.22)**
Arizona	598	17% (2.42)	47% (3.25)	12% (2.12)	24% (2.79)
Colorado	502	12% (2.33)	45% (3.54)	16% (2.63)	27% (3.15)
Idaho	162	16% (2.30)	51% (3.11)	10% (1.85)	22% (2.58)
Montana	125	18% (2.47)	46% (3.23)	12% (2.13)	24% (2.79)
Nevada	194	19% (2.60)	28% (3.00)	15% (2.41)	38% (3.24)
New Mexico	363	15% (1.84)	56% (2.56)	11% (1.60)	19% (2.01)
Utah	164	16% (2.99)	49% (4.09)	8% (2.24)	27% (3.65)
Wyoming	59	20% (3.43)	34% (4.04)	16% (3.11)	29% (3.88)
PACIFIC	**6,254**	**16%** **(0.83)**	**42%** **(1.12)**	**10%** **(0.69)**	**32%** **(1.06)**
Alaska	99	16% (2.09)	36% (2.73)	15% (2.02)	33% (2.68)
California	5,154	15% (0.92)	44% (1.29)	10% (0.78)	31% (1.20)
Hawaii	90	26% (4.16)	35% (4.54)	9% (2.66)	31% (4.42)
Oregon	376	18% (2.98)	39% (3.80)	15% (2.76)	28% (3.49)
Washington	535	25% (3.38)	30% (3.57)	6% (1.93)	39% (3.82)

Source: Three-year merged March CPS, 1989, 1990, and 1991.

TABLE C4

UNINSURED UNDER AGE 65: BY WORK STATUS OF SPOUSE AND HEAD

	Number (000s)	Full-time	Part-time	Not Working
UNITED STATES	33,202	71% (0.28)	15% (0.22)	14% (0.21)
NEW ENGLAND	1,211	72% (1.13)	15% (0.90)	13% (0.84)
Connecticut	272	76% (3.17)	16% (2.69)	9% (2.07)
Maine	118	73% (2.74)	15% (2.20)	12% (2.01)
Massachusetts	517	68% (1.60)	15% (1.23)	17% (1.28)
New Hampshire	157	80% (2.26)	12% (1.82)	8% (1.56)
Rhode Island	91	76% (2.96)	12% (2.27)	12% (2.24)
Vermont	55	68% (3.11)	21% (2.71)	11% (2.09)
MIDDLE ATLANTIC	3,935	69% (0.76)	14% (0.57)	17% (0.62)
New Jersey	723	72% (1.45)	13% (1.10)	15% (1.14)
New York	2,148	66% (1.09)	16% (0.85)	18% (0.88)
Pennsylvania	1,064	72% (1.45)	10% (0.98)	17% (1.23)
SOUTH ATLANTIC	6,146	72% (0.65)	15% (0.52)	13% (0.49)
Delaware	90	80% (2.22)	8% (1.56)	11% (1.77)
District of Columbia	101	69% (2.42)	12% (1.69)	19% (2.07)
Florida	2,239	75% (0.96)	14% (0.76)	11% (0.70)
Georgia	947	68% (2.23)	21% (1.94)	11% (1.52)
Maryland	437	69% (3.04)	16% (2.42)	15% (2.32)
North Carolina	808	75% (1.19)	14% (0.95)	11% (0.86)
South Carolina	463	68% (2.17)	17% (1.75)	15% (1.67)
Virginia	836	71% (2.05)	14% (1.59)	14% (1.58)
West Virginia	225	64% (2.59)	12% (1.78)	24% (2.29)
EAST SOUTH CENTRAL	2,243	67% (1.16)	15% (0.88)	18% (0.94)
Alabama	701	62% (2.19)	16% (1.66)	21% (1.85)
Kentucky	436	64% (2.64)	18% (2.12)	18% (2.10)
Mississippi	455	67% (2.00)	16% (1.57)	17% (1.59)
Tennessee	651	74% (2.17)	11% (1.55)	15% (1.76)
WEST SOUTH CENTRAL	5,444	73% (0.72)	16% (0.60)	11% (0.52)
Arkansas	426	68% (2.05)	18% (1.69)	14% (1.54)
Louisiana	811	65% (2.13)	17% (1.69)	17% (1.69)
Oklahoma	560	74% (1.95)	15% (1.59)	11% (1.38)
Texas	3,648	75% (0.90)	15% (0.75)	10% (0.61)

	Number (000s)	Full-time	Part-time	Not Working
EAST NORTH CENTRAL	4,017	65% (0.84)	17% (0.66)	18% (0.67)
Illinois	1,182	67% (1.47)	14% (1.08)	19% (1.23)
Indiana	670	67% (2.65)	21% (2.30)	12% (1.82)
Michigan	828	60% (1.62)	17% (1.26)	22% (1.38)
Ohio	980	63% (1.57)	18% (1.24)	20% (1.29)
Wisconsin	358	71% (2.96)	19% (2.58)	9% (1.90)
WEST NORTH CENTRAL	1,785	71% (1.21)	18% (1.04)	10% (0.82)
Iowa	208	64% (3.23)	22% (2.77)	14% (2.37)
Kansas	218	68% (2.86)	23% (2.60)	8% (1.70)
Minnesota	437	75% (2.64)	19% (2.38)	6% (1.49)
Missouri	616	71% (2.54)	16% (2.08)	12% (1.85)
Nebraska	161	76% (2.42)	13% (1.90)	11% (1.78)
North Dakota	54	73% (2.70)	17% (2.28)	10% (1.83)
South Dakota	91	73% (2.06)	18% (1.80)	9% (1.31)
MOUNTAIN	2,168	74% (0.89)	15% (0.73)	11% (0.63)
Arizona	598	75% (2.02)	14% (1.63)	10% (1.43)
Colorado	502	71% (2.32)	16% (1.88)	13% (1.71)
Idaho	162	79% (1.82)	16% (1.62)	5% (1.01)
Montana	125	75% (2.02)	18% (1.81)	6% (1.15)
Nevada	194	72% (2.17)	16% (1.74)	13% (1.60)
New Mexico	363	73% (1.66)	16% (1.35)	12% (1.20)
Utah	164	74% (2.59)	13% (1.97)	13% (2.01)
Wyoming	59	77% (2.59)	13% (2.10)	10% (1.83)
PACIFIC	6,254	75% (0.71)	13% (0.55)	12% (0.52)
Alaska	99	75% (1.79)	14% (1.42)	11% (1.31)
California	5,154	76% (0.80)	12% (0.61)	12% (0.60)
Hawaii	90	68% (3.20)	22% (2.85)	10% (2.04)
Oregon	376	70% (2.57)	20% (2.23)	10% (1.71)
Washington	535	73% (2.51)	14% (1.95)	13% (1.92)

Source: Three-year merged March CPS, 1989, 1990, and 1991.

TABLE C5
UNINSURED UNDER AGE 65: BY INCOME RELATIVE TO POVERTY

	Number (000s)	<100%	100-149%	150-199%	200+%
UNITED STATES	33,202	27% (0.53)	18% (0.46)	15% (0.42)	41% (0.59)
NEW ENGLAND	1,211	15% (1.75)	11% (1.52)	11% (1.53)	63% (2.36)
Connecticut	272	9% (4.18)	8% (3.87)	8% (3.84)	75% (6.21)
Maine	118	20% (4.80)	20% (4.74)	13% (3.96)	47% (5.96)
Massachusetts	517	17% (2.47)	12% (2.17)	10% (1.95)	62% (3.22)
New Hampshire	157	16% (4.02)	6% (2.67)	13% (3.72)	64% (5.23)
Rhode Island	91	15% (4.72)	7% (3.37)	15% (4.78)	63% (6.43)
Vermont	55	16% (4.72)	12% (4.18)	22% (5.34)	50% (6.45)
MIDDLE ATLANTIC	3,935	22% (1.29)	15% (1.11)	12% (1.03)	52% (1.57)
New Jersey	723	18% (2.38)	11% (1.98)	10% (1.84)	61% (3.04)
New York	2,148	23% (1.86)	14% (1.53)	12% (1.45)	51% (2.21)
Pennsylvania	1,064	21% (2.55)	18% (2.41)	14% (2.16)	47% (3.12)
SOUTH ATLANTIC	6,146	26% (1.24)	19% (1.09)	15% (1.00)	40% (1.38)
Delaware	90	15% (3.81)	13% (3.68)	12% (3.56)	59% (5.29)
District of Columbia	101	22% (4.18)	12% (3.28)	15% (3.65)	51% (5.06)
Florida	2,239	25% (1.86)	20% (1.70)	16% (1.58)	39% (2.08)
Georgia	947	32% (4.30)	17% (3.44)	16% (3.40)	35% (4.42)
Maryland	437	17% (4.73)	17% (4.71)	11% (3.97)	56% (6.29)
North Carolina	808	24% (2.26)	20% (2.10)	16% (1.95)	41% (2.60)
South Carolina	463	38% (4.37)	20% (3.61)	12% (2.89)	30% (4.10)
Virginia	836	25% (3.77)	18% (3.34)	13% (2.96)	45% (4.36)
West Virginia	225	31% (4.81)	24% (4.43)	12% (3.41)	32% (4.85)
EAST SOUTH CENTRAL	2,243	37% (2.30)	21% (1.92)	16% (1.73)	26% (2.10)
Alabama	701	44% (4.32)	16% (3.20)	15% (3.14)	25% (3.77)
Kentucky	436	31% (4.94)	24% (4.52)	21% (4.32)	24% (4.57)
Mississippi	455	38% (3.98)	23% (3.45)	13% (2.81)	26% (3.60)
Tennessee	651	34% (4.53)	22% (3.96)	14% (3.34)	30% (4.38)
WEST SOUTH CENTRAL	5,444	35% (1.51)	19% (1.24)	14% (1.10)	31% (1.46)
Arkansas	426	36% (4.06)	21% (3.46)	15% (3.00)	29% (3.84)
Louisiana	811	39% (4.20)	19% (3.37)	13% (2.93)	29% (3.92)
Oklahoma	560	29% (3.90)	21% (3.49)	16% (3.11)	34% (4.05)
Texas	3,648	36% (1.92)	19% (1.56)	14% (1.39)	31% (1.86)

UNINSURED UNDER AGE 65: BY INCOME RELATIVE TO POVERTY

	Number (000s)	<100%	100-149%	150-199%	200+%
EAST NORTH CENTRAL	**4,017**	**26%** **(1.49)**	**17%** **(1.28)**	**15%** **(1.20)**	**42%** **(1.67)**
Illinois	1,182	25% (2.60)	15% (2.18)	16% (2.20)	44% (3.00)
Indiana	670	35% (5.17)	20% (4.36)	10% (3.24)	34% (5.14)
Michigan	828	30% (2.94)	16% (2.33)	13% (2.14)	41% (3.15)
Ohio	980	21% (2.55)	19% (2.44)	17% (2.34)	43% (3.10)
Wisconsin	358	18% (4.86)	16% (4.59)	19% (4.95)	47% (6.30)
WEST NORTH CENTRAL	**1,785**	**25%** **(2.24)**	**20%** **(2.07)**	**17%** **(1.97)**	**38%** **(2.52)**
Iowa	208	27% (5.77)	19% (5.11)	16% (4.76)	38% (6.30)
Kansas	218	32% (5.54)	18% (4.55)	15% (4.21)	35% (5.65)
Minnesota	437	18% (4.55)	15% (4.23)	19% (4.60)	48% (5.87)
Missouri	616	24% (4.65)	26% (4.76)	18% (4.16)	32% (5.07)
Nebraska	161	26% (4.78)	15% (3.82)	17% (4.03)	43% (5.37)
North Dakota	54	25% (5.09)	21% (4.80)	21% (4.76)	33% (5.53)
South Dakota	91	33% (4.25)	17% (3.39)	17% (3.35)	33% (4.23)
MOUNTAIN	**2,168**	**29%** **(1.78)**	**20%** **(1.57)**	**14%** **(1.37)**	**37%** **(1.89)**
Arizona	598	28% (4.05)	21% (3.68)	14% (3.17)	37% (4.38)
Colorado	502	31% (4.57)	21% (4.01)	16% (3.59)	33% (4.66)
Idaho	162	28% (3.89)	22% (3.57)	16% (3.15)	34% (4.10)
Montana	125	29% (4.07)	20% (3.61)	13% (3.06)	38% (4.38)
Nevada	194	25% (4.00)	14% (3.18)	11% (2.94)	51% (4.65)
New Mexico	363	38% (3.48)	19% (2.81)	14% (2.46)	30% (3.29)
Utah	164	17% (4.27)	25% (4.95)	13% (3.81)	45% (5.66)
Wyoming	59	31% (5.50)	17% (4.42)	19% (4.66)	33% (5.55)
PACIFIC	**6,254**	**21%** **(1.29)**	**17%** **(1.17)**	**16%** **(1.16)**	**46%** **(1.57)**
Alaska	99	28% (3.53)	18% (3.02)	13% (2.65)	42% (3.90)
California	5,154	21% (1.46)	17% (1.35)	16% (1.32)	46% (1.79)
Hawaii	90	26% (5.81)	14% (4.57)	16% (4.81)	45% (6.61)
Oregon	376	25% (4.65)	20% (4.36)	17% (4.05)	38% (5.26)
Washington	535	19% (4.28)	12% (3.48)	16% (4.02)	53% (5.43)

Source: Three-year merged March CPS, 1989, 1990, and 1991.

TABLE C6
UNINSURED ADULTS AGES 18-64: BY OWN WORK STATUS

	Number (000s)	Full-time	Part-time	Not Working
UNITED STATES	24,501	24% (0.31)	53% (0.36)	23% (0.30)
NEW ENGLAND	939	23% (1.20)	58% (1.42)	20% (1.14)
Connecticut	207	22% (3.54)	60% (4.15)	17% (3.21)
Maine	94	24% (2.97)	58% (3.41)	17% (2.62)
Massachusetts	414	22% (1.59)	56% (1.90)	22% (1.58)
New Hampshire	103	23% (2.94)	54% (3.48)	23% (2.95)
Rhode Island	77	21% (3.05)	64% (3.60)	15% (2.70)
Vermont	44	26% (3.30)	58% (3.70)	16% (2.74)
MIDDLE ATLANTIC	3,159	21% (0.75)	51% (0.91)	27% (0.81)
New Jersey	570	21% (1.48)	56% (1.81)	24% (1.55)
New York	1,769	21% (1.03)	50% (1.27)	29% (1.15)
Pennsylvania	820	23% (1.54)	51% (1.85)	27% (1.63)
SOUTH ATLANTIC	4,502	24% (0.73)	55% (0.84)	20% (0.68)
Delaware	66	20% (2.59)	63% (3.14)	18% (2.48)
District of Columbia	83	22% (2.40)	56% (2.87)	22% (2.40)
Florida	1,626	22% (1.07)	56% (1.29)	22% (1.08)
Georgia	707	30% (2.54)	51% (2.76)	18% (2.14)
Maryland	353	25% (3.18)	57% (3.61)	17% (2.75)
North Carolina	597	25% (1.38)	58% (1.57)	17% (1.20)
South Carolina	323	27% (2.47)	50% (2.79)	23% (2.36)
Virginia	571	25% (2.38)	58% (2.71)	17% (2.05)
West Virginia	175	20% (2.43)	46% (3.04)	34% (2.89)
EAST SOUTH CENTRAL	1,609	23% (1.23)	49% (1.45)	28% (1.30)
Alabama	488	23% (2.27)	48% (2.70)	29% (2.45)
Kentucky	326	28% (2.87)	43% (3.16)	29% (2.90)
Mississippi	333	24% (2.13)	52% (2.49)	24% (2.13)
Tennessee	462	20% (2.36)	52% (2.94)	28% (2.63)
WEST SOUTH CENTRAL	3,725	22% (0.82)	53% (0.98)	24% (0.85)
Arkansas	286	25% (2.33)	54% (2.67)	21% (2.18)
Louisiana	562	21% (2.20)	47% (2.68)	32% (2.50)
Oklahoma	405	22% (2.14)	56% (2.58)	22% (2.16)
Texas	2,472	22% (1.04)	54% (1.25)	24% (1.07)

	Number (000s)	Full-time	Part-time	Not Working
EAST NORTH CENTRAL	**3,155**	**26%** **(0.87)**	**49%** **(0.99)**	**25%** **(0.85)**
Illinois	940	22% (1.45)	49% (1.75)	29% (1.59)
Indiana	477	27% (2.94)	51% (3.32)	22% (2.77)
Michigan	665	25% (1.60)	47% (1.85)	28% (1.66)
Ohio	783	29% (1.64)	48% (1.81)	23% (1.53)
Wisconsin	292	34% (3.43)	55% (3.60)	11% (2.23)
WEST NORTH CENTRAL	**1,301**	**29%** **(1.43)**	**56%** **(1.56)**	**15%** **(1.11)**
Iowa	166	32% (3.51)	55% (3.75)	14% (2.59)
Kansas	167	29% (3.20)	56% (3.48)	15% (2.49)
Minnesota	319	34% (3.39)	57% (3.53)	9% (2.00)
Missouri	429	27% (2.98)	55% (3.36)	18% (2.61)
Nebraska	119	23% (2.74)	59% (3.21)	18% (2.50)
North Dakota	40	29% (3.21)	59% (3.49)	12% (2.34)
South Dakota	60	29% (2.59)	56% (2.84)	15% (2.04)
MOUNTAIN	**1,474**	**26%** **(1.08)**	**54%** **(1.23)**	**20%** **(0.98)**
Arizona	394	25% (2.51)	53% (2.88)	21% (2.36)
Colorado	334	27% (2.79)	51% (3.14)	22% (2.60)
Idaho	112	27% (2.40)	60% (2.64)	13% (1.79)
Montana	88	32% (2.62)	56% (2.78)	12% (1.81)
Nevada	146	22% (2.30)	59% (2.72)	19% (2.17)
New Mexico	242	25% (1.96)	53% (2.27)	23% (1.91)
Utah	113	28% (3.19)	51% (3.55)	21% (2.89)
Wyoming	44	27% (3.15)	59% (3.49)	14% (2.47)
PACIFIC	**4,638**	**22%** **(0.79)**	**56%** **(0.94)**	**22%** **(0.79)**
Alaska	75	23% (2.00)	59% (2.32)	18% (1.80)
California	3,801	21% (0.88)	56% (1.08)	23% (0.92)
Hawaii	66	25% (3.48)	49% (4.02)	26% (3.52)
Oregon	268	31% (3.06)	52% (3.31)	17% (2.49)
Washington	428	26% (2.75)	56% (3.13)	18% (2.43)

Source: Three-year merged March CPS, 1989, 1990, and 1991.

TABLE C7
UNINSURED WORKERS AGES 18-64: BY FIRM SIZE

	Number (000s)	Under 25 Workers	25-99 Workers	100+ Workers
UNITED STATES	18,894	49% (0.41)	15% (0.30)	36% (0.39)
NEW ENGLAND	755	50% (1.60)	16% (1.17)	34% (1.52)
Connecticut	171	50% (4.66)	16% (3.43)	34% (4.41)
Maine	78	52% (3.80)	23% (3.20)	25% (3.31)
Massachusetts	324	46% (2.16)	15% (1.53)	40% (2.12)
New Hampshire	79	58% (3.93)	13% (2.68)	29% (3.60)
Rhode Island	65	49% (4.07)	19% (3.20)	32% (3.81)
Vermont	37	66% (3.86)	12% (2.68)	21% (3.35)
MIDDLE ATLANTIC	2,296	46% (1.07)	17% (0.80)	37% (1.03)
New Jersey	435	46% (2.08)	17% (1.57)	36% (2.00)
New York	1,258	48% (1.50)	17% (1.14)	35% (1.43)
Pennsylvania	603	42% (2.13)	16% (1.57)	42% (2.12)
SOUTH ATLANTIC	3,589	48% (0.95)	14% (0.66)	38% (0.92)
Delaware	55	48% (3.58)	10% (2.11)	42% (3.54)
District of Columbia	65	33% (3.08)	12% (2.14)	55% (3.26)
Florida	1,267	54% (1.47)	14% (1.02)	32% (1.38)
Georgia	577	44% (3.04)	12% (1.99)	44% (3.03)
Maryland	293	41% (3.94)	20% (3.19)	40% (3.92)
North Carolina	496	43% (1.73)	16% (1.27)	42% (1.73)
South Carolina	247	49% (3.18)	15% (2.28)	36% (3.06)
Virginia	475	45% (2.99)	11% (1.91)	43% (2.98)
West Virginia	115	53% (3.75)	16% (2.77)	30% (3.45)
EAST SOUTH CENTRAL	1,165	49% (1.71)	12% (1.10)	39% (1.67)
Alabama	347	48% (3.21)	14% (2.23)	38% (3.12)
Kentucky	231	56% (3.77)	8% (2.10)	36% (3.64)
Mississippi	253	43% (2.83)	13% (1.92)	44% (2.83)
Tennessee	334	51% (3.45)	11% (2.15)	38% (3.36)
WEST SOUTH CENTRAL	2,812	49% (1.14)	14% (0.79)	37% (1.10)
Arkansas	226	49% (3.02)	13% (2.03)	37% (2.92)
Louisiana	382	45% (3.24)	14% (2.24)	41% (3.21)
Oklahoma	315	50% (2.95)	17% (2.21)	34% (2.79)
Texas	1,889	49% (1.44)	14% (1.00)	37% (1.39)

UNINSURED WORKERS AGES 18-64: BY FIRM SIZE

	Number (000s)	Under 25 Workers	25-99 Workers	100+ Workers
EAST NORTH CENTRAL	**2,377**	**44%** **(1.13)**	**17%** **(0.85)**	**40%** **(1.12)**
Illinois	666	42% (2.06)	17% (1.55)	42% (2.06)
Indiana	370	44% (3.75)	16% (2.78)	39% (3.68)
Michigan	480	46% (2.17)	17% (1.65)	37% (2.10)
Ohio	601	42% (2.04)	16% (1.53)	41% (2.04)
Wisconsin	260	46% (3.82)	16% (2.79)	38% (3.72)
WEST NORTH CENTRAL	**1,112**	**49%** **(1.70)**	**16%** **(1.26)**	**35%** **(1.63)**
Iowa	143	44% (4.03)	19% (3.21)	36% (3.91)
Kansas	142	47% (3.79)	18% (2.94)	35% (3.62)
Minnesota	292	53% (3.72)	14% (2.60)	33% (3.50)
Missouri	350	46% (3.72)	16% (2.75)	38% (3.62)
Nebraska	98	49% (3.60)	15% (2.60)	35% (3.44)
North Dakota	35	53% (3.78)	17% (2.87)	29% (3.44)
South Dakota	51	52% (3.10)	14% (2.15)	34% (2.94)
MOUNTAIN	**1,181**	**51%** **(1.37)**	**16%** **(1.00)**	**34%** **(1.30)**
Arizona	310	46% (3.25)	18% (2.51)	36% (3.12)
Colorado	261	49% (3.55)	13% (2.36)	38% (3.46)
Idaho	98	51% (2.88)	19% (2.28)	30% (2.64)
Montana	77	61% (2.90)	14% (2.04)	25% (2.58)
Nevada	119	45% (3.06)	19% (2.40)	36% (2.95)
New Mexico	188	55% (2.58)	15% (1.87)	30% (2.37)
Utah	89	55% (3.97)	12% (2.61)	33% (3.75)
Wyoming	38	59% (3.76)	14% (2.67)	27% (3.39)
PACIFIC	**3,607**	**54%** **(1.07)**	**16%** **(0.80)**	**30%** **(0.99)**
Alaska	61	54% (2.59)	12% (1.70)	34% (2.46)
California	2,925	54% (1.24)	17% (0.93)	29% (1.13)
Hawaii	49	44% (4.64)	13% (3.17)	42% (4.61)
Oregon	222	58% (3.60)	12% (2.33)	31% (3.36)
Washington	350	53% (3.48)	15% (2.46)	32% (3.26)

Source: Three-year merged March CPS, 1989, 1990, and 1991.

TABLE C8
UNINSURED WORKERS AGES 18-64: BY SECTOR

	Number (000s)	Private	Government	Self-Employed
UNITED STATES	18,894	80% (0.33)	7% (0.21)	13% (0.28)
NEW ENGLAND	755	79% (1.32)	6% (0.75)	16% (1.16)
Connecticut	171	78% (3.89)	4% (1.73)	19% (3.65)
Maine	78	72% (3.41)	6% (1.76)	22% (3.17)
Massachusetts	324	81% (1.70)	8% (1.19)	11% (1.35)
New Hampshire	79	77% (3.34)	1% (0.85)	22% (3.27)
Rhode Island	65	80% (3.25)	7% (2.07)	13% (2.73)
Vermont	37	75% (3.51)	4% (1.67)	20% (3.27)
MIDDLE ATLANTIC	2,296	81% (0.85)	7% (0.56)	12% (0.70)
New Jersey	435	79% (1.69)	8% (1.12)	13% (1.39)
New York	1,258	81% (1.18)	8% (0.79)	11% (0.95)
Pennsylvania	603	80% (1.72)	7% (1.08)	13% (1.45)
SOUTH ATLANTIC	3,589	80% (0.76)	7% (0.49)	12% (0.63)
Delaware	55	81% (2.82)	7% (1.79)	13% (2.37)
District of Columbia	65	75% (2.82)	19% (2.56)	6% (1.52)
Florida	1,267	80% (1.17)	4% (0.61)	15% (1.06)
Georgia	577	83% (2.32)	8% (1.65)	10% (1.80)
Maryland	293	77% (3.38)	13% (2.73)	10% (2.37)
North Carolina	496	80% (1.41)	8% (0.94)	13% (1.16)
South Carolina	247	80% (2.57)	8% (1.70)	13% (2.12)
Virginia	475	81% (2.37)	8% (1.65)	11% (1.89)
West Virginia	115	84% (2.79)	7% (1.90)	10% (2.21)
EAST SOUTH CENTRAL	1,165	81% (1.33)	7% (0.86)	12% (1.11)
Alabama	347	86% (2.22)	5% (1.41)	9% (1.82)
Kentucky	231	80% (3.00)	7% (1.90)	13% (2.53)
Mississippi	253	78% (2.38)	10% (1.70)	13% (1.90)
Tennessee	334	80% (2.78)	6% (1.66)	14% (2.41)
WEST SOUTH CENTRAL	2,812	80% (0.90)	7% (0.57)	13% (0.76)
Arkansas	226	73% (2.67)	11% (1.86)	16% (2.23)
Louisiana	382	81% (2.55)	10% (1.93)	9% (1.88)
Oklahoma	315	76% (2.52)	7% (1.53)	17% (2.21)
Texas	1,889	82% (1.11)	6% (0.66)	13% (0.96)

	Number (000s)	Private	Government	Self-Employed
EAST NORTH CENTRAL	**2,377**	**80%**	**8%**	**12%**
		(0.91)	**(0.61)**	**(0.74)**
Illinois	666	81%	7%	12%
		(1.64)	(1.08)	(1.35)
Indiana	370	83%	7%	10%
		(2.83)	(1.91)	(2.27)
Michigan	480	82%	6%	12%
		(1.67)	(1.06)	(1.39)
Ohio	601	78%	10%	12%
		(1.71)	(1.25)	(1.33)
Wisconsin	260	77%	8%	15%
		(3.23)	(2.13)	(2.71)
WEST NORTH CENTRAL	**1,112**	**79%**	**7%**	**14%**
		(1.39)	**(0.87)**	**(1.18)**
Iowa	143	79%	7%	15%
		(3.33)	(2.05)	(2.87)
Kansas	142	81%	7%	12%
		(2.96)	(1.92)	(2.45)
Minnesota	292	77%	7%	16%
		(3.11)	(1.87)	(2.72)
Missouri	350	82%	6%	12%
		(2.87)	(1.80)	(2.41)
Nebraska	98	77%	8%	16%
		(3.05)	(1.91)	(2.63)
North Dakota	35	71%	13%	16%
		(3.43)	(2.56)	(2.75)
South Dakota	51	69%	12%	20%
		(2.87)	(1.98)	(2.47)
MOUNTAIN	**1,181**	**78%**	**8%**	**13%**
		(1.13)	**(0.76)**	**(0.94)**
Arizona	310	84%	7%	9%
		(2.39)	(1.63)	(1.90)
Colorado	261	78%	10%	12%
		(2.94)	(2.09)	(2.35)
Idaho	98	79%	7%	15%
		(2.36)	(1.43)	(2.05)
Montana	77	70%	13%	17%
		(2.72)	(2.01)	(2.22)
Nevada	119	84%	5%	11%
		(2.26)	(1.34)	(1.92)
New Mexico	188	71%	11%	18%
		(2.34)	(1.62)	(1.98)
Utah	89	73%	8%	19%
		(3.52)	(2.13)	(3.12)
Wyoming	38	77%	6%	17%
		(3.24)	(1.84)	(2.89)
PACIFIC	**3,607**	**79%**	**6%**	**16%**
		(0.88)	**(0.50)**	**(0.78)**
Alaska	61	64%	20%	16%
		(2.49)	(2.06)	(1.92)
California	2,925	80%	5%	15%
		(0.98)	(0.54)	(0.87)
Hawaii	49	69%	15%	16%
		(4.33)	(3.36)	(3.43)
Oregon	222	72%	7%	21%
		(3.28)	(1.86)	(2.98)
Washington	350	73%	7%	19%
		(3.09)	(1.81)	(2.76)

Source: Three-year merged March CPS, 1989, 1990, and 1991.

TABLE C9
PRIVATE-SECTOR UNINSURED WORKERS AGES 18-64: BY INDUSTRY

	Number (000s)	Manufacturing	Services	Wholesale/ Retail	Other
UNITED STATES	15,081	15% (0.33)	28% (0.41)	31% (0.43)	26% (0.40)
NEW ENGLAND	593	18% (1.40)	28% (1.62)	28% (1.62)	26% (1.59)
Connecticut	133	21% (4.28)	32% (4.93)	23% (4.44)	25% (4.59)
Maine	56	17% (3.37)	23% (3.80)	35% (4.29)	24% (3.83)
Massachusetts	263	17% (1.83)	28% (2.16)	28% (2.15)	27% (2.14)
New Hampshire	61	18% (3.49)	24% (3.87)	30% (4.17)	28% (4.05)
Rhode Island	52	24% (3.87)	22% (3.75)	30% (4.15)	25% (3.94)
Vermont	28	7% (2.42)	31% (4.34)	30% (4.29)	32% (4.39)
MIDDLE ATLANTIC	1,849	16% (0.87)	30% (1.10)	31% (1.10)	23% (1.01)
New Jersey	345	18% (1.81)	27% (2.08)	32% (2.18)	23% (1.96)
New York	1,021	16% (1.22)	31% (1.55)	30% (1.53)	23% (1.40)
Pennsylvania	483	14% (1.66)	31% (2.22)	31% (2.23)	25% (2.07)
SOUTH ATLANTIC	2,883	15% (0.75)	27% (0.94)	30% (0.98)	28% (0.95)
Delaware	44	9% (2.25)	31% (3.69)	32% (3.71)	29% (3.60)
District of Columbia	49	4% (1.43)	43% (3.73)	31% (3.49)	22% (3.13)
Florida	1,017	10% (0.97)	29% (1.49)	32% (1.53)	29% (1.49)
Georgia	476	20% (2.69)	25% (2.93)	34% (3.20)	20% (2.72)
Maryland	225	7% (2.32)	33% (4.29)	23% (3.82)	38% (4.43)
North Carolina	395	25% (1.69)	19% (1.55)	28% (1.77)	28% (1.76)
South Carolina	197	17% (2.71)	24% (3.07)	28% (3.22)	30% (3.27)
Virginia	383	17% (2.54)	26% (2.92)	29% (3.03)	28% (3.01)
West Virginia	96	14% (2.88)	22% (3.40)	33% (3.87)	31% (3.79)
EAST SOUTH CENTRAL	947	20% (1.52)	22% (1.57)	34% (1.79)	24% (1.62)
Alabama	299	18% (2.68)	22% (2.86)	35% (3.30)	25% (2.98)
Kentucky	186	17% (3.19)	25% (3.65)	36% (4.05)	22% (3.50)
Mississippi	196	23% (2.72)	19% (2.56)	34% (3.08)	24% (2.76)
Tennessee	266	22% (3.20)	22% (3.23)	31% (3.57)	25% (3.35)
WEST SOUTH CENTRAL	2,258	13% (0.84)	28% (1.14)	30% (1.17)	29% (1.15)
Arkansas	165	19% (2.74)	22% (2.94)	32% (3.30)	27% (3.12)
Louisiana	309	11% (2.22)	28% (3.26)	33% (3.40)	28% (3.24)
Oklahoma	240	16% (2.46)	30% (3.12)	25% (2.93)	29% (3.08)
Texas	1,544	12% (1.03)	29% (1.44)	30% (1.47)	29% (1.45)

PRIVATE-SECTOR UNINSURED WORKERS AGES 18-64: BY INDUSTRY

	Number (000s)	Manufacturing	Services	Wholesale/ Retail	Other
EAST NORTH CENTRAL	**1,910**	**15%** **(0.92)**	**29%** **(1.15)**	**34%** **(1.21)**	**21%** **(1.04)**
Illinois	539	17% (1.75)	28% (2.08)	34% (2.19)	21% (1.89)
Indiana	307	16% (3.06)	29% (3.76)	32% (3.85)	23% (3.47)
Michigan	394	17% (1.79)	30% (2.21)	34% (2.27)	19% (1.89)
Ohio	470	12% (1.51)	31% (2.17)	35% (2.23)	22% (1.94)
Wisconsin	200	15% (3.10)	23% (3.68)	40% (4.27)	23% (3.66)
WEST NORTH CENTRAL	**876**	**16%** **(1.40)**	**30%** **(1.75)**	**34%** **(1.82)**	**20%** **(1.54)**
Iowa	113	19% (3.62)	32% (4.27)	29% (4.14)	20% (3.65)
Kansas	116	13% (2.83)	32% (3.92)	31% (3.88)	25% (3.64)
Minnesota	226	15% (3.04)	34% (4.01)	32% (3.95)	19% (3.32)
Missouri	287	18% (3.15)	26% (3.62)	38% (4.00)	18% (3.17)
Nebraska	75	14% (2.86)	28% (3.68)	39% (4.02)	19% (3.24)
North Dakota	25	8% (2.49)	25% (3.89)	38% (4.35)	29% (4.07)
South Dakota	35	13% (2.52)	28% (3.37)	31% (3.47)	27% (3.33)
MOUNTAIN	**924**	**8%** **(0.86)**	**29%** **(1.41)**	**33%** **(1.46)**	**29%** **(1.41)**
Arizona	261	9% (2.01)	34% (3.36)	31% (3.30)	26% (3.11)
Colorado	204	9% (2.32)	24% (3.46)	34% (3.80)	33% (3.78)
Idaho	77	11% (2.01)	22% (2.69)	37% (3.14)	31% (2.99)
Montana	54	8% (1.93)	31% (3.27)	36% (3.40)	26% (3.10)
Nevada	100	4% (1.36)	35% (3.20)	29% (3.05)	32% (3.13)
New Mexico	134	8% (1.65)	26% (2.71)	37% (2.96)	29% (2.79)
Utah	66	11% (2.95)	33% (4.38)	29% (4.22)	27% (4.13)
Wyoming	29	6% (2.04)	21% (3.56)	37% (4.22)	36% (4.20)
PACIFIC	**2,840**	**15%** **(0.86)**	**29%** **(1.10)**	**30%** **(1.11)**	**27%** **(1.08)**
Alaska	39	5% (1.38)	28% (2.91)	30% (2.99)	37% (3.14)
California	2,351	15% (1.00)	28% (1.25)	29% (1.26)	27% (1.23)
Hawaii	---	--- ---	--- ---	--- ---	--- ---
Oregon	159	15% (3.05)	33% (4.04)	31% (3.96)	22% (3.55)
Washington	256	12% (2.65)	27% (3.63)	33% (3.83)	28% (3.64)

Source: Three-year merged March CPS, 1989, 1990, and 1991.

Notes for tables C3–C9

C3   The distribution listed is the number of individuals in families of a given type. One family of the type "single" will have fewer persons than one family of the type "married with children."

C4   This table includes all persons under age 65 by the work status of the head or spouse. The work status of other adults in the family is not considered.

        Full-time workers are defined as individuals who reported that their usual number of hours of work per week in the previous year was more than 35. This column includes all persons in families where either the head or the spouse or both is a full-time worker.

        Part-time workers are defined as individuals who reported that their usual number of hours of work per week in the previous year was 35 or less.

        Nonworkers are defined as individuals who reported that their usual hours of work per week in the previous year was zero. This column includes all persons in families where neither the head nor the spouse is working.

C5   Poverty is defined using the federal poverty guidelines from the U.S. Department of Health and Human Services.

C6   Work status is defined using the reported number of usual hours per week worked in the previous year. Full-time is defined as more than 35 hours, part-time is defined as 35 or fewer hours, and nonworker is defined as zero hours.

C7–C9   Workers are defined as individuals who reported a positive number of usual hours of work per week in the previous year.

C8   Sector is based upon the longest job held in the previous year.

C9   This table includes only private-sector workers. Industry is based upon the longest job held in the previous year. The category "Other" includes agriculture, forestry, fisheries, mining, construction, transportation, communication, other public utilities, finance, insurance, and real estate.

Medicaid

This section provides data on Medicaid eligibility and enrollment for each state. As mentioned, not all persons eligible for government assistance actually enroll and receive benefits. The estimates of persons eligible for Medicaid presented here were developed using a microsimulation model that incorporates each state's Medicaid program rules. The model examines the characteristics of each person on the CPS to determine whether that person falls into at least one of the state's categorical eligibility categories, whether the person's assets fall below the limits defined for that eligibility group, and whether the person's income falls below the state's maximum threshold. Persons who actually *enroll* in Medicaid are chosen from the *eligible* population using reported Medicaid status from the CPS adjusted to match states' administrative records on enrollees. (See Appendix Two.) This section also provides data on Medicaid expenditures per enrollee and per capita for each state. These expenditures will reflect different provider-payment policies in the states as well as different health care costs. Finally, information is provided on Medicaid fees relative to Medicare and private fees in each state. These data highlight differences in provider-payment policies across the states.

ELIGIBILITY AND ENROLLMENT

Table D1 provides data on the percentage of the population eligible for Medicaid, as well as the enrollment rate, which is defined as the percentage of eligibles who enroll. The percentage of the population eligible for Medicaid varies from 5 percent in New Hampshire to 21 percent in Mississippi and Louisiana. The percentage eligible reflects the number of low-income people in the state meeting Medicaid eligibility criteria and the generosity of state Medicaid programs. (Some states are more restrictive and follow mandated federal eligibility standards; others take full advantage of all of the optional eligibility rules.) For example, New York and California, relatively high economic status states, have eligibility rates of 18 percent and 19 percent, respectively, reflecting their liberal eligibility rules. Many of the poorer states have eligibility rates of around 18–21 percent (for example, Mississippi, Arkansas, and Louisiana), even though their eligibility standards are more restrictive.

The percentage of Medicaid eligibles who enroll in Medicaid, also shown in table D1, depends on such factors as attitudes toward welfare and Medicaid, as well as eligibility processing systems and outreach efforts by the states. The enrollment rate varies from 50 percent in Florida to 95 percent in West Virginia and Washington. The differences between states' Medicaid eligible and enrollee populations give policymakers some indication as to the number of additional persons who could potentially enroll in Medicaid under eligibility rules in effect during the 1988–90 period. In some areas (such as the West South Central), full program participation could increase the Medicaid rolls dramatically. On the other hand, full program participation would also significantly reduce the number of uninsured in these areas.

Table D2 shows Medicaid enrollment as a percentage of those eligible by the three age groups: 0 to 5, 6 to 17, and 18 to 64. This information is important because some Medicaid expansion policies focus on particular age groups. The estimates of the percentage enrolled are limited by the number of observations, especially for the 6–17-year-old age group and, in general, for the New England region. The estimates we show indicate that, again, states' enrollment rates vary considerably within age groups. In general, adults have lower enrollment rates than children, but adults in the East Central and Pacific regions are more likely to enroll than adults living elsewhere. Children in the Middle Atlantic and East North Central Regions have higher enrollment rates than children living elsewhere in the country.

Figures from the three-year merged CPS data reflect average enrollment over the 1988–90 period. However, during this period changes in Medicaid eligibility and other factors led to growth in enrollment and expenditures. Medicaid enrollment for the nonelderly grew at a rate of over 8 percent annually. Table D3 shows average annual growth rates for Medicaid enrollment, expenditures, and expenditures per enrollee. These numbers are for the entire population, including the elderly.

Growth in enrollment nationwide was over 5 percent per year. This rate varied substantially by region, from 1.7 percent in the Middle Atlantic region to over 12 percent in the West South Central region. Growth in expenditures was even greater than growth in enrollment due to increasing health care costs generally. This high expenditure growth led to an annual increase in expenditures per enrollee of 10.1 percent.

EXPENDITURES

Tables D4 through D8 provide information on Medicaid enrollment and expenditures for all Medicaid enrollees, all adult enrollees, blind and disabled enrollees, child enrollees, and aged enrollees, respectively. The ratio of enrollees to 1,000 population reflects both eligibility and enrollment rates. Thus, it measures program generosity, the relative size of the low-income population in each state, and the propensity of the states' Medicaid-eligible population to apply for Medicaid coverage. Expenditures per enrollee reflect the value of benefits, including the cost of health care in the state and the effects of cost-containment efforts such as limitations on benefits and reimbursement policies. Expenditures per enrollee also reflect variations across states in the importance of different health care services. Finally, this measure includes the impact of variations in turnover in the Medicaid population. Expenditures per capita combines the impacts of variations in expenditures per enrollee and enrollees per capita.

As shown in table D4, for the whole Medicaid population, the number of enrollees varies from 47 per 1,000 persons in New Hampshire to 193 per 1,000 in Mississippi. Expenditures per enrollee vary from $4,662 in New York to $1,482 in California. These amounts reflect the high level of benefits in New York, broad coverage of relatively inexpensive children in California, and strong cost-containment measures implemented in California. Finally, expenditures per capita vary from $853 in New York to $171 in Nevada.

PAYMENT POLICIES

Table D9 provides data on Medicaid fees relative to fees under the new Medicare Fee Schedule established by the Health Care Financing Administration in 1992. In order for these fees to reflect the same year as the Medicaid fee data, we calculated Medicare fees as though the new 1992 schedule had been fully implemented in 1990. Table D9 shows the ratio of actual 1990 Medicaid fees to the Medicare fee schedule for each of six services to indicate differences in Medicaid payment policies across states and service categories. The results show that some states pay providers fees that are very close to those required under the new Medicare few schedule. Other states pay substantially below the Medicare fee schedule. It is important to note, however, that Medicaid obstetrical fees exceed the Medicare Fee Schedule in all but 14 states. On the other hand, most states pay less for primary care services and hospital visits under Medicaid than they would pay under the Medicare fee schedule. This is not surprising, given that the new Medicare Fee Schedule increased fees substantially for these services relative to other services.

Table D10 gives information on the ratio of Medicaid fees to private fees. For many services, this ratio may be a better indicator of access and comparisons than the ratio of Medicaid fees to Medicare fees. In almost all cases, private fees are above Medicare fees; thus, the ratios of Medicaid to private fees are even lower than those of Medicaid to Medicare. The information in tables D9 and D10 should give states preliminary information to initiate consideration of physician payment systems that would affect all payers.

TABLE D1
TOTAL POPULATION UNDER AGE 65: BY MEDICAID ELIGIBILITY AND ENROLLMENT

	Number (000s)	Eligibles (000s)	Eligibility Rate	Enrollees (000s)	Enrollment Rate
NEW ENGLAND	**11,157**	**1,213**	**11%**	**960**	**79%**
Connecticut	2,761	206	7%	171	83%
Maine	1,055	164	16%	127	77%
Massachusetts	5,062	646	13%	509	79%
New Hampshire	972	48	5%	30	63%
Rhode Island	823	97	12%	81	83%
Vermont	485	52	11%	43	83%
MIDDLE ATLANTIC	**32,415**	**4,769**	**15%**	**3,789**	**79%**
New Jersey	6,631	689	10%	516	75%
New York	15,507	2,779	18%	2,178	78%
Pennsylvania	10,277	1,301	13%	1,095	84%
SOUTH ATLANTIC	**36,005**	**4,961**	**14%**	**3,202**	**65%**
Delaware	574	41	7%	39	93%
District of Columbia	493	94	19%	87	92%
Florida	10,334	1,624	16%	815	50%
Georgia	5,475	795	15%	552	69%
Maryland	3,977	475	12%	370	78%
North Carolina	5,469	753	14%	511	68%
South Carolina	2,932	373	13%	246	66%
Virginia	5,166	540	10%	329	61%
West Virginia	1,586	266	17%	252	95%
EAST SOUTH CENTRAL	**13,214**	**2,079**	**16%**	**1,664**	**80%**
Alabama	3,570	385	11%	313	81%
Kentucky	3,123	522	17%	458	88%
Mississippi	2,285	475	21%	403	85%
Tennessee	4,236	696	16%	490	70%
EAST NORTH CENTRAL	**36,786**	**4,643**	**13%**	**4,178**	**90%**
Illinois	10,171	1,428	14%	1,231	86%
Indiana	4,773	345	7%	302	88%
Michigan	8,201	1,380	17%	1,215	88%
Ohio	9,537	1,114	12%	1,091	98%
Wisconsin	4,104	376	9%	340	90%
WEST SOUTH CENTRAL	**23,455**	**3,523**	**15%**	**2,184**	**62%**
Arkansas	2,103	374	18%	220	59%
Louisiana	3,701	782	21%	521	67%
Oklahoma	2,679	370	14%	245	66%
Texas	14,973	1,997	13%	1,199	60%
WEST NORTH CENTRAL	**15,279**	**1,741**	**11%**	**1,283**	**74%**
Iowa	2,386	216	9%	183	84%
Kansas	2,078	230	11%	196	86%
Minnesota	3,849	634	16%	384	61%
Missouri	4,475	440	10%	345	78%
Nebraska	1,361	137	10%	97	71%
North Dakota	546	42	8%	38	90%
South Dakota	585	42	7%	40	94%
MOUNTAIN	**11,712**	**1,227**	**10%**	**839**	**68%**
Arizona	3,016	380	13%	229	60%
Colorado	2,836	292	10%	183	63%
Idaho	896	71	8%	46	64%
Montana	711	102	14%	64	63%
Nevada	1,010	66	7%	44	66%
New Mexico	1,302	136	10%	118	86%
Utah	1,525	150	10%	129	86%
Wyoming	414	30	7%	27	90%
PACIFIC	**33,556**	**5,809**	**17%**	**4,619**	**80%**
Alaska	435	49	11%	42	86%
California	25,588	4,888	19%	3,855	79%
Hawaii	850	115	14%	94	82%
Oregon	2,464	304	12%	199	65%
Washington	4,219	452	11%	428	95%
UNITED STATES	**213,580**	**29,963**	**14%**	**22,718**	**76%**

Source: Three-year merged March CPS, 1989, 1990, and 1991.

MEDICAID ELIGIBILITY AND ENROLLMENT: BY AGE FOR PERSONS UNDER AGE 65

	Eligibles Ages 0-5 (000s)	Enrollment Rate	Eligibles Ages 6-17 (000s)	Enrollment Rate	Eligibles Ages 18-64 (000s)	Enrollment Rate
NEW ENGLAND	**296**	**83%**	**335**	**85%**	**582**	**74%**
Connecticut	---	---	---	---	---	---
Maine	---	---	48	90%	80	72%
Massachusetts	142	85%	195	85%	310	72%
New Hampshire	---	---	---	---	---	---
Rhode Island	---	---	---	---	49	72%
Vermont	---	---	---	---	25	82%
MIDDLE ATLANTIC	**1,075**	**89%**	**1,455**	**92%**	**2,239**	**67%**
New Jersey	168	76%	212	83%	308	69%
New York	619	91%	828	92%	1,333	64%
Pennsylvania	288	92%	415	95%	598	72%
SOUTH ATLANTIC	**1,323**	**64%**	**1,579**	**62%**	**2,059**	**67%**
Delaware	---	---	---	---	---	---
District of Columbia	23	92%	29	99%	42	88%
Florida	452	50%	547	45%	625	55%
Georgia	210	71%	281	65%	304	72%
Maryland	---	---	---	---	225	68%
North Carolina	194	68%	214	70%	345	66%
South Carolina	109	59%	127	58%	137	80%
Virginia	130	52%	178	63%	232	65%
West Virginia	66	97%	66	97%	133	93%
EAST SOUTH CENTRAL	**649**	**73%**	**563**	**84%**	**867**	**83%**
Alabama	167	65%	---	---	147	93%
Kentucky	117	91%	137	91%	268	85%
Mississippi	164	81%	148	86%	163	88%
Tennessee	200	63%	207	74%	289	73%
EAST NORTH CENTRAL	**1,216**	**92%**	**1,432**	**95%**	**1,995**	**85%**
Illinois	357	95%	460	94%	612	75%
Indiana	---	---	---	---	---	---
Michigan	333	91%	400	93%	647	84%
Ohio	285	97%	406	99%	422	98%
Wisconsin	---	---	113	95%	180	85%
WEST SOUTH CENTRAL	**1,019**	**59%**	**1,322**	**56%**	**1,182**	**71%**
Arkansas	118	56%	144	47%	111	77%
Louisiana	187	62%	265	71%	329	66%
Oklahoma	97	75%	113	71%	161	57%
Texas	617	57%	799	50%	581	78%
WEST NORTH CENTRAL	**502**	**72%**	**502**	**78%**	**736**	**71%**
Iowa	---	---	---	---	99	79%
Kansas	74	81%	---	---	94	85%
Minnesota	152	60%	206	67%	277	56%
Missouri	158	72%	---	---	174	82%
Nebraska	39	73%	---	---	58	66%
North Dakota	---	---	15	90%	17	86%
South Dakota	---	---	---	---	---	---
MOUNTAIN	**447**	**61%**	**353**	**69%**	**427**	**76%**
Arizona	135	51%	141	56%	103	78%
Colorado	107	57%	---	---	112	66%
Idaho	32	49%	---	---	---	---
Montana	27	66%	27	70%	47	58%
Nevada	---	---	---	---	---	---
New Mexico	56	80%	---	---	55	88%
Utah	45	86%	54	83%	50	90%
Wyoming	---	---	---	---	---	---
PACIFIC	**1,455**	**78%**	**1,862**	**78%**	**2,492**	**82%**
Alaska	17	81%	17	92%	16	84%
California	1,179	76%	1,608	77%	2,100	82%
Hawaii	37	76%	---	---	50	81%
Oregon	---	---	---	---	131	66%
Washington	135	98%	---	---	195	90%
UNITED STATES	**7,982**	**75%**	**9,402**	**77%**	**12,579**	**75%**

Source: Three-year merged March CPS, 1989, 1990, and 1991.

TABLE D3
GROWTH IN MEDICAID ENROLLMENT AND EXPENDITURES:
FISCAL YEAR 1988-1990

	Average Annual Growth in Enrollees	Average Annual Growth in Expenditures	Average Annual Growth in Expenditures per Enrollee
NEW ENGLAND	**6.23**	**22.63**	**15.44**
Connecticut	6.23	22.63	15.44
Maine	7.66	21.36	12.73
Massachusetts	7.86	15.34	6.94
New Hampshire	5.94	26.31	19.23
Rhode Island	13.08	15.68	2.29
Vermont	-0.15	15.04	15.21
MIDDLE ATLANTIC	**1.71**	**12.84**	**10.95**
New Jersey	1.71	12.84	10.95
New York	3.17	16.83	13.24
Pennsylvania	2.50	12.65	9.91
SOUTH ATLANTIC	**9.89**	**19.72**	**8.95**
Delaware	9.89	19.72	8.95
District of Columbia	4.24	11.07	6.55
Florida	-2.05	2.42	4.55
Georgia	13.56	27.05	11.88
Maryland	9.08	16.50	6.80
North Carolina	3.78	13.45	9.32
South Carolina	15.54	22.97	6.43
Virginia	9.50	33.56	21.97
West Virginia	9.01	14.56	5.09
EAST SOUTH CENTRAL	**7.55**	**20.44**	**11.99**
Alabama	7.55	20.44	11.99
Kentucky	7.37	30.57	21.61
Mississippi	0.74	18.36	17.49
Tennessee	8.63	18.34	8.94
EAST NORTH CENTRAL	**2.60**	**14.74**	**11.83**
Illinois	2.60	14.74	11.83
Indiana	2.45	13.40	10.69
Michigan	2.14	18.86	16.38
Ohio	1.92	13.32	11.19
Wisconsin	4.73	16.22	10.98
WEST SOUTH CENTRAL	**12.27**	**17.83**	**4.95**
Arkansas	12.27	17.83	4.95
Louisiana	4.74	19.20	13.81
Oklahoma	9.86	16.76	6.28
Texas	5.49	9.16	3.48
WEST NORTH CENTRAL	**6.30**	**12.91**	**6.22**
Iowa	6.30	12.91	6.22
Kansas	3.89	14.93	10.63
Minnesota	9.47	20.51	10.09
Missouri	4.96	10.14	4.93
Nebraska	7.68	13.72	5.61
North Dakota	5.35	14.06	8.27
South Dakota	1.97	4.17	2.16
MOUNTAIN	**8.42**	**13.02**	**4.24**
Colorado	8.42	13.02	4.24
Idaho	6.53	8.07	1.45
Montana	7.30	14.79	6.98
Nevada	5.49	11.77	5.95
New Mexico	9.40	23.94	13.29
Utah	11.38	12.80	1.27
Wyoming	8.99	17.04	7.38
PACIFIC	**2.08**	**14.39**	**12.06**
Alaska	2.08	14.39	12.06
California	7.73	20.55	11.91
Hawaii	1.82	13.67	11.64
Oregon	-2.90	13.14	16.52
Washington	8.06	19.28	10.38
UNITED STATES	**5.20**	**15.84**	**10.11**

Source: Health Care Financing Administration Form 64 and Form 2082.

TABLE D4
MEDICAID ENROLLEES AND EXPENDITURES: TOTAL POPULATION, 1990

	Total Number	All Enrollees	Enrollees per 1000 Population	Expenditures (000s)	Expenditures per Capita	Expenditures per Enrollee
NEW ENGLAND	**13,206,943**	**1,357,899**	**103**	**$5,661,354**	**$429**	**$4,169**
Connecticut	3,287,116	269,053	82	$1,238,522	$377	$4,603
Maine	1,227,928	156,324	127	$437,833	$357	$2,801
Massachusetts	6,016,425	689,424	115	$3,159,356	$525	$4,583
New Hampshire	1,109,252	51,762	47	$226,310	$204	$4,372
Rhode Island	1,003,464	122,508	122	$445,709	$444	$3,638
Vermont	562,758	68,828	122	$153,624	$273	$2,232
MIDDLE ATLANTIC	**37,602,286**	**4,559,412**	**121**	**$17,610,263**	**$468**	**$3,862**
New Jersey	7,730,188	641,608	83	$2,389,735	$309	$3,725
New York	17,990,455	2,614,339	145	$12,187,015	$677	$4,662
Pennsylvania	11,881,643	1,303,465	110	$3,033,513	$255	$2,327
SOUTH ATLANTIC	**43,566,853**	**4,253,689**	**98**	**$9,615,549**	**$221**	**$2,261**
Delaware	666,168	54,231	81	$125,922	$189	$2,322
District of Columbia	606,900	108,232	178	$406,356	$670	$3,754
Florida	12,937,926	1,186,304	92	$2,534,842	$196	$2,137
Georgia	6,478,216	715,610	110	$1,566,007	$242	$2,188
Maryland	4,781,468	440,631	92	$1,181,626	$247	$2,682
North Carolina	6,628,637	635,487	96	$1,498,778	$226	$2,358
South Carolina	3,486,703	354,220	102	$856,722	$246	$2,419
Virginia	6,187,358	440,612	71	$1,036,095	$167	$2,351
West Virginia	1,793,477	318,362	178	$409,201	$228	$1,285
EAST SOUTH CENTRAL	**15,176,284**	**2,144,425**	**141**	**$3,879,637**	**$256**	**$1,809**
Alabama	4,040,587	431,238	107	$803,688	$199	$1,864
Kentucky	3,685,296	523,388	142	$1,012,980	$275	$1,935
Mississippi	2,573,216	495,991	193	$623,583	$242	$1,257
Tennessee	4,877,185	693,808	142	$1,439,386	$295	$2,075
EAST NORTH CENTRAL	**42,008,942**	**4,889,636**	**116**	**$11,327,883**	**$270**	**$2,317**
Illinois	11,430,602	1,438,141	126	$2,479,272	$217	$1,724
Indiana	5,544,159	378,819	68	$1,486,917	$268	$3,925
Michigan	9,295,297	1,173,384	126	$2,617,681	$282	$2,231
Ohio	10,847,115	1,337,395	123	$3,262,020	$301	$2,439
Wisconsin	4,891,769	561,897	115	$1,481,993	$303	$2,637
WEST SOUTH CENTRAL	**26,702,793**	**3,029,034**	**113**	**$5,738,786**	**$215**	**$1,895**
Arkansas	2,350,725	289,903	123	$618,179	$263	$2,132
Louisiana	4,219,973	649,302	154	$1,402,326	$332	$2,160
Oklahoma	3,145,585	330,940	105	$723,282	$230	$2,186
Texas	16,986,510	1,758,889	104	$2,994,999	$176	$1,703
WEST NORTH CENTRAL	**17,659,690**	**1,680,048**	**95**	**$4,244,381**	**$240**	**$2,526**
Iowa	2,776,755	267,375	96	$642,740	$231	$2,404
Kansas	2,477,574	232,895	94	$492,583	$199	$2,115
Minnesota	4,375,099	401,806	92	$1,471,967	$336	$3,663
Missouri	5,117,073	530,467	104	$947,918	$185	$1,787
Nebraska	1,578,385	132,097	84	$319,222	$202	$2,417
North Dakota	638,800	55,375	87	$199,402	$312	$3,601
South Dakota	696,004	60,033	86	$170,550	$245	$2,841
MOUNTAIN	**13,658,776**	**777,053**	**57**	**$1,677,752**	**$123**	**$2,159**
Arizona	3,665,228	N/A	N/A	N/A	N/A	N/A
Colorado	3,294,394	239,878	73	$540,533	$164	$2,253
Idaho	1,006,749	65,824	65	$156,761	$156	$2,382
Montana	799,065	73,790	92	$193,121	$242	$2,617
Nevada	1,201,833	62,957	52	$149,822	$125	$2,380
New Mexico	1,515,069	158,477	105	$294,373	$194	$1,858
Utah	1,722,850	139,993	81	$275,779	$160	$1,970
Wyoming	453,588	36,134	80	$67,364	$149	$1,864
PACIFIC	**39,127,306**	**5,692,068**	**145**	**$9,170,097**	**$234**	**$1,611**
Alaska	550,043	49,839	91	$153,054	$278	$3,071
California	29,760,021	4,756,243	160	$7,047,049	$237	$1,482
Hawaii	1,108,229	93,366	84	$206,523	$186	$2,212
Oregon	2,842,321	262,273	92	$536,556	$189	$2,046
Washington	4,866,692	530,347	109	$1,226,915	$252	$2,313
UNITED STATES	**248,709,873**	**28,383,264**	**114**	**$68,925,702**	**$277**	**$2,428**

Source: Health Care Financing Administration Form 64 and Form 2082.

TABLE D5
MEDICAID ENROLLEES AND EXPENDITURES: ADULTS AGES 18-65, 1990

	Adults Ages 18-65	Adult Enrollees	Enrollees per 1000 Population	Expenditures (000s)	Expenditures per capita	Expenditures per enrollee
NEW ENGLAND	**8,271,003**	**312,366**	**38**	**$414,884**	**$50**	**$1,328**
Connecticut	2,070,492	53,769	26	$59,288	$29	$1,103
Maine	753,558	36,680	49	$38,185	$51	$1,041
Massachusetts	3,781,468	157,625	42	$251,576	$67	$1,596
New Hampshire	699,464	20,604	29	$14,011	$20	$680
Rhode Island	616,028	25,148	41	$30,660	$50	$1,219
Vermont	349,992	18,540	53	$21,165	$60	$1,142
MIDDLE ATLANTIC	**23,338,680**	**903,627**	**39**	**$1,586,816**	**$68**	**$1,756**
New Jersey	4,869,904	144,780	30	$311,875	$64	$2,154
New York	11,261,078	491,218	44	$1,001,006	$89	$2,038
Pennsylvania	7,207,698	267,629	37	$273,935	$38	$1,024
SOUTH ATLANTIC	**26,999,096**	**982,276**	**36**	**$1,382,858**	**$51**	**$1,408**
Delaware	416,381	12,951	31	$12,370	$30	$955
District of Columbia	400,092	23,661	59	$44,654	$112	$1,887
Florida	7,655,479	261,290	34	$328,577	$43	$1,258
Georgia	4,071,909	156,847	39	$323,657	$79	$2,064
Maryland	3,072,553	94,904	31	$136,803	$45	$1,441
North Carolina	4,173,344	155,091	37	$204,778	$49	$1,320
South Carolina	2,155,456	69,478	32	$130,468	$61	$1,878
Virginia	3,969,314	96,435	24	$126,986	$32	$1,317
West Virginia	1,084,567	111,619	103	$74,567	$69	$668
EAST SOUTH CENTRAL	**9,245,311**	**425,459**	**46**	**$588,711**	**$64**	**$1,384**
Alabama	2,453,555	81,050	33	$114,834	$47	$1,417
Kentucky	2,258,096	124,586	55	$159,021	$70	$1,276
Mississippi	1,505,488	88,340	59	$98,168	$65	$1,111
Tennessee	3,028,173	131,483	43	$216,688	$72	$1,648
EAST NORTH CENTRAL	**25,646,251**	**1,169,987**	**46**	**$1,319,405**	**$51**	**$1,128**
Illinois	7,009,403	321,588	46	$263,321	$38	$819
Indiana	3,378,767	91,538	27	$173,932	$51	$1,900
Michigan	5,705,029	322,666	57	$426,958	$75	$1,323
Ohio	6,616,331	314,074	47	$362,839	$55	$1,155
Wisconsin	2,936,722	120,121	41	$92,355	$31	$769
WEST SOUTH CENTRAL	**16,178,360**	**654,415**	**40**	**$895,528**	**$55**	**$1,368**
Arkansas	1,382,140	50,426	36	$44,278	$32	$878
Louisiana	2,518,619	139,429	55	$225,743	$90	$1,619
Oklahoma	1,882,077	68,229	36	$102,046	$54	$1,496
Texas	10,395,523	396,331	38	$523,461	$50	$1,321
WEST NORTH CENTRAL	**10,504,282**	**414,686**	**39**	**$483,479**	**$46**	**$1,166**
Iowa	1,625,141	65,700	40	$88,259	$54	$1,343
Kansas	1,465,480	70,162	48	$82,542	$56	$1,176
Minnesota	2,648,132	95,025	36	$160,244	$61	$1,686
Missouri	3,073,784	132,003	43	$90,696	$30	$687
Nebraska	925,474	27,139	29	$30,761	$33	$1,133
North Dakota	370,686	11,921	32	$17,615	$48	$1,478
South Dakota	395,585	12,736	32	$13,363	$34	$1,049
MOUNTAIN	**8,239,825**	**190,122**	**23**	**$235,236**	**$29**	**$1,237**
Arizona	2,191,245	N/A	N/A	N/A	N/A	N/A
Colorado	2,092,548	57,136	27	$52,659	$25	$922
Idaho	581,193	15,883	27	$18,214	$31	$1,147
Montana	473,660	16,369	35	$22,560	$48	$1,378
Nevada	771,783	13,947	18	$18,633	$24	$1,336
New Mexico	907,439	34,982	39	$50,411	$56	$1,441
Utah	948,656	42,527	45	$58,253	$61	$1,370
Wyoming	273,300	9,278	34	$14,506	$53	$1,563
PACIFIC	**24,445,066**	**1,578,161**	**65**	**$1,658,726**	**$68**	**$1,051**
Alaska	354,348	12,390	35	$29,589	$84	$2,388
California	18,656,246	1,322,605	71	$1,316,588	$71	$995
Hawaii	696,213	22,793	33	$31,497	$45	$1,382
Oregon	1,724,707	73,003	42	$71,364	$41	$978
Washington	3,013,552	147,370	49	$209,688	$70	$1,423
UNITED STATES	**152,867,873**	**6,636,305**	**43**	**$8,565,644**	**$56**	**$1,291**

Source: Health Care Financing Administration Form 64 and Form 2082.

TABLE D6
MEDICAID ENROLLEES AND EXPENDITURES: BLIND AND DISABLED AGES 18-65, 1990

	Adults Ages 18-65	Blind and Disabled Enrollees	Enrollees per 1000 Population	Expenditures (000s)	Expenditures per Capita	Expenditures per Enrollee
NEW ENGLAND	**8,271,003**	**208,336**	**25**	**$2,097,751**	**$254**	**$10,069**
Connecticut	2,070,492	38,920	19	$414,512	$200	$10,650
Maine	753,558	25,030	33	$155,596	$206	$6,216
Massachusetts	3,781,468	103,291	27	$1,193,566	$316	$11,555
New Hampshire	699,464	6,852	10	$83,031	$119	$12,118
Rhode Island	616,028	25,310	41	$198,006	$321	$7,823
Vermont	349,992	8,933	26	$53,039	$152	$5,937
MIDDLE ATLANTIC	**23,338,680**	**664,474**	**28**	**$6,373,954**	**$273**	**$9,592**
New Jersey	4,869,904	99,887	21	$999,456	$205	$10,006
New York	11,261,078	372,792	33	$4,395,335	$390	$11,790
Pennsylvania	7,207,698	191,795	27	$979,164	$136	$5,105
SOUTH ATLANTIC	**26,999,096**	**664,412**	**25**	**$3,366,558**	**$125**	**$5,067**
Delaware	416,381	8,074	19	$51,588	$124	$6,389
District of Columbia	400,092	17,665	44	$151,355	$378	$8,568
Florida	7,655,479	183,334	24	$779,720	$102	$4,253
Georgia	4,071,909	134,742	33	$595,784	$146	$4,422
Maryland	3,072,553	63,200	21	$419,157	$136	$6,632
North Carolina	4,173,344	74,505	18	$510,285	$122	$6,849
South Carolina	2,155,456	73,350	34	$364,916	$169	$4,975
Virginia	3,969,314	66,646	17	$372,645	$94	$5,591
West Virginia	1,084,567	42,896	40	$121,108	$112	$2,823
EAST SOUTH CENTRAL	**9,245,311**	**427,879**	**46**	**$1,435,003**	**$155**	**$3,354**
Alabama	2,453,555	96,743	39	$303,257	$124	$3,135
Kentucky	2,258,096	103,302	46	$395,205	$175	$3,826
Mississippi	1,505,488	86,363	57	$209,003	$139	$2,420
Tennessee	3,028,173	141,471	47	$527,538	$174	$3,729
EAST NORTH CENTRAL	**25,646,251**	**629,998**	**25**	**$4,418,932**	**$172**	**$7,014**
Illinois	7,009,403	188,711	27	$1,172,182	$167	$6,212
Indiana	3,378,767	58,598	17	$599,171	$177	$10,225
Michigan	5,705,029	140,917	25	$1,000,125	$175	$7,097
Ohio	6,616,331	161,204	24	$1,126,235	$170	$6,986
Wisconsin	2,936,722	80,568	27	$521,219	$177	$6,469
WEST SOUTH CENTRAL	**16,178,360**	**355,384**	**22**	**$1,806,631**	**$112**	**$5,084**
Arkansas	1,382,140	57,131	41	$225,537	$163	$3,948
Louisiana	2,518,619	89,472	36	$510,779	$203	$5,709
Oklahoma	1,882,077	39,196	21	$212,907	$113	$5,432
Texas	10,395,523	169,585	16	$857,407	$82	$5,056
WEST NORTH CENTRAL	**10,504,282**	**209,377**	**20**	**$1,461,517**	**$139**	**$6,980**
Iowa	1,625,141	35,523	22	$233,538	$144	$6,574
Kansas	1,465,480	24,241	17	$167,777	$114	$6,921
Minnesota	2,648,132	42,317	16	$506,515	$191	$11,970
Missouri	3,073,784	77,032	25	$302,484	$98	$3,927
Nebraska	925,474	14,315	15	$102,545	$111	$7,163
North Dakota	370,686	6,495	18	$78,944	$213	$12,155
South Dakota	395,585	9,454	24	$69,714	$176	$7,374
MOUNTAIN	**8,239,825**	**102,630**	**12**	**$671,760**	**$82**	**$6,545**
Arizona	2,191,245	N/A	N/A	N/A	N/A	N/A
Colorado	2,092,548	33,039	16	$220,785	$106	$6,683
Idaho	581,193	9,995	17	$70,258	$121	$7,029
Montana	473,660	10,155	21	$71,291	$151	$7,020
Nevada	771,783	8,752	11	$63,471	$82	$7,252
New Mexico	907,439	25,060	28	$119,174	$131	$4,756
Utah	948,656	12,294	13	$111,255	$117	$9,050
Wyoming	273,300	3,335	12	$15,525	$57	$4,655
PACIFIC	**24,445,066**	**732,293**	**30**	**$3,218,557**	**$132**	**$4,395**
Alaska	354,348	4,198	12	$43,053	$121	$10,256
California	18,656,246	622,891	33	$2,449,634	$131	$3,933
Hawaii	696,213	8,895	13	$51,074	$73	$5,742
Oregon	1,724,707	31,347	18	$231,572	$134	$7,387
Washington	3,013,552	64,962	22	$443,224	$147	$6,823
UNITED STATES	**152,867,873**	**3,994,783**	**26**	**$24,850,664**	**$163**	**$6,221**

Source: Health Care Financing Administration Form 64 and Form 2082.

TABLE D7
MEDICAID ENROLLEES AND EXPENDITURES: CHILDREN AGES 0-18, 1990

	Children Ages 0-18	Child Enrollees	Enrollees per 1000 Population	Expenditures (000s)	Expenditures per capita	Expenditures per enrollee
NEW ENGLAND	**3,165,637**	**613,941**	**194**	**$487,949**	**$154**	**$795**
Connecticut	770,717	117,958	153	$84,789	$110	$719
Maine	310,997	72,596	233	$37,910	$122	$522
Massachusetts	1,415,673	330,594	234	$310,726	$219	$940
New Hampshire	284,759	13,985	49	$7,611	$27	$544
Rhode Island	236,889	47,885	202	$31,904	$135	$666
Vermont	146,603	30,923	211	$15,010	$102	$485
MIDDLE ATLANTIC	**9,038,753**	**2,412,647**	**267**	**$2,034,648**	**$225**	**$843**
New Jersey	1,828,259	317,290	174	$224,630	$123	$708
New York	4,365,655	1,397,066	320	$1,449,206	$332	$1,037
Pennsylvania	2,844,840	698,291	245	$360,812	$127	$517
SOUTH ATLANTIC	**10,733,349**	**2,040,830**	**190**	**$1,425,064**	**$133**	**$698**
Delaware	169,052	28,412	168	$14,890	$88	$524
District of Columbia	128,961	55,365	429	$54,002	$419	$975
Florida	2,913,017	574,305	197	$426,142	$146	$742
Georgia	1,752,037	341,098	195	$209,176	$119	$613
Maryland	1,191,433	238,865	200	$199,182	$167	$834
North Carolina	1,650,952	301,613	183	$226,629	$137	$751
South Carolina	934,312	159,399	171	$129,367	$138	$812
Virginia	1,553,574	207,818	134	$124,675	$80	$600
West Virginia	440,013	133,955	304	$41,000	$93	$306
EAST SOUTH CENTRAL	**4,001,037**	**994,148**	**248**	**$665,584**	**$166**	**$670**
Alabama	1,064,043	177,243	167	$112,530	$106	$635
Kentucky	960,355	235,587	245	$146,595	$153	$622
Mississippi	746,444	255,520	342	$103,775	$139	$406
Tennessee	1,230,194	325,798	265	$302,684	$246	$929
EAST NORTH CENTRAL	**11,063,307**	**2,648,389**	**239**	**$1,639,651**	**$148**	**$619**
Illinois	2,984,654	782,092	262	$382,591	$128	$489
Indiana	1,469,196	184,490	126	$154,890	$105	$840
Michigan	2,481,807	625,949	252	$406,997	$164	$650
Ohio	2,823,823	760,253	269	$574,204	$203	$755
Wisconsin	1,303,826	295,605	227	$120,969	$93	$409
WEST SOUTH CENTRAL	**7,564,595**	**1,580,035**	**209**	**$996,608**	**$132**	**$631**
Arkansas	618,527	134,959	218	$112,593	$182	$834
Louisiana	1,232,363	329,381	267	$238,438	$193	$724
Oklahoma	839,295	169,081	201	$117,394	$140	$694
Texas	4,874,411	946,614	194	$528,182	$108	$558
WEST NORTH CENTRAL	**4,705,662**	**841,299**	**179**	**$571,633**	**$121**	**$679**
Iowa	725,509	130,581	180	$100,889	$139	$773
Kansas	669,523	110,786	165	$60,194	$90	$543
Minnesota	1,180,034	217,836	185	$177,614	$151	$815
Missouri	1,325,608	253,726	191	$136,684	$103	$539
Nebraska	429,843	73,115	170	$51,362	$119	$702
North Dakota	177,059	26,777	151	$22,751	$128	$850
South Dakota	198,088	28,478	144	$22,138	$112	$777
MOUNTAIN	**3,895,126**	**400,304**	**103**	**$223,633**	**$57**	**$559**
Arizona	995,209	N/A	N/A	N/A	N/A	N/A
Colorado	872,403	116,619	134	$63,370	$73	$543
Idaho	304,291	32,516	107	$18,000	$59	$554
Montana	218,908	40,304	184	$22,697	$104	$563
Nevada	302,419	31,368	104	$21,213	$70	$676
New Mexico	444,568	82,937	187	$47,996	$108	$579
Utah	624,236	76,386	122	$39,793	$64	$521
Wyoming	133,093	20,174	152	$10,563	$79	$524
PACIFIC	**10,432,702**	**2,791,439**	**268**	**$1,337,041**	**$128**	**$479**
Alaska	173,326	30,031	173	$46,573	$269	$1,551
California	7,968,223	2,309,858	290	$1,036,994	$130	$449
Hawaii	287,012	49,232	172	$32,096	$112	$652
Oregon	726,290	132,238	182	$57,189	$79	$432
Washington	1,277,852	270,080	211	$164,189	$128	$608
UNITED STATES	**64,600,169**	**14,317,826**	**222**	**$9,381,811**	**$145**	**$655**

Source: Health Care Financing Administration Form 64 and Form 2082.

TABLE D8
MEDICAID ENROLLEES AND EXPENDITURES: AGES 65 AND OVER, 1990

	Aged Ages 65+	Aged Enrollees	Enrollees per 1000 Population	Expenditures (000s)	Expenditures per capita	Expenditures per enrollee
NEW ENGLAND	**1,770,303**	**223,256**	**126**	**$2,473,162**	**$1,397**	**$11,078**
Connecticut	445,907	58,406	131	$636,310	$1,427	$10,895
Maine	163,373	22,018	135	$195,175	$1,195	$8,864
Massachusetts	819,284	97,914	120	$1,289,698	$1,574	$13,172
New Hampshire	125,029	10,321	83	$113,233	$906	$10,971
Rhode Island	150,547	24,165	161	$177,056	$1,176	$7,327
Vermont	66,163	10,432	158	$61,690	$932	$5,914
MIDDLE ATLANTIC	**5,224,853**	**578,664**	**111**	**$6,184,447**	**$1,184**	**$10,687**
New Jersey	1,032,025	79,651	77	$774,691	$751	$9,726
New York	2,363,722	353,263	149	$4,400,230	$1,862	$12,456
Pennsylvania	1,829,106	145,750	80	$1,009,526	$552	$6,926
SOUTH ATLANTIC	**5,834,408**	**566,171**	**97**	**$3,094,382**	**$530**	**$5,465**
Delaware	80,735	4,794	59	$44,226	$548	$9,225
District of Columbia	77,847	11,541	148	$115,859	$1,488	$10,039
Florida	2,369,431	167,375	71	$923,599	$390	$5,518
Georgia	654,270	82,923	127	$422,973	$646	$5,101
Maryland	517,482	43,662	84	$355,618	$687	$8,145
North Carolina	804,341	104,278	130	$492,682	$613	$4,725
South Carolina	396,935	51,993	131	$200,320	$505	$3,853
Virginia	664,470	69,713	105	$377,806	$569	$5,419
West Virginia	268,897	29,892	111	$161,299	$600	$5,396
EAST SOUTH CENTRAL	**1,929,936**	**296,939**	**154**	**$1,087,549**	**$564**	**$3,663**
Alabama	522,989	76,202	146	$261,866	$501	$3,436
Kentucky	466,845	59,913	128	$270,629	$580	$4,517
Mississippi	321,284	65,768	205	$208,477	$649	$3,170
Tennessee	618,818	95,056	154	$346,576	$560	$3,646
EAST NORTH CENTRAL	**5,299,384**	**441,262**	**83**	**$3,050,283**	**$576**	**$6,913**
Illinois	1,436,545	145,750	101	$558,781	$389	$3,834
Indiana	696,196	44,193	63	$415,353	$597	$9,399
Michigan	1,108,461	83,852	76	$507,189	$458	$6,049
Ohio	1,406,961	101,864	72	$973,638	$692	$9,558
Wisconsin	651,221	65,603	101	$595,322	$914	$9,075
WEST SOUTH CENTRAL	**2,959,838**	**439,200**	**148**	**$1,857,316**	**$628**	**$4,229**
Arkansas	350,058	47,387	135	$216,456	$618	$4,568
Louisiana	468,991	91,020	194	$367,886	$784	$4,042
Oklahoma	424,213	54,434	128	$239,906	$566	$4,407
Texas	1,716,576	246,359	144	$1,033,068	$602	$4,193
WEST NORTH CENTRAL	**2,449,746**	**214,686**	**88**	**$1,538,466**	**$628**	**$7,166**
Iowa	426,106	35,571	83	$202,494	$475	$5,693
Kansas	342,571	27,706	81	$156,157	$456	$5,636
Minnesota	546,934	46,628	85	$526,059	$962	$11,282
Missouri	717,681	67,706	94	$391,335	$545	$5,780
Nebraska	223,068	17,528	79	$128,241	$575	$7,316
North Dakota	91,055	10,182	112	$74,853	$822	$7,351
South Dakota	102,331	9,365	92	$59,329	$580	$6,335
MOUNTAIN	**1,523,825**	**83,997**	**55**	**$501,209**	**$329**	**$5,967**
Arizona	478,774	N/A	N/A	N/A	N/A	N/A
Colorado	329,443	33,084	100	$179,413	$545	$5,423
Idaho	121,265	7,430	61	$49,205	$406	$6,622
Montana	106,497	6,962	65	$65,663	$617	$9,432
Nevada	127,631	8,890	70	$43,620	$342	$4,907
New Mexico	163,062	15,498	95	$76,552	$469	$4,939
Utah	149,958	8,786	59	$60,399	$403	$6,875
Wyoming	47,195	3,347	71	$26,357	$558	$7,875
PACIFIC	**4,249,538**	**590,175**	**139**	**$2,369,209**	**$558**	**$4,014**
Alaska	22,369	3,220	144	$32,868	$1,469	$10,208
California	3,135,552	500,889	160	$1,737,393	$554	$3,469
Hawaii	125,005	12,446	100	$87,871	$703	$7,060
Oregon	391,324	25,685	66	$137,265	$351	$5,344
Washington	575,288	47,935	83	$373,812	$650	$7,798
UNITED STATES	**31,241,831**	**3,434,350**	**110**	**$22,156,022**	**$709**	**$6,451**

Source: Health Care Financing Administration Form 64 and Form 2082.

TABLE D9
RATIO OF MEDICAID MAXIMUM FEES TO NEW MEDICARE FEE SCHEDULE LEVELS, 1990

	Primary Care	Hospital Visits	Surgery	Obstetrical Care	Laboratory Tests	Imaging	All Services
NEW ENGLAND	**0.77**	**0.56**	**0.92**	**1.29**	**0.79**	**0.58**	**0.77**
Connecticut	0.52	0.52	0.94	1.07	0.74	0.59	0.62
Maine	0.51	0.38	0.58	1.06	0.87	0.53	0.56
Massachusetts	0.95	0.64	1.04	1.43	0.77	0.58	0.90
New Hampshire	0.68	0.32	0.60	1.32	0.66	0.51	0.62
Rhode Island	N/A	N/A	N/A	N/A	N/A	N/A	N/A
Vermont	0.55	0.52	0.66	1.18	1.02	0.70	0.65
MIDDLE ATLANTIC	**0.33**	**0.24**	**0.49**	**0.92**	**0.29**	**0.55**	**0.37**
New Jersey	0.37	0.22	0.44	0.58	0.36	0.45	0.37
New York	0.29	0.14	0.32	1.12	0.17	0.46	0.30
Pennsylvania	0.40	0.43	0.86	0.70	0.50	0.78	0.49
SOUTH ATLANTIC	**0.65**	**0.68**	**1.18**	**1.35**	**0.99**	**0.92**	**0.78**
Delaware	0.48	0.64	0.99	0.97	0.80	0.86	0.62
District of Columbia	0.56	0.41	0.75	1.62	0.44	0.71	0.64
Florida	0.70	0.85	1.04	1.08	0.96	1.32	0.84
Georgia	0.78	0.96	1.90	1.76	1.14	0.93	0.98
Maryland	0.49	0.26	0.54	1.70	0.83	0.46	0.51
North Carolina	0.67	0.66	1.26	1.24	0.96	0.84	0.79
South Carolina	0.73	0.53	0.97	1.62	1.07	0.94	0.82
Virginia	0.68	0.77	1.65	1.32	1.17	0.82	0.83
West Virginia	0.27	0.26	0.59	0.86	0.86	0.46	0.35
EAST SOUTH CENTRAL	**0.65**	**0.49**	**1.11**	**1.21**	**0.94**	**0.90**	**0.71**
Alabama	0.61	0.54	1.12	1.30	0.81	0.76	0.72
Kentucky	0.58	0.53	1.23	1.37	0.87	0.92	0.71
Mississippi	0.43	0.29	0.66	1.25	0.72	0.85	0.51
Tennessee	0.87	0.56	1.33	0.99	1.23	1.01	0.86
EAST NORTH CENTRAL	**0.57**	**0.44**	**0.98**	**0.94**	**0.77**	**0.64**	**0.61**
Illinois	0.54	0.37	0.91	1.10	0.69	0.36	0.56
Indiana	0.89	0.88	1.86	1.14	1.31	0.92	0.98
Michigan	0.57	0.38	0.75	0.79	0.51	0.60	0.57
Ohio	0.53	0.38	0.88	0.88	0.89	0.75	0.58
Wisconsin	0.54	0.62	1.23	0.82	0.87	1.01	0.66
WEST SOUTH CENTRAL	**0.81**	**0.78**	**1.47**	**1.56**	**1.33**	**1.23**	**0.96**
Arkansas	0.93	0.93	1.27	1.01	0.89	0.93	0.96
Louisiana	0.78	0.80	1.01	1.73	0.98	0.83	0.92
Oklahoma	0.62	0.64	1.32	1.06	1.01	0.99	0.74
Texas	0.84	0.78	1.69	1.69	1.60	1.47	1.02
WEST NORTH CENTRAL	**0.63**	**0.52**	**1.00**	**0.96**	**0.85**	**0.93**	**0.69**
Iowa	0.67	0.60	1.37	1.11	0.80	0.92	0.77
Kansas	0.67	0.30	0.98	1.03	0.91	1.19	0.65
Minnesota	0.72	0.74	1.29	0.99	0.75	0.95	0.82
Missouri	0.46	0.32	0.54	0.82	0.80	0.60	0.50
Nebraska	0.79	0.65	1.06	1.04	1.15	1.55	0.87
North Dakota	0.62	0.66	1.08	1.12	1.03	1.20	0.76
South Dakota	0.70	0.81	1.36	0.85	1.01	1.16	0.81
MOUNTAIN	**0.71**	**0.66**	**1.03**	**1.10**	**0.87**	**0.70**	**0.77**
Arizona	N/A	N/A	N/A	N/A	N/A	N/A	N/A
Colorado	0.68	0.56	0.80	1.18	1.08	0.72	0.74
Idaho	0.71	0.62	1.01	1.57	0.88	0.83	0.82
Montana	0.69	0.69	0.94	0.93	1.03	0.71	0.75
Nevada	0.87	0.76	1.51	1.41	0.92	0.75	0.94
New Mexico	0.70	0.63	1.21	1.02	0.44	0.63	0.74
Utah	0.66	0.78	1.00	0.79	0.82	0.55	0.70
Wyoming	0.89	0.73	1.24	1.16	1.12	1.16	0.95
PACIFIC	**0.57**	**0.56**	**0.90**	**0.94**	**0.87**	**0.68**	**0.65**
Alaska	1.08	1.23	2.27	1.22	0.93	1.01	1.15
California	0.55	0.56	0.89	0.93	0.87	0.67	0.64
Hawaii	0.78	0.82	1.42	0.70	0.76	0.87	0.79
Oregon	0.66	0.55	0.99	1.16	0.86	0.76	0.73
Washington	0.66	0.44	0.78	0.97	0.86	0.68	0.67
UNITED STATES	**0.59**	**0.52**	**0.98**	**1.11**	**0.83**	**0.78**	**0.67**

Sources: Health Care Financing Administration, 1991, "Federal Register: The Fee Schedule for Physicians' Services"
and The Urban Institute, 1991, "Survey of 1990 State Medicaid Physician Payment".

TABLE D10
RATIO OF MEDICAID MAXIMUM FEES TO PRIVATE FEE LEVELS, 1990

	Primary Care	Hospital Visits	Surgery	Obstetrical Care	Laboratory Tests	Imaging	All Services
NEW ENGLAND	**0.72**	**0.54**	**0.44**	**0.60**	**0.43**	**0.48**	**0.62**
Connecticut	0.48	0.47	0.41	0.42	0.37	0.38	0.45
Maine	0.63	0.38	0.29	0.61	0.55	0.56	0.56
Massachusetts	0.84	0.61	0.48	0.65	0.41	0.49	0.70
New Hampshire	0.66	0.30	0.30	0.82	0.39	0.61	0.61
Rhode Island	N/A	N/A	N/A	N/A	N/A	N/A	N/A
Vermont	0.75	0.71	0.59	0.58	0.60	0.49	0.67
MIDDLE ATLANTIC	**0.37**	**0.22**	**0.21**	**0.35**	**0.23**	**0.37**	**0.35**
New Jersey	0.41	0.22	0.19	0.22	0.28	0.32	0.33
New York	0.27	0.14	0.12	0.38	0.15	0.34	0.28
Pennsylvania	0.53	0.38	0.38	0.37	0.36	0.44	0.46
SOUTH ATLANTIC	**0.68**	**0.61**	**0.57**	**0.66**	**0.60**	**0.66**	**0.66**
Delaware	0.54	0.52	0.50	0.50	0.48	0.53	0.52
District of Columbia	0.48	0.32	0.31	0.47	0.26	0.49	0.44
Florida	0.66	0.71	0.56	0.49	0.60	0.95	0.66
Georgia	0.83	0.86	0.83	0.78	0.73	0.67	0.83
Maryland	0.55	0.21	0.24	0.87	0.47	0.29	0.54
North Carolina	0.73	0.59	0.62	0.64	0.61	0.64	0.68
South Carolina	0.78	0.55	0.53	0.94	0.51	0.69	0.76
Virginia	0.74	0.70	0.73	0.66	0.74	0.62	0.71
West Virginia	0.34	0.27	0.29	0.53	0.47	0.26	0.36
EAST SOUTH CENTRAL	**0.74**	**0.53**	**0.58**	**0.67**	**0.64**	**0.74**	**0.69**
Alabama	0.64	0.57	0.58	0.68	0.58	0.66	0.64
Kentucky	0.68	0.58	0.62	0.82	0.59	0.66	0.69
Mississippi	0.57	0.36	0.36	0.62	0.46	0.81	0.56
Tennessee	0.96	0.60	0.70	0.59	0.84	0.79	0.81
EAST NORTH CENTRAL	**0.67**	**0.48**	**0.52**	**0.55**	**0.53**	**0.51**	**0.60**
Illinois	0.64	0.38	0.44	0.54	0.42	0.27	0.55
Indiana	1.08	0.99	0.97	0.81	1.14	0.76	1.00
Michigan	0.68	0.45	0.48	0.47	0.34	0.47	0.56
Ohio	0.64	0.42	0.46	0.54	0.62	0.57	0.58
Wisconsin	0.56	0.59	0.63	0.55	0.55	0.87	0.62
WEST SOUTH CENTRAL	**0.87**	**0.71**	**0.74**	**0.70**	**0.79**	**0.90**	**0.84**
Arkansas	0.87	0.78	0.67	0.73	0.58	0.68	0.80
Louisiana	0.93	0.81	0.49	0.31	0.60	0.59	0.85
Oklahoma	0.65	0.64	0.66	0.66	0.65	0.87	0.68
Texas	0.88	0.67	0.86	0.85	0.92	1.06	0.88
WEST NORTH CENTRAL	**0.69**	**0.50**	**0.56**	**0.65**	**0.57**	**0.75**	**0.66**
Iowa	0.81	0.61	0.78	0.73	0.49	0.80	0.77
Kansas	0.73	0.34	0.55	0.58	0.58	0.90	0.65
Minnesota	0.68	0.59	0.73	0.78	0.45	0.88	0.71
Missouri	0.56	0.34	0.29	0.48	0.59	0.46	0.49
Nebraska	0.98	0.84	0.65	0.98	0.96	1.18	0.96
North Dakota	0.51	0.46	0.53	0.31	0.57	0.59	0.68
South Dakota	0.79	0.74	0.70	0.69	0.62	0.88	0.76
MOUNTAIN	**0.72**	**0.61**	**0.54**	**0.60**	**0.64**	**0.62**	**0.67**
Arizona	N/A	N/A	N/A	N/A	N/A	N/A	N/A
Colorado	0.66	0.51	0.43	0.60	0.73	0.62	0.64
Idaho	0.74	0.65	0.55	1.02	0.56	0.80	0.78
Montana	0.70	0.63	0.51	0.54	0.82	0.61	0.64
Nevada	0.80	0.62	0.69	0.84	0.78	0.57	0.76
New Mexico	0.69	0.62	0.61	0.34	0.43	0.67	0.59
Utah	0.75	0.71	0.59	0.58	0.60	0.49	0.67
Wyoming	0.99	0.78	0.67	0.70	0.72	0.69	0.84
PACIFIC	**0.50**	**0.45**	**0.43**	**0.57**	**0.48**	**0.47**	**0.51**
Alaska	0.94	1.05	1.15	0.79	0.58	1.07	0.94
California	0.48	0.44	0.41	0.56	0.46	0.44	0.49
Hawaii	0.58	0.57	0.61	0.63	0.66	1.02	0.63
Oregon	0.60	0.52	0.54	0.66	0.59	0.57	0.59
Washington	0.61	0.40	0.42	0.61	0.52	0.50	0.57
UNITED STATES	**0.62**	**0.49**	**0.49**	**0.57**	**0.52**	**0.58**	**0.59**

Sources: Health Insurance Association of America, 1990, "Prevailing Healthcare Charges System"
and The Urban Institute, 1991, "Survey of 1990 State Medicaid Physician Payment".

Notes for tables D1–D10

D1–D2 The eligible population is an estimate of all individuals under age 65 that would qualify for Medicaid if they applied. Eligibility for Medicaid was calculated using the Urban Institute's Transfer Income Model (TRIM2). Using income and demographic information from the March CPS and applying state Medicaid eligibility rules, individuals were determined to be eligible for Medicaid. For more information, see Appendix Two.

The enrolled population is an estimate of the number of individuals under age 65 that actually enrolled in the Medicaid program. The TRIM2 simulation model is used to correct for underrporting of Medicaid benefits on the CPS. See Appendix Two for more details. The enrollment rate is the percentage of eligibles that are enrolled in the program.

D4 Numbers of enrollees in Medicaid differ from those reported in table D1, for several reasons. First, the numbers in D1 are based on the CPS, which includes only noninstitutionalized individuals. Also, the CPS numbers are an average over three years—1988 through 1990—and Medicaid enrollment was increasing over these years. The numbers in this table are for 1990 alone. Finally, there may also be some error introduced by simulation in the numbers in table D1.

D4–D8 Expenditures per capita are per the population group listed in column one.

D6 Since accurate population counts for blind and disabled persons are not available, the entire adult population 18 through 65 years of age is presented.

D9 Medicare fee values were calculated assuming that the Medicare Fee Schedule (MFS), published in 1992, was introduced in 1990. A series of adjustments to the actual published MFS were made to calculate the 1990 fee values.

D9–D10 Data for Arizona and Rhode Island are not included. Arizona does not have a Medicaid program, and owing to state budget problems, Rhode Island did not respond to the Urban Institute's Medicaid Fee Survey.

Texas data provided to the Urban Institute's Medicaid Fee Survey were for Harris County (Houston) only, and therefore are not representative of the whole state. The ratio for Texas in both tables, however, are comparisons to Medicare and private fees in Harris county.

Indices of Health Status

This section's tables provide information on health status indicators within each state. Attention is concentrated on three subpopulations—pregnant women and infants, the total population, and selected populations including individuals infected with the AIDS virus as well as those with disabilities that prevent or limit working.

PREGNANT WOMEN AND INFANTS

Newborn infants and pregnant women are the focus of most of the data in this subsection. Table E1 provides information on infant mortality rates per 1,000 births by race (white and black). Infant mortality is widely used as a measure of infant health status. The data show important variation between white and black infant mortality rates. On average there are twice as many black infant deaths as white infant deaths per 1,000 live births, a result that is fairly consistent across states.

Recent policy reforms have stressed the need to provide quality health care to pregnant women and infants. These data give some indication of the quality of care received. Table E2 lists the number of neonatal deaths, the number of births in which the mother received late or no prenatal care, and the number of low-weight births. Births in which the mother did not receive any prenatal care before the seventh month of pregnancy are classified as births receiving late prenatal care. Births under 2,500 grams are classified as low-weight births. The percentage of births in which the mother receives late or no prenatal care varies among the states. The rates in Texas, the District of Columbia, and New Mexico, for example, are at least twice the national average of 5.9 percent.

Table E3 highlights racial differences in the number of births to unmarried women. Births to unmarried black women as a percent of all black births range from 15 percent in Hawaii to 77 percent in Wisconsin, whereas the percentage for white women ranges from 12 percent in North Carolina to 27 percent in California. The variation between the races can be seen clearly when comparing national averages; the percentage of births to unmarried white women is 18 percent, whereas the percentage of births to unmarried black women is 60 percent.

Total population

Table E4 shows birthrates and death rates per 1,000 population. States with birthrates higher than the national average tend to have death rates below the national average. The opposite of this is also true. For example, California's birthrate per 1,000 population of 18.8 was almost 20 percent higher than the national average, while its death rate per 1,000 population of 7.6 was about 15 percent lower than the national average. The information presented here along with the population characteristics found in section G indicate relatively younger or older state populations.

Death rates by selected causes are presented in table E5. These six leading causes of death account for over three-quarters of all deaths in the United States. In all of the states, heart disease is the leading cause of death and malignant neoplasms is second. However, there is variation across states in the rates of death due to these factors. For example, death rates from heart disease vary from 218.8 per 100,000 in the West North Central region to 379.8 per 100,000 in the Middle Atlantic region. Differences in death rates across states reflect, among other factors, differences in population characteristics such as age and income (tables G1 and G5) and differences in state health care system.

SELECTED POPULATIONS

Table E6 provides information on the number of AIDS deaths in 1988, AIDS cases as a percent of total U.S. AIDS cases since 1981, and the number of AIDS cases since 1981 per 100,000 population. This information is important since people afflicted with the AIDS virus are high-cost users of our health care system as well as being individuals likely to have difficulty obtaining or retaining health insurance. These data show that since 1981 six states—New York, California, Florida, Texas, New Jersey, and Illinois—have accounted for over 65 percent of the AIDS cases in this country. The number of AIDS cases per 100,000 population shows that the AIDS virus affects all of the states. However, there is wide variation in the number of cases per population across the states. For example, the number of AIDS cases per 100,000 ranges from 4 in North Dakota to 592 in the District of Columbia.

Table E7 provides information on the distribution of the population aged 18 through 64 with self-reported disabilities that prevent or limit working. This is not a representative measure of the number of disabled people within a state because the statistics are self-reported and only cover the adult population. Table E7 shows that the adult population reporting disabilities that prevent or limit the ability to work ranges from 4 percent in Connecticut to 11 percent in Kentucky and Mississippi, with most states falling within the range of 5 percent to 9 percent.

TABLE E1
INFANT MORTALITY: BY RACE, 1988

	Total Infant Deaths under Age 1	Infant Deaths per 1000 Births under Age 1	White Infant Deaths under Age 1	White Infant Deaths per 1000 White Births under Age 1	Black Infant Deaths under Age 1	Black Infant Deaths per 1000 Black Births under Age 1
NEW ENGLAND	**1,572**	**8.14**	**1,297**	**7.60**	**251**	**15.15**
Connecticut	426	8.86	323	7.96	101	15.50
Maine	136	7.92	135	8.04	0	0.00
Massachuetts	695	7.88	550	7.25	132	15.38
New Hampshire	144	8.29	141	8.37	2	13.42
Rhode Island	116	8.16	94	7.51	16	13.76
Vermont	55	6.78	54	6.75	0	0.00
MIDDLE ATLANTIC	**5,828**	**10.33**	**3,634**	**8.43**	**2102**	**18.57**
New Jersey	1,168	9.92	705	7.86	439	18.48
New York	3,017	10.75	1,813	8.88	1150	18.09
Pennsylvania	1,643	9.92	1,116	8.14	513	19.82
SOUTH ATLANTIC	**7,561**	**11.55**	**3,968**	**8.84**	**3526**	**18.47**
Delaware	123	11.82	71	9.07	51	21.13
District of Columbia	245	23.24	33	19.87	212	25.96
Florida	1,952	10.60	1,166	8.54	777	17.38
Georgia	1,331	12.57	609	9.17	716	18.92
Maryland	854	11.27	415	8.48	424	17.82
North Carolina	1,215	12.45	631	9.57	563	19.49
South Carolina	677	12.28	318	9.60	357	16.61
Virginia	967	10.38	548	8.13	406	17.92
West Virginia	197	9.02	177	8.51	20	21.60
EAST SOUTH CENTRAL	**2,557**	**11.39**	**1,445**	**9.06**	**1086**	**17.24**
Alabama	736	12.12	366	9.33	361	17.20
Kentucky	544	10.65	453	9.95	89	17.38
Mississippi	516	12.26	189	8.70	320	16.12
Tennessee	761	10.76	437	8.23	316	18.56
EAST NORTH CENTRAL	**6,686**	**10.49**	**4,466**	**8.68**	**2143**	**19.55**
Illinois	2,083	11.27	1,193	8.67	869	20.72
Indiana	899	11.01	709	9.95	188	19.89
Michigan	1,544	11.05	954	8.59	571	21.91
Ohio	1,565	9.75	1,150	8.64	406	15.92
Wisconsin	595	8.40	460	7.46	109	16.37
WEST SOUTH CENTRAL	**4,341**	**9.44**	**3,027**	**8.49**	**1262**	**14.44**
Arkansas	374	10.68	229	8.73	145	17.39
Louisiana	814	11.01	381	9.00	429	14.29
Oklahoma	429	9.05	332	9.26	66	12.64
Texas	2,724	8.98	2,085	8.27	622	14.19
WEST NORTH CENTRAL	**2,368**	**8.92**	**1,892**	**8.11**	**374**	**17.06**
Iowa	331	8.68	301	8.29	23	19.88
Kansas	309	7.97	237	6.98	60	16.54
Minnesota	521	7.81	434	7.19	54	19.49
Missouri	773	10.11	564	8.99	205	16.15
Nebraska	215	8.99	177	8.13	32	22.36
North Dakota	106	10.49	90	10.02	0	0.00
South Dakota	113	10.09	89	9.70	0	0.00
MOUNTAIN	**2,160**	**9.20**	**1,847**	**9.00**	**147**	**15.45**
Arizona	637	9.71	516	9.43	55	17.91
Colorado	510	9.56	466	9.64	38	12.02
Idaho	138	8.77	128	8.47	2	25.00
Montana	102	8.72	87	8.82	1	12.82
Nevada	152	8.44	110	7.47	37	18.72
New Mexico	270	9.99	214	9.75	10	14.18
Utah	287	7.96	267	7.86	2	6.21
Wyoming	64	8.94	59	8.84	2	16.81
PACIFIC	**5,837**	**8.63**	**4,349**	**8.26**	**949**	**15.85**
Alaska	130	11.57	71	9.78	13	20.22
California	4,573	8.58	3,386	8.15	854	15.92
Hawaii	137	7.19	33	7.20	8	8.96
Oregon	343	8.56	314	8.54	16	14.67
Washington	654	9.02	545	8.71	58	16.09
UNITED STATES	**38,910**	**9.95**	**25,925**	**8.51**	**11840**	**17.62**

Source: National Center for Health Statistics, 1988, "Vital Statistics of the United States: Volume II Mortality".

TABLE E2
INFANT HEALTH STATUS INDICATORS, 1988

	Neonatal Deaths Ages 1-27 Days	Neonatal Deaths per 1000 Births Ages 1-27 Days	Births with Late or No Prenatal Care	Percentage with Late or No Prenatal Care	Low-Weight Births	Percentage Low-Weight Births
NEW ENGLAND	**409**	**2.12**	**5,974**	**3.09%**	**11,453**	**5.93%**
Connecticut	126	2.62	1,652	3.44%	3,238	6.74%
Maine	39	2.27	474	2.76%	832	4.85%
Massachuetts	155	1.76	2,623	2.97%	5,286	5.99%
New Hampshire	37	2.13	516	2.97%	837	4.82%
Rhode Island	37	2.60	421	2.96%	854	6.00%
Vermont	15	1.85	288	3.55%	406	5.01%
MIDDLE ATLANTIC	**1,623**	**2.88**	**30,839**	**5.47%**	**41,476**	**7.35%**
New Jersey	343	2.91	6,164	5.23%	8,285	7.04%
New York	855	3.05	18,245	6.50%	21,774	7.76%
Pennsylvania	425	2.57	6,430	3.88%	11,417	6.89%
SOUTH ATLANTIC	**1,915**	**2.93**	**42,777**	**6.54%**	**52,081**	**7.96%**
Delaware	30	2.88	425	4.08%	765	7.35%
District of Columbia	56	5.31	1,167	11.07%	1,507	14.30%
Florida	528	2.87	14,910	8.10%	14,119	7.67%
Georgia	333	3.14	7,179	6.78%	8,858	8.36%
Maryland	206	2.72	3,008	3.97%	6,136	8.10%
North Carolina	261	2.67	5,428	5.56%	7,823	8.02%
South Carolina	195	3.54	5,506	9.99%	4,935	8.95%
Virginia	259	2.78	3,897	4.18%	6,549	7.03%
West Virginia	47	2.15	1,257	5.75%	1,389	6.36%
EAST SOUTH CENTRAL	**719**	**3.20**	**11,683**	**5.20%**	**17,511**	**7.80%**
Alabama	221	3.64	3,823	6.29%	4,866	8.01%
Kentucky	138	2.70	2,525	4.95%	3,421	6.70%
Mississippi	145	3.45	1,698	4.04%	3,668	8.72%
Tennessee	215	3.04	3,637	5.14%	5,556	7.86%
EAST NORTH CENTRAL	**1,675**	**2.63**	**26,822**	**4.21%**	**44,223**	**6.94%**
Illinois	536	2.90	9,452	5.11%	13,793	7.46%
Indiana	195	2.39	3,909	4.79%	5,365	6.57%
Michigan	387	2.77	5,115	3.66%	10,192	7.29%
Ohio	420	2.62	5,989	3.73%	11,017	6.86%
Wisconsin	137	1.93	2,357	3.33%	3,856	5.45%
WEST SOUTH CENTRAL	**1,228**	**2.67**	**44,301**	**9.64%**	**33,203**	**7.22%**
Arkansas	115	3.28	2,447	6.98%	2,870	8.19%
Louisiana	216	2.92	5,080	6.87%	6,504	8.80%
Oklahoma	121	2.55	2,728	5.75%	3,102	6.54%
Texas	776	2.56	34,046	11.22%	20,727	6.83%
WEST NORTH CENTRAL	**578**	**2.18**	**10,068**	**3.79%**	**15,321**	**5.77%**
Iowa	77	2.02	952	2.50%	2,072	5.44%
Kansas	65	1.68	1,438	3.71%	2,379	6.13%
Minnesota	112	1.68	2,641	3.96%	3,322	4.98%
Missouri	202	2.64	3,337	4.36%	5,221	6.83%
Nebraska	59	2.47	774	3.24%	1,319	5.52%
North Dakota	34	3.37	281	2.78%	485	4.80%
South Dakota	29	2.59	645	5.76%	523	4.67%
MOUNTAIN	**534**	**2.28**	**17,793**	**7.58%**	**15,638**	**6.66%**
Arizona	168	2.56	6,521	9.94%	4,088	6.23%
Colorado	138	2.59	2,824	5.29%	4,186	7.84%
Idaho	30	1.91	845	5.37%	808	5.13%
Montana	27	2.31	587	5.02%	696	5.95%
Nevada	19	1.06	1,684	9.35%	1,358	7.54%
New Mexico	76	2.81	4,030	14.92%	1,950	7.22%
Utah	62	1.72	973	2.70%	2,048	5.68%
Wyoming	14	1.95	329	4.59%	504	7.04%
PACIFIC	**1,778**	**2.63**	**39,685**	**5.87%**	**39,775**	**5.88%**
Alaska	25	2.23	445	3.96%	558	4.97%
California	1,472	2.76	32,238	6.05%	32,001	6.00%
Hawaii	44	2.31	960	5.04%	1,311	6.88%
Oregon	90	2.25	2,546	6.36%	2,101	5.25%
Washington	147	2.03	3,496	4.82%	3,804	5.25%
UNITED STATES	**10,459**	**2.68**	**229,942**	**5.88%**	**270,681**	**6.92%**

Sources: Cols.1 and 2--National Center for Health Statistics, 1988, "Vital Statistics of the United States: Volume II Mortality";
Cols.3-6--National Center for Health Statistics, 1988, "Vital Statistics of the United States: Volume I Natality".

TABLE E3
BIRTHS TO UNMARRIED WOMEN: TOTALS AND RATIOS BY RACE, 1988

	Total Births to Unmarried Women	Percentage of Total Births to Unmarried Women	White Births to Unmarried Women	Percentage of White Births to Unmarried Women	Black Births to Unmarried Women	Percentage of Black Births to Unmarried Women
NEW ENGLAND	**41,783**	**21.63%**	**30530**	**17.90%**	**9908**	**59.81%**
Connecticut	11,460	23.84%	6933	17.09%	4297	65.94%
Maine	3,489	20.32%	3404	20.28%	24	20.00%
Massachuetts	19,559	22.18%	13928	18.36%	4850	56.50%
New Hampshire	2,503	14.41%	2357	14.00%	41	27.52%
Rhode Island	3,262	22.93%	2427	19.38%	683	58.73%
Vermont	1,510	18.62%	1481	18.51%	13	38.24%
MIDDLE ATLANTIC	**156,880**	**27.81%**	**79582**	**18.47%**	**75151**	**66.39%**
New Jersey	28,580	24.27%	13177	14.70%	15073	63.44%
New York	84,381	30.07%	42330	20.72%	40605	63.89%
Pennsylvania	43,919	26.51%	24075	17.57%	19473	75.24%
SOUTH ATLANTIC	**187,675**	**28.68%**	**66586**	**14.84%**	**118504**	**62.08%**
Delaware	2,819	27.09%	1213	15.50%	1599	66.24%
District of Columbia	6,507	61.74%	227	13.67%	5973	73.15%
Florida	52,867	28.71%	23614	17.30%	28850	64.53%
Georgia	31,348	29.60%	7926	11.93%	23283	61.51%
Maryland	24,716	32.62%	8589	17.56%	15469	65.00%
North Carolina	25,622	26.26%	7682	11.65%	17193	59.53%
South Carolina	16,722	30.34%	4088	12.35%	12575	58.49%
Virginia	22,126	23.76%	8883	13.17%	12986	57.32%
West Virginia	4,948	22.65%	4364	20.98%	576	62.20%
EAST SOUTH CENTRAL	**63,475**	**28.26%**	**22311**	**13.99%**	**40875**	**64.90%**
Alabama	16,934	27.88%	4150	10.58%	12744	60.72%
Kentucky	11,206	21.95%	7855	17.26%	3315	64.75%
Mississippi	15,824	37.61%	2483	11.44%	13195	66.47%
Tennessee	19,511	27.59%	7823	14.74%	11621	68.25%
EAST NORTH CENTRAL	**161,150**	**25.28%**	**81930**	**15.92%**	**77576**	**70.77%**
Illinois	54,436	29.45%	22421	16.30%	31561	75.25%
Indiana	18,543	22.71%	11907	16.70%	6532	69.11%
Michigan	30,195	21.61%	13804	12.43%	16166	62.03%
Ohio	42,448	26.44%	23981	18.01%	18222	71.45%
Wisconsin	15,528	21.93%	9817	15.91%	5095	76.54%
WEST SOUTH CENTRAL	**104,265**	**22.68%**	**51554**	**14.46%**	**50475**	**57.74%**
Arkansas	9,273	26.47%	3745	14.28%	5476	65.68%
Louisiana	24,572	33.25%	5470	12.91%	19074	63.55%
Oklahoma	10,600	22.36%	5777	16.11%	3133	60.00%
Texas	59,820	19.72%	36562	14.50%	22792	51.99%
WEST NORTH CENTRAL	**53,365**	**20.11%**	**34718**	**14.88%**	**14869**	**67.82%**
Iowa	6,736	17.67%	5798	15.97%	800	69.14%
Kansas	7,025	18.11%	4714	13.89%	2084	57.46%
Minnesota	12,235	18.33%	8977	14.87%	1883	67.98%
Missouri	19,124	25.00%	9926	15.83%	9079	71.54%
Nebraska	4,333	18.12%	3053	14.01%	977	68.27%
North Dakota	1,578	15.62%	1038	11.55%	23	16.79%
South Dakota	2,334	20.85%	1212	13.21%	23	20.54%
MOUNTAIN	**51,485**	**21.94%**	**38360**	**18.68%**	**4762**	**50.05%**
Arizona	18,815	28.67%	13302	24.31%	1670	54.38%
Colorado	10,431	19.55%	8691	17.99%	1436	45.41%
Idaho	2,216	14.08%	2062	13.65%	18	22.50%
Montana	2,430	20.78%	1443	14.63%	29	37.18%
Nevada	3,432	19.06%	2184	14.83%	1089	55.08%
New Mexico	8,711	32.25%	5937	27.04%	324	45.96%
Utah	4,221	11.71%	3668	10.80%	152	47.20%
Wyoming	1,229	17.16%	1073	16.08%	44	36.97%
PACIFIC	**185,041**	**27.37%**	**134125**	**25.48%**	**34545**	**57.70%**
Alaska	2,627	23.39%	1016	13.99%	183	28.46%
California	152,607	28.62%	111706	26.90%	31804	59.29%
Hawaii	4,222	22.17%	592	12.92%	137	15.34%
Oregon	9,435	23.56%	8238	22.42%	679	62.24%
Washington	16,150	22.27%	12573	20.09%	1742	48.34%
UNITED STATES	**1,005,119**	**25.71%**	**539696**	**17.72%**	**426665**	**63.49%**

Source: National Center for Health Statistics, 1988, "Vital Statistics of the United States: Volume I Natality".

TABLE E4
TOTAL BIRTHS AND DEATHS, 1988

	Births (000s)	Birthrate per 1000 Population	Deaths (000s)	Death Rate per 1000 Population
NEW ENGLAND	**193**	**14.9**	**120**	**9.2**
Connecticut	48	14.9	29	8.8
Maine	17	14.3	12	9.6
Massachuetts	88	15.0	56	9.6
New Hampshire	17	16.0	9	8.1
Rhode Island	14	14.3	10	9.8
Vermont	8	14.6	5	8.8
MIDDLE ATLANTIC	**564**	**15.0**	**376**	**10.0**
New Jersey	118	15.3	73	9.5
New York	281	15.7	176	9.8
Pennsylvania	166	13.8	126	10.5
SOUTH ATLANTIC	**654**	**15.4**	**389**	**9.2**
Delaware	10	15.8	6	8.7
District of Columbia	11	17.1	8	12.4
Florida	184	14.9	131	10.6
Georgia	106	16.7	52	8.1
Maryland	76	16.4	39	8.4
North Carolina	98	15.0	58	8.9
South Carolina	55	15.9	29	8.5
Virginia	93	15.5	48	7.9
West Virginia	22	11.6	20	10.6
EAST SOUTH CENTRAL	**225**	**14.6**	**145**	**9.5**
Alabama	61	14.8	39	9.5
Kentucky	51	13.7	36	9.6
Mississippi	42	16.1	25	9.5
Tennessee	71	14.4	46	9.4
EAST NORTH CENTRAL	**638**	**15.1**	**379**	**9.0**
Illinois	185	15.9	105	9.1
Indiana	82	14.7	50	9.0
Michigan	140	15.1	80	8.7
Ohio	161	14.8	100	9.2
Wisconsin	71	14.6	43	8.9
WEST SOUTH CENTRAL	**460**	**17.1**	**215**	**8.0**
Arkansas	35	14.6	25	10.4
Louisiana	74	16.8	38	8.5
Oklahoma	47	14.6	30	9.3
Texas	303	18.0	123	7.3
WEST NORTH CENTRAL	**265**	**14.9**	**164**	**9.3**
Iowa	38	13.5	28	9.8
Kansas	39	15.5	23	9.2
Minnesota	67	15.5	35	8.2
Missouri	76	14.9	51	9.9
Nebraska	24	14.9	15	9.3
North Dakota	10	15.1	6	8.5
South Dakota	11	15.7	7	9.2
MOUNTAIN	**235**	**17.6**	**95**	**7.1**
Arizona	66	18.8	28	7.9
Colorado	53	16.2	21	6.5
Idaho	16	15.7	8	7.7
Montana	12	14.5	7	8.4
Nevada	18	17.1	8	8.0
New Mexico	27	17.9	10	6.9
Utah	36	21.3	9	5.5
Wyoming	7	15.0	3	6.8
PACIFIC	**676**	**18.1**	**285**	**7.6**
Alaska	11	21.4	2	3.9
California	533	18.8	215	7.6
Hawaii	19	17.3	6	5.5
Oregon	40	14.5	25	9.0
Washington	73	15.6	36	7.8
UNITED STATES	**3,910**	**15.9**	**2,168**	**8.8**

Sources: Cols.1 and 2--National Center for Health Statistics, 1988, "Vital Statistics of the United States: Volume I Natality"; Cols.3 and 4--National Center for Health Statistics, 1988, "Vital Statistics of the United States: Volume II Mortality".

TABLE E5
DEATH RATES: BY CAUSE, 1988
(per 100,000 population)

	Diseases of Heart	Malignant Neoplasms	Cerebrovascular Disease	Accidents and Adverse effects	Chronic Abstructive Pulmonary Disease	Pneumonia
NEW ENGLAND	**329.3**	**218.2**	**60.4**	**31.2**	**34.6**	**36.6**
Connecticut	318.8	211.9	53.9	30.7	29.3	34.1
Maine	330.4	226.6	64.5	39.5	46.1	29.5
Massachuetts	343.9	233.4	63.5	29.7	34.4	43.0
New Hampshire	278.3	195.2	56.2	27.6	33.5	28.2
Rhode Island	353.6	242.0	64.0	29.7	34.3	26.1
Vermont	289.4	183.3	56.9	41.8	45.2	33.4
MIDDLE ATLANTIC	**379.8**	**224.2**	**58.4**	**33.7**	**32.2**	**35.4**
New Jersey	356.1	223.5	54.9	31.5	29.3	31.1
New York	376.2	216.0	54.0	32.1	31.0	38.7
Pennsylvania	400.6	237.1	67.3	37.6	36.0	33.3
SOUTH ATLANTIC	**316.0**	**209.1**	**66.3**	**44.5**	**34.2**	**27.9**
Delaware	309.8	217.7	44.7	43.8	30.2	22.9
District of Columbia	355.9	263.9	64.5	39.1	23.5	44.7
Florida	380.4	253.0	71.5	43.7	43.1	27.3
Georgia	266.7	171.2	63.7	49.6	29.0	26.1
Maryland	276.2	201.0	51.3	33.3	30.4	27.9
North Carolina	299.4	195.8	73.6	49.5	32.3	29.7
South Carolina	293.9	177.1	74.7	55.9	27.4	21.5
Virginia	268.6	184.5	58.5	37.1	27.3	29.0
West Virginia	397.1	231.7	69.8	47.7	48.1	36.7
EAST SOUTH CENTRAL	**333.4**	**206.0**	**73.1**	**50.9**	**35.9**	**31.6**
Alabama	323.5	206.2	71.2	54.5	35.1	28.8
Kentucky	338.0	215.3	68.9	46.1	41.1	35.9
Mississippi	352.7	201.4	76.1	54.8	30.7	27.1
Tennessee	327.7	201.1	76.2	49.4	35.6	33.2
EAST NORTH CENTRAL	**333.5**	**203.2**	**62.3**	**36.2**	**33.6**	**31.3**
Illinois	340.8	202.3	59.9	37.9	30.4	33.1
Indiana	318.0	204.3	70.0	39.0	37.4	28.8
Michigan	327.2	193.8	56.8	35.1	31.4	29.1
Ohio	344.6	212.1	62.1	34.6	37.5	29.9
Wisconsin	320.7	202.1	69.8	34.8	32.7	37.1
WEST SOUTH CENTRAL	**274.6**	**171.6**	**56.5**	**41.5**	**27.2**	**26.7**
Arkansas	359.4	225.8	88.9	51.7	36.2	41.7
Louisiana	303.0	190.8	58.4	44.5	25.9	23.2
Oklahoma	339.6	197.3	71.1	44.2	37.2	36.0
Texas	242.5	153.8	48.5	38.8	24.3	23.7
WEST NORTH CENTRAL	**328.9**	**202.8**	**71.9**	**39.7**	**37.3**	**39.0**
Iowa	359.2	218.4	78.1	41.4	42.5	44.4
Kansas	322.8	199.6	71.3	40.2	40.4	38.1
Minnesota	276.5	188.2	69.9	34.7	30.1	35.7
Missouri	359.3	212.7	71.1	43.6	40.5	37.7
Nebraska	321.4	197.6	72.3	38.5	36.4	45.7
North Dakota	308.5	192.7	64.6	35.8	30.4	31.5
South Dakota	364.0	189.9	73.2	40.4	33.7	43.2
MOUNTAIN	**218.8**	**153.7**	**44.2**	**44.3**	**38.6**	**28.2**
Arizona	251.5	180.0	43.9	48.6	41.9	28.6
Colorado	196.2	134.9	40.1	34.4	39.3	29.8
Idaho	237.1	158.8	60.1	54.6	40.2	34.2
Montana	257.3	191.7	57.0	46.7	47.6	30.9
Nevada	258.3	193.3	39.5	42.7	52.8	25.0
New Mexico	189.8	144.7	42.0	56.7	31.3	24.3
Utah	175.3	101.1	40.8	35.0	22.1	24.3
Wyoming	191.9	145.7	48.9	53.2	41.1	31.1
PACIFIC	**247.5**	**171.0**	**57.1**	**38.3**	**34.8**	**31.7**
Alaska	88.7	85.7	16.4	74.4	13.5	8.8
California	249.5	168.5	56.5	37.4	34.2	33.0
Hawaii	167.3	139.3	39.2	28.7	17.5	17.9
Oregon	281.1	210.6	72.5	45.4	43.2	33.4
Washington	252.7	179.3	60.2	37.5	39.7	28.3
UNITED STATES	**311.3**	**197.3**	**61.2**	**39.5**	**33.7**	**31.6**

Source: National Center for Health Statistics, 1988, "Vital Statistics of the United States: Volume II Mortality".

TABLE E6
AIDS DEATHS AND CASES

	AIDS Deaths, 1988	AIDS Cases as Percent of Total U.S. AIDS Cases (1981-92)	U.S. AIDS Cases since 1981 per 100,000 Population
NEW ENGLAND	**606**	**3.90%**	**62**
Connecticut	199	1.21%	78
Maine	17	0.14%	23
Massachusetts	318	2.15%	76
New Hampshire	24	0.12%	23
Rhode Island	42	0.24%	50
Vermont	6	0.05%	17
MIDDLE ATLANTIC	**5615**	**30.01%**	**169**
New Jersey	1157	6.28%	172
New York	3990	20.90%	246
Pennsylvania	468	2.83%	50
SOUTH ATLANTIC	**2979**	**20.00%**	**97**
Delaware	26	0.20%	64
District of Columbia	247	1.70%	592
Florida	1449	9.85%	161
Georgia	401	2.86%	93
Maryland	248	2.07%	91
North Carolina	220	1.13%	36
South Carolina	115	0.71%	43
Virginia	257	1.37%	47
West Virginia	16	0.12%	14
EAST SOUTH CENTRAL	**317**	**2.19%**	**30**
Alabama	92	0.66%	34
Kentucky	46	0.34%	19
Mississippi	74	0.45%	37
Tennessee	105	0.74%	32
EAST NORTH CENTRAL	**1081**	**7.18%**	**36**
Illinois	459	3.17%	59
Indiana	113	0.71%	27
Michigan	217	1.39%	32
Ohio	233	1.49%	29
Wisconsin	59	0.43%	18
WEST SOUTH CENTRAL	**1544**	**9.58%**	**76**
Arkansas	53	0.33%	30
Louisiana	247	1.57%	78
Oklahoma	79	0.47%	32
Texas	1165	7.21%	90
WEST NORTH CENTRAL	**370**	**2.38%**	**29**
Iowa	24	0.16%	12
Kansas	55	0.30%	26
Minnesota	72	0.50%	24
Missouri	183	1.27%	52
Nebraska	28	0.12%	17
North Dakota	3	0.01%	4
South Dakota	5	0.01%	4
MOUNTIAN	**466**	**2.84%**	**44**
Arizona	151	0.78%	45
Colorado	167	1.02%	65
Idaho	11	0.06%	12
Montana	5	0.04%	11
Nevada	64	0.45%	78
New Mexico	31	0.23%	32
Utah	34	0.24%	29
Wyoming	3	0.03%	12
PACIFIC	**3552**	**21.93%**	**118**
Alaska	7	0.06%	23
California	3180	19.42%	138
Hawaii	61	0.41%	79
Oregon	99	0.64%	48
Washington	205	1.39%	60
UNITED STATES	**16530**	**100%**	**85**

Sources: Col.1--National Center for Health Statistics, 1988, "Vital Statistics of the United States:
Volume II Mortality"; Cols.2 and 3--Centers for Disease Control, 1992, "HIV/AIDS Surveillance".

TABLE E7

**ADULTS AGES 18-64: PERCENTAGE WITH HEALTH PROBLEM
OR DISABILITY THAT PREVENTS OR LIMITS WORKING**

	Number (000s)	Percent Disabled	Percent Not Disabled
UNITED STATES	150,318	7% (0.07)	93% (0.07)
NEW ENGLAND	8,163	6% (0.24)	94% (0.24)
Connecticut	2,022	4% (0.55)	96% (0.55)
Maine	747	8% (0.68)	92% (0.68)
Massachusetts	3,731	7% (0.32)	93% (0.32)
New Hampshire	701	6% (0.62)	94% (0.62)
Rhode Island	607	8% (0.70)	92% (0.70)
Vermont	355	6% (0.64)	94% (0.64)
MIDDLE ATLANTIC	23,262	6% (0.16)	94% (0.16)
New Jersey	4,855	4% (0.25)	96% (0.25)
New York	11,077	7% (0.25)	93% (0.25)
Pennsylvania	7,330	7% (0.31)	93% (0.31)
SOUTH ATLANTIC	25,967	7% (0.19)	93% (0.19)
Delaware	417	6% (0.62)	94% (0.62)
District of Columbia	369	7% (0.70)	93% (0.70)
Florida	7,518	7% (0.31)	93% (0.31)
Georgia	3,865	8% (0.66)	92% (0.66)
Maryland	2,936	7% (0.63)	93% (0.63)
North Carolina	3,998	7% (0.32)	93% (0.32)
South Carolina	2,087	8% (0.61)	92% (0.61)
Virginia	3,669	7% (0.55)	93% (0.55)
West Virginia	1,110	10% (0.73)	90% (0.73)
EAST SOUTH CENTRAL	9,213	10% (0.36)	90% (0.36)
Alabama	2,469	9% (0.70)	91% (0.70)
Kentucky	2,233	11% (0.76)	89% (0.76)
Mississippi	1,513	11% (0.72)	89% (0.72)
Tennessee	2,997	9% (0.65)	91% (0.65)
WEST SOUTH CENTRAL	15,962	7% (0.25)	93% (0.25)
Arkansas	1,410	9% (0.70)	91% (0.70)
Louisiana	2,528	9% (0.73)	91% (0.73)
Oklahoma	1,882	8% (0.67)	92% (0.67)
Texas	10,142	7% (0.31)	93% (0.31)

ADULTS AGES 18-64: PERCENTAGE WITH HEALTH PROBLEM
OR DISABILITY THAT PREVENTS OR LIMITS WORKING

	Number (000s)	Percent Disabled	Percent Not Disabled
EAST NORTH CENTRAL	**25,836**	**7%** **(0.18)**	**93%** **(0.18)**
Illinois	7,174	6% (0.31)	94% (0.31)
Indiana	3,391	6% (0.57)	94% (0.57)
Michigan	5,755	9% (0.36)	91% (0.36)
Ohio	6,617	7% (0.33)	93% (0.33)
Wisconsin	2,898	6% (0.55)	94% (0.55)
WEST NORTH CENTRAL	**10,548**	**7%** **(0.28)**	**93%** **(0.28)**
Iowa	1,655	6% (0.58)	94% (0.58)
Kansas	1,444	6% (0.56)	94% (0.56)
Minnesota	2,657	7% (0.62)	93% (0.62)
Missouri	3,100	7% (0.66)	93% (0.66)
Nebraska	927	6% (0.55)	94% (0.55)
North Dakota	366	7% (0.60)	93% (0.60)
South Dakota	399	7% (0.56)	93% (0.56)
MOUNTAIN	**7,871**	**7%** **(0.27)**	**93%** **(0.27)**
Arizona	2,078	7% (0.62)	93% (0.62)
Colorado	1,938	6% (0.63)	94% (0.63)
Idaho	582	8% (0.65)	92% (0.65)
Montana	480	9% (0.68)	91% (0.68)
Nevada	725	5% (0.56)	95% (0.56)
New Mexico	878	8% (0.65)	92% (0.65)
Utah	909	5% (0.55)	95% (0.55)
Wyoming	281	8% (0.74)	92% (0.74)
PACIFIC	**23,495**	**7%** **(0.22)**	**93%** **(0.22)**
Alaska	295	6% (0.55)	94% (0.55)
California	17,870	7% (0.25)	93% (0.25)
Hawaii	626	5% (0.56)	95% (0.56)
Oregon	1,714	9% (0.74)	91% (0.74)
Washington	2,990	8% (0.64)	92% (0.64)

Source: Three-year merged March CPS, 1989, 1990, and 1991.

Notes for tables E1–E7

E1   Rate per 1,000 births is the number of total infant deaths under one year of age per 1,000 live births. Rate per 1,000 white births is the number of white infant deaths under one year of age per 1,000 white births. Rate per 1,000 black births is the number of total black infant deaths under one year of age per 1,000 black births.

E2   Rate per 1,000 births ages 1–27 days is the number of total neonatal deaths (ages 1–27 days) per 1,000 total births.

Late or no prenatal care is defined as pregnant women who did not receive any prenatal care before their seventh month of pregnancy, as well as those who reported receiving no prenatal care throughout the pregnancy. "Percentage with Late or No Prenatal Care" is a percentage of all births.

On average, 2.5 percent of the mothers did not state the month in which they received prenatal care. The percentage reported is out of all births, including those with missing answers.

Low-weight births are defined as infants that weigh under 2,500 grams at birth.

E3   Percentage of total births to unmarried women is the number of total births to unmarried women divided by the number of total births.

Percentage of white births to unmarried women is the number of white births to unmarried women divided by the number of white births.

Percentage of black births to unmarried women is the number of black births to unmarried women divided by the number of black births.

E4   Death rates per 1,000 are the total number of deaths per 1,000 total population count.

Birthrates per 1,000 are the total number of births per 1,000 total population count.

E5   Death rates are the total number of deaths for a given cause per 1,000 total population count.

E6   AIDS cases per state are reported as percentage of total U.S. cases spanning the 11-year period from 1981 to 1992. This is calculated by dividing the number of AIDS cases in this period for a particular state by the total cases nationwide for the same period.

E7   Individuals included are those who reported that they have a disability that prevents work or limits their ability to work. Children with a disability are not included. These numbers do not necessarily reflect the handicapped population where disability is based on a medical standard.

Health Care Costs, Access, and Utilization

This section provides a set of broad-based indicators of health care costs, access, and utilization. The tables include information about hospital and physician costs, hospital utilization, and numbers of nursing homes, physicians, and health maintenance organizations (HMOs).

HOSPITAL AND PHYSICIAN COSTS

Table F1 provides, first of all, information on short-term general hospital costs per patient day, per admission, and per capita. These data reflect variations across states in cost of hospital care. The data generally show that costs per admission are highest in the Middle Atlantic and Pacific regions and lowest in the East South Central region.

The next three columns provide data on variations in the costs of physician practices, private physician fees, and the Medicaid hospital payment index. The geographic practice cost index reflects variations in all the input costs to a physician's practice. The index, developed by the Urban Institute and the Center for Health Economics Research, includes measures of professional earnings, employee wages, office rents, and malpractice premiums. A variant of this index is used in the new Medicare Fee Schedule. The costs of physicians' practices are also highest in the

Middle Atlantic and Pacific regions. The Normalized Private Fee Index indicates how private physician fees vary across geographic areas. Any physician payment reform policy would have to consider both variations in cost as well as in current charges.

The last column shows the Medicaid hospital payment index, which is defined as Medicaid hospital payments multiplied by the ratio of hospital costs to charges. The higher the index, the more Medicaid payments are compensating hospitals for the costs of serving Medicaid patients.

HOSPITALS AND NURSING HOMES

Table F2 provides data on hospital utilization. The table includes data on hospital beds as well as admissions and lengths of stay. The number of hospital beds per 1,000 population is highest in the East South Central region and lowest in the Pacific region, 4.8 compared to 2.7, respectively. The rate of hospital admissions is also highest in the East South Central states (about 160 per 1,000 population) and lowest in the Pacific region (about 107 per 1,000 population). Length of stays, measured by inpatient days per admission, are longest in the Middle Atlantic region (8.5 days) and shortest in the Mountain states (5.5 days) on average.

Table F3 provides data on the availability of nursing home beds per capita. It also provides the proportion of nursing home beds that are proprietary, public, or nonprofit. There is high variation across states in the ratio of nursing home beds per 1,000 elderly, from 2.2 beds in Alaska to 13.1 beds in Nebraska. Ownership also varies, with more than 70 percent of the beds in homes owned by for-profit firms in the majority of states. However, public and nonprofit facilities account for over one-third of the beds in 21 states.

PHYSICIANS AND HMOs

Table F4 provides data on physician availability across states. Both the total number of physicians per 100,000 population as well as patient-care physicians per 100,000 population are provided.

The availability of physicians tends to be greatest in New England and the Middle Atlantic states and lowest in many of the southern and Mountain states.

Table F5 provides data on the number of HMOs as well as HMO membership per 1,000 population. The importance of HMOs varies considerably across the country. HMOs have become particularly important in California, Minnesota and Massachusetts, whereas penetration in most of the southern states is minimal.

TABLE F1
RELATIVE HOSPITAL AND PHYSICIAN COSTS, 1990

	Short-term General Hospital Cost per Patient Day	Short-term General Hospital Cost per Admission	Short-term General Hospital Cost per Capita	Geographic Practice Cost Index	Normalized Private Fee Index	Medicaid Hospital Payment Index
NEW ENGLAND	**$765**	**$5,507**	**$669**	**1.004**	**1.06**	**0.828**
Connecticut	$832	$6,201	$682	1.071	1.05	0.711
Maine	$658	$4,486	$533	0.845	0.92	0.850
Massachusetts	$775	$5,647	$743	1.037	1.11	0.871
New Hampshire	$757	$4,488	$508	0.900	0.95	0.846
Rhode Island	$657	$5,073	$601	1.003	1.19	0.946
Vermont	$658	$4,340	$469	0.825	0.95	0.755
MIDDLE ATLANTIC	**$680**	**$5,507**	**$759**	**1.104**	**1.16**	**0.848**
New Jersey	$614	$4,511	$667	1.126	1.12	1.048
New York	$696	$6,503	$831	1.163	1.24	0.889
Pennsylvania	$705	$5,064	$743	1.000	1.06	0.656
SOUTH ATLANTIC	**$737**	**$4,819**	**$640**	**0.938**	**0.98**	**0.821**
Delaware	$741	$4,809	$623	1.044	0.93	0.808
District of Columbia	$915	$7,804	$2,210	1.191	1.11	0.695
Florida	$800	$5,341	$699	0.969	0.99	0.826
Georgia	$736	$4,333	$620	0.876	0.94	0.861
Maryland	$691	$4,616	$575	1.097	1.07	1.063
North Carolina	$669	$4,632	$578	0.846	0.96	0.617
South Carolina	$682	$4,324	$553	0.854	0.90	0.835
Virginia	$724	$4,551	$554	0.945	1.00	0.795
West Virginia	$650	$4,142	$670	0.878	0.98	0.848
EAST SOUTH CENTRAL	**$639**	**$3,933**	**$629**	**0.869**	**0.86**	**0.899**
Alabama	$691	$4,357	$662	0.886	0.89	0.731
Kentucky	$612	$3,783	$576	0.884	0.86	0.937
Mississippi	$519	$3,138	$533	0.839	0.82	1.041
Tennessee	$686	$4,180	$698	0.858	0.86	0.935
EAST NORTH CENTRAL	**$760**	**$4,918**	**$635**	**1.015**	**0.96**	**0.805**
Illinois	$799	$5,340	$716	1.083	1.04	0.568
Indiana	$703	$4,480	$589	0.917	0.90	0.951
Michigan	$804	$5,400	$626	1.106	0.90	0.862
Ohio	$747	$4,723	$648	0.954	0.96	0.944
Wisconsin	$683	$4,156	$506	0.934	0.91	0.776
WEST SOUTH CENTRAL	**$726**	**$4,424**	**$572**	**0.899**	**0.95**	**0.823**
Arkansas	$568	$3,552	$543	0.817	0.88	0.720
Louisiana	$748	$4,755	$694	0.930	0.96	0.884
Oklahoma	$680	$4,336	$574	0.871	0.84	0.833
Texas	$758	$4,508	$547	0.907	0.98	0.821
WEST NORTH CENTRAL	**$735**	**$4,743**	**$641**	**0.907**	**0.87**	**0.813**
Iowa	$624	$4,511	$631	0.888	0.86	0.881
Kansas	$675	$4,361	$564	0.879	0.85	0.870
Minnesota	$841	$4,975	$599	0.971	0.91	0.880
Missouri	$781	$5,198	$751	0.915	0.87	0.683
Nebraska	$678	$4,319	$535	0.835	0.75	0.734
North Dakota	$699	$4,408	$722	0.864	0.99	0.959
South Dakota	$680	$4,249	$686	0.818	0.92	0.911
MOUNTAIN	**$892**	**$4,560**	**$513**	**0.969**	**0.93**	**0.793**
Arizona	$943	$4,781	$569	0.996	1.00	0.988
Colorado	$915	$4,887	$530	0.976	0.88	0.564
Idaho	$803	$3,762	$374	0.893	0.85	0.821
Montana	$768	$4,067	$573	0.883	0.84	0.906
Nevada	$908	$5,598	$563	1.092	1.15	0.468
New Mexico	$897	$4,304	$518	0.916	0.96	0.962
Utah	$863	$3,930	$401	0.950	0.83	0.787
Wyoming	$785	$3,995	$451	0.928	0.85	0.928
PACIFIC	**$972**	**$5,236**	**$557**	**1.133**	**1.07**	**0.688**
Alaska	$1,416	$7,179	$746	1.336	1.09	0.878
California	$993	$5,449	$580	1.167	1.10	0.667
Hawaii	$986	$6,444	$591	1.046	1.23	0.736
Oregon	$895	$4,272	$471	0.959	0.91	0.625
Washington	$873	$4,574	$495	1.026	0.92	0.818
UNITED STATES	**$749**	**$4,885**	**$628**	**1.000**	**1.00**	**0.805**

Sources: Cols.1-3 and 6--Urban Institute analysis of American Hospital Association's 1990 Annual Survey of Hospitals; Col.4--Stephen Zuckerman and Stephen Norton, 1991, "Refining the Malpractice Geographic Practice Cost Index, Urban Institute Working Paper 3839-02-03"; Col.5--Urban Institute analysis of Health Insurance Association of America's Prevailing Healthcare Charges System, Sept. 1990.

TABLE F2
HOSPITAL UTILIZATION, 1990

	Hospital Beds	Hospital Beds per 1000 Population	Hospital Admissions	Admissions per 1000 Population	Inpatient Days	Inpatient Days per Admission
NEW ENGLAND	**44,397**	**3.36**	**1,604,703**	**121.50**	**11,900,481**	**7.42**
Connecticut	9,888	3.01	361,527	109.98	2,781,101	7.69
Maine	4,029	3.28	145,785	118.72	1,007,487	6.91
Massachusetts	22,260	3.70	792,197	131.67	6,007,763	7.58
New Hampshire	3,211	2.89	125,487	113.13	756,285	6.03
Rhode Island	3,250	3.24	118,873	118.46	927,616	7.80
Vermont	1,759	3.13	60,834	108.10	420,229	6.91
MIDDLE ATLANTIC	**151,695**	**4.03**	**5,184,822**	**137.89**	**43,851,193**	**8.46**
New Jersey	30,352	3.93	1,142,747	147.83	8,811,548	7.71
New York	71,542	3.98	2,297,823	127.72	21,981,854	9.57
Pennsylvania	49,801	4.19	1,744,252	146.80	13,057,791	7.49
SOUTH ATLANTIC	**162,090**	**3.72**	**5,789,791**	**132.89**	**39,318,066**	**6.79**
Delaware	2,090	3.14	86,277	129.51	587,451	6.81
District of Columbia	5,469	9.01	171,895	283.23	1,518,323	8.83
Florida	52,075	4.02	1,692,026	130.78	11,668,045	6.90
Georgia	25,564	3.95	927,297	143.14	5,866,677	6.33
Maryland	14,196	2.97	595,550	124.55	4,021,000	6.75
North Carolina	22,211	3.35	827,577	124.85	5,806,785	7.02
South Carolina	11,462	3.29	446,103	127.94	2,911,368	6.53
Virginia	20,508	3.31	752,833	121.67	5,021,074	6.67
West Virginia	8,515	4.75	290,233	161.83	1,917,343	6.61
EAST SOUTH CENTRAL	**72,630**	**4.79**	**2,426,583**	**159.89**	**16,214,731**	**6.68**
Alabama	18,432	4.56	613,962	151.95	4,099,414	6.68
Kentucky	16,162	4.39	561,227	152.29	3,640,616	6.49
Mississippi	13,696	5.32	437,206	169.91	2,868,433	6.56
Tennessee	24,340	4.99	814,188	166.94	5,606,268	6.89
EAST NORTH CENTRAL	**158,462**	**3.77**	**5,422,608**	**129.08**	**36,692,745**	**6.77**
Illinois	46,202	4.04	1,531,996	134.03	10,914,331	7.12
Indiana	21,373	3.86	729,242	131.53	4,696,443	6.44
Michigan	31,925	3.43	1,077,367	115.90	7,407,317	6.88
Ohio	42,051	3.88	1,488,287	137.21	9,908,968	6.66
Wisconsin	16,911	3.46	595,716	121.78	3,765,686	6.32
WEST SOUTH CENTRAL	**104,285**	**3.91**	**3,451,419**	**129.25**	**22,187,628**	**6.43**
Arkansas	10,903	4.64	359,040	152.74	2,432,788	6.78
Louisiana	18,820	4.46	615,888	145.95	3,981,615	6.46
Oklahoma	12,952	4.12	416,152	132.30	2,729,474	6.56
Texas	61,610	3.63	2,060,339	121.29	13,043,751	6.33
WEST NORTH CENTRAL	**78,166**	**4.43**	**2,387,748**	**135.21**	**16,298,350**	**6.83**
Iowa	12,913	4.65	388,170	139.79	2,670,582	6.88
Kansas	11,799	4.76	320,556	129.38	2,314,316	7.22
Minnesota	15,130	3.46	526,957	120.44	3,236,731	6.14
Missouri	23,674	4.63	739,609	144.54	5,234,704	7.08
Nebraska	7,219	4.57	195,520	123.87	1,371,955	7.02
North Dakota	3,460	5.42	104,572	163.70	696,365	6.66
South Dakota	3,971	5.71	112,364	161.44	773,697	6.89
MOUNTAIN	**40,783**	**2.99**	**1,536,357**	**112.48**	**8,481,390**	**5.52**
Arizona	10,757	2.93	435,946	118.94	2,396,860	5.50
Colorado	9,522	2.89	357,391	108.48	2,085,055	5.83
Idaho	2,734	2.72	100,050	99.38	489,517	4.89
Montana	3,524	4.41	112,609	140.93	653,479	5.80
Nevada	3,489	2.90	120,901	100.60	752,721	6.23
New Mexico	4,664	3.08	182,453	120.43	940,094	5.15
Utah	4,338	2.52	175,764	102.02	893,370	5.08
Wyoming	1,755	3.87	51,243	112.97	270,294	5.27
PACIFIC	**106,265**	**2.72**	**4,166,026**	**106.47**	**24,215,214**	**5.81**
Alaska	1,569	2.85	57,190	103.97	275,384	4.82
California	81,118	2.73	3,167,156	106.42	18,661,188	5.89
Hawaii	2,500	2.26	101,570	91.65	736,575	7.25
Oregon	8,111	2.85	313,495	110.30	1,647,911	5.26
Washington	12,967	2.66	526,615	108.21	2,894,156	5.50
UNITED STATES	**918,773**	**3.69**	**31,970,057**	**128.54**	**219,159,798**	**6.86**

Source: Urban Institute analysis of American Hospital Association's 1990 Annual Survey of Hospitals.

TABLE F3
NURSING HOME BED DISTRIBUTION, 1986

	Total Nursing Home Beds	Nursing Home Beds per 1000 Population	Percent Proprietary	Percent Government	Percent Nonprofit
NEW ENGLAND	**119,604**	**9.06**	**77%**	**5%**	**18%**
Connecticut	29,709	9.04	80%	3%	17%
Maine	11,860	9.66	77%	4%	20%
Massachusetts	54,621	9.08	78%	4%	18%
New Hampshire	8,567	7.72	52%	27%	22%
Rhode Island	10,339	10.30	80%	3%	17%
Vermont	4,508	8.01	76%	3%	21%
MIDDLE ATLANTIC	**271,835**	**7.23**	**54%**	**14%**	**32%**
New Jersey	44,937	5.81	66%	12%	22%
New York	125,715	6.99	54%	11%	35%
Pennsylvania	101,183	8.52	49%	17%	34%
SOUTH ATLANTIC	**236,852**	**5.44**	**75%**	**5%**	**20%**
Delaware	4,165	6.25	53%	21%	26%
District of Columbia	3,033	5.00	39%	32%	29%
Florida	70,487	5.45	78%	2%	20%
Georgia	35,209	5.43	83%	5%	12%
Maryland	25,714	5.38	66%	5%	29%
North Carolina	38,984	5.88	81%	2%	17%
South Carolina	16,020	4.59	73%	12%	14%
Virginia	33,421	5.40	71%	5%	24%
West Virginia	9,819	5.47	71%	6%	23%
EAST SOUTH CENTRAL	**96,893**	**6.38**	**75%**	**9%**	**16%**
Alabama	23,559	5.83	84%	6%	10%
Kentucky	28,294	7.68	74%	2%	24%
Mississippi	14,123	5.49	80%	12%	8%
Tennessee	30,917	6.34	68%	16%	16%
EAST NORTH CENTRAL	**355,547**	**8.46**	**67%**	**10%**	**23%**
Illinois	99,375	8.69	67%	7%	26%
Indiana	48,480	8.74	76%	6%	18%
Michigan	67,994	7.31	70%	10%	20%
Ohio	85,733	7.90	72%	7%	21%
Wisconsin	53,965	11.03	45%	24%	31%
WEST SOUTH CENTRAL	**196,548**	**7.36**	**87%**	**2%**	**11%**
Arkansas	22,678	9.65	85%	6%	8%
Louisiana	35,674	8.45	86%	4%	10%
Oklahoma	31,445	10.00	86%	3%	11%
Texas	106,751	6.28	87%	1%	12%
WEST NORTH CENTRAL	**203,214**	**11.51**	**56%**	**8%**	**36%**
Iowa	36,563	13.17	62%	6%	31%
Kansas	26,544	10.71	64%	7%	29%
Minnesota	48,526	11.09	44%	13%	43%
Missouri	54,429	10.64	70%	4%	26%
Nebraska	20,681	13.10	44%	17%	38%
North Dakota	8,192	12.82	20%	3%	77%
South Dakota	8,279	11.90	42%	2%	56%
MOUNTAIN	**64,900**	**4.75**	**68%**	**8%**	**24%**
Arizona	13,410	3.66	70%	5%	26%
Colorado	20,432	6.20	70%	4%	26%
Idaho	6,235	6.19	70%	15%	14%
Montana	6,114	7.65	46%	22%	32%
Nevada	3,329	2.77	92%	3%	5%
New Mexico	6,093	4.02	56%	10%	34%
Utah	6,736	3.91	88%	5%	7%
Wyoming	2,551	5.62	38%	25%	37%
PACIFIC	**224,813**	**5.75**	**82%**	**3%**	**15%**
Alaska	1,203	2.19	0%	57%	43%
California	168,149	5.65	85%	2%	13%
Hawaii	3,617	3.26	55%	18%	27%
Oregon	18,390	6.47	78%	2%	20%
Washington	33,454	6.87	76%	2%	22%
UNITED STATES	**1,770,206**	**7.12**	**70%**	**7%**	**23%**

Source: National Center for Health Statistics, 1986 Inventory of Long-Term Care Plans.

TABLE F4
TOTAL AND PATIENT CARE PHYSICIANS, 1989

	Total Physicians	Total Physicians per 100,000 Population	Patient Care Physicians	Patient Care Physicians per 100,000 Population
NEW ENGLAND	**37,273**	**293**	**32,384**	**254**
Connecticut	9,643	309	8,468	271
Maine	2,147	176	1,995	163
Massachusetts	19,517	336	16,547	285
New Hampshire	2,101	193	1,953	179
Rhode Island	2,468	260	2,193	231
Vermont	1,397	251	1,228	221
MIDDLE ATLANTIC	**102,016**	**272**	**90,736**	**242**
New Jersey	18,515	243	16,765	220
New York	55,730	312	48,886	274
Pennsylvania	27,771	230	25,085	207
SOUTH ATLANTIC	**88,861**	**215**	**79,815**	**193**
Delaware	1,271	195	1,168	179
District of Columbia	3,651	651	2,943	525
Florida	25,376	204	23,435	188
Georgia	10,765	175	9,960	162
Maryland	15,167	340	12,560	282
North Carolina	11,847	191	10,700	173
South Carolina	5,446	162	5,059	150
Virginia	12,222	212	11,105	192
West Virginia	3,116	173	2,885	160
EAST SOUTH CENTRAL	**25,173**	**169**	**23,432**	**157**
Alabama	6,356	157	5,877	145
Kentucky	6,105	174	5,721	163
Mississippi	3,352	132	3,182	125
Tennessee	9,360	194	8,652	180
EAST NORTH CENTRAL	**80,053**	**192**	**73,157**	**176**
Illinois	24,576	214	22,263	194
Indiana	8,580	159	7,964	147
Michigan	16,836	181	15,336	165
Ohio	21,066	196	19,273	180
Wisconsin	8,995	192	8,321	178
WEST SOUTH CENTRAL	**45,259**	**173**	**41,590**	**159**
Arkansas	3,492	146	3,282	137
Louisiana	8,198	201	7,565	185
Oklahoma	4,696	151	4,361	140
Texas	28,873	174	26,382	159
WEST NORTH CENTRAL	**32,623**	**186**	**29,859**	**170**
Iowa	4,218	149	3,826	135
Kansas	4,312	180	4,010	167
Minnesota	9,344	219	8,560	200
Missouri	9,941	191	8,975	173
Nebraska	2,715	176	2,512	163
North Dakota	1,102	179	1,044	170
South Dakota	991	144	932	135
MOUNTAIN	**24,023**	**182**	**22,155**	**168**
Arizona	6,759	195	6,257	180
Colorado	6,763	212	6,141	193
Idaho	1,218	120	1,173	116
Montana	1,244	154	1,194	148
Nevada	1,657	150	1,556	141
New Mexico	2,665	179	2,425	163
Utah	3,047	182	2,776	165
Wyoming	670	148	633	140
PACIFIC	**86,857**	**229**	**78,351**	**207**
Alaska	710	157	660	146
California	68,519	237	61,596	213
Hawaii	2,394	246	2,216	228
Oregon	5,564	191	5,151	177
Washington	9,670	210	8,728	189
UNITED STATES	**522,138**	**215**	**471,479**	**194**

Source: American Medical Association, Master File 1990.

TABLE F5
NUMBER OF HMOs AND HMO MEMBERSHIP, 1990

	HMOs	HMO Membership	HMO Membership per 1000
NEW ENGLAND	**41**	**2,621,802**	**198.52**
Connecticut	12	654,629	199.15
Maine	3	32,048	26.10
Massachusetts	19	1,569,364	260.85
New Hampshire	2	106,742	96.23
Rhode Island	4	222,449	221.68
Vermont	1	36,570	64.98
MIDDLE ATLANTIC	**72**	**5,130,702**	**136.45**
New Jersey	14	948,642	122.72
New York	37	2,774,167	154.20
Pennsylvania	21	1,407,893	118.49
SOUTH ATLANTIC	**88**	**3,911,441**	**89.78**
Delaware	6	121,218	181.96
District of Columbia	4	486,039	800.86
Florida	29	1,395,856	107.89
Georgia	8	327,918	50.62
Maryland	11	731,597	153.01
North Carolina	12	320,111	48.29
South Carolina	4	71,005	20.36
Virginia	13	385,402	62.29
West Virginia	1	72,295	40.31
EAST SOUTH CENTRAL	**24**	**711,274**	**46.87**
Alabama	8	217,179	53.75
Kentucky	7	299,112	81.16
Mississippi	0	0	0
Tennessee	9	194,983	39.98
EAST NORTH CENTRAL	**117**	**5,774,447**	**137.46**
Illinois	26	1,472,455	128.82
Indiana	12	339,026	61.15
Michigan	17	1,435,284	154.41
Ohio	34	1,461,580	134.74
Wisconsin	28	1,066,102	217.94
WEST SOUTH CENTRAL	**45**	**1,754,315**	**65.70**
Arkansas	4	54,464	23.17
Louisiana	9	243,469	57.69
Oklahoma	6	176,159	56.00
Texas	26	1,280,223	75.37
WEST NORTH CENTRAL	**51**	**2,266,356**	**128.33**
Iowa	7	286,365	103.13
Kansas	8	199,963	80.71
Minnesota	11	1,094,014	250.05
Missouri	17	564,155	110.25
Nebraska	5	87,166	55.22
North Dakota	2	11,010	17.24
South Dakota	1	23,683	34.03
MOUNTAIN	**47**	**1,840,544**	**134.75**
Arizona	13	580,899	158.49
Colorado	18	678,749	206.03
Idaho	1	17,804	17.68
Montana	1	5,200	6.51
Nevada	3	101,274	84.27
New Mexico	5	195,058	128.75
Utah	6	261,560	151.82
Wyoming	0	0	0
PACIFIC	**68**	**10,591,994**	**270.71**
Alaska	0	0	0
California	46	8,945,358	300.58
Hawaii	5	240,477	216.99
Oregon	9	709,133	249.49
Washington	8	697,026	143.22
UNITED STATES	**553**	**37,653,870**	**151.40**

Source: 1990 Health Maintenance Organization Census.

Notes for tables F1–F5

F1   Short-term general hospital (STGH) cost per patient day is total payroll and nonpayroll expenses divided by total adjusted patient days. Only hospitals without long-term care units are included in totals. Total adjusted patient days reflect inpatient days as well as outpatient visits.

    Short-term general hospital cost per admission is total payroll and nonpayroll expenses divided by total adjusted admissions. Only hospitals without long-term care units are included in totals. Total adjusted admissions reflect inpatient admissions as well as outpatient visits.

    The Geographic Practice Cost Index is an index of physician practice input prices developed by The Urban Institute.

    The Normalized Private Fee Index is a weighted average of private fees reported to the Health Insurance Association of America. The weighted averages are normalized to the U.S. average.

F2   Beds, admissions, and inpatient days are for all short-term general hospitals. Beds, admissions, and inpatient days associated with long-term care are omitted for hospitals that have long-term care units.

F4   Total physicians includes, in addition to practicing physicians, physicians who work as professors and administrators.

F5   HMO membership per 1,000 represents the portion of a state's population that is enrolled in an HMO. It is total HMO membership divided by the total population.

    HMO membership per 1,000 population in areas where a plan services multiple states may be misstated, since this measure is based on the state population in which the plan's headquarters is located. For example, the high membership rate for the District of Columbia reflects residents of neighboring states who are members of plans with headquarters in the District.

SECTION G

State Demographic and Economic Profiles

T he tables in this section provide background information on the demographic and economic characteristics of each state. The tables are broken down into five subsections encompassing general population characteristics, family income characteristics, worker characteristics, establishment characteristics, and state finances. Information in this section may also be used in conjunction with the tables in the health insurance coverage of specific groups of individuals in sections A and B.

POPULATION CHARACTERISTICS

T ables G1 through G3 show distributions for the nonelderly population by age (under 18, 18 to 34, 35 to 53, and 54 through 64), race and sex, and family type (married with no children, married with children, single with children, and single). This information is important because various health policy initiatives focus on these population subgroups.

FAMILY INCOME CHARACTERISTICS

Data on family income characteristics give states information about the distribution of family income in their state and allow comparisons with other states. Table G4 shows the upper limits for the 25th, median, and 75th income percentiles in each state. These data are derived by sorting families into four income groups, each of which includes one-quarter of the population. Thus, the income distribution for families in the United States is: lowest quarter, up to $14,000; second quarter, $14,000 to $28,167; third quarter, $28,167 to $47,229; and upper quarter, all families with incomes above $47,229. The median, $28,167, marks the income level that 50 percent of families earn more than and 50 percent of families earn less than.

These distributions indicate that the income ranges within quartiles of the population are uneven. That is, the range of income for the second quartile of the income distribution is much smaller than the range between the median and upper end of the third income quartile. This indicates that the income spread gets larger in higher-income quartiles. In addition, these data show that there are large differences in the distribution of income across states. For example, family income at the upper end of the first income quartile is $8,600 in Mississippi, compared to $23,435 in Connecticut (table G4). In general, families in the New England and Middle Atlantic regions have higher-than-average median incomes, and families in the other regions have lower-than-average median incomes. As with access to health insurance, important differences in family income also exist across states within regions. For example, families in Virginia have a $32,300 median income, compared to $27,060 for the entire South Atlantic region.

Tables G5 through G9 provide information on family income relative to poverty (below 100 percent of poverty, 100–149 percent of poverty, 150–199 percent of poverty, 200–399 percent of poverty, and above 400 percent of poverty). The population counts presented in each of the tables represent all persons included in that family type. The four family types are: married couples with children, married couples with no children, single parents with children, and single persons. This information is useful for two reasons. First, the number of low-income individuals in the different family types provides information on persons potentially eligible for specific programs or subsidies that vary by income level. Second, the number of individuals in family types at high income levels gives some indication of the ability of states to finance new programs.

Table G5 shows all persons by their family's income relative to the poverty line. These data can be used in conjunction with data on insured status by income relative to poverty presented in sections A and C. In addition, they stress that this measure of income well-being varies across states. For example, the percentage of persons below poverty ranges from 5 percent in Connecticut to 25 percent in Louisiana. Some of the states with the highest rates of uninsurance also have the highest poverty rates: for example, New Mexico has an uninsured rate of 28 percent, and 22 percent of its population falls below poverty.

Tables G6 through G9 provide information on all persons within each of the four family types by their family's income relative to poverty. As shown, poverty rates vary greatly across family types. For example, table G7 shows that nationally, 4 percent of the persons in married-couple families have incomes below 100 percent of poverty, while table G8 shows that nationally, 47 percent of persons in single-person-with children families have incomes below 100 percent of poverty. This information also varies greatly among the states. For example, table G6 shows that the percentage of persons in married-couple-with-children families who have incomes below 100 percent of poverty ranges from zero percent in Connecticut to 16 percent in Mississippi.

Worker Characteristics

Table G10 provides information on labor force participation and unemployment rates for the working population. The participation and unemployment rates indicate the employment environment that exists in each of the states. The information presented in this table is an average for 1988, 1989, and 1990 and therefore does not reflect the effects of the recent recession. However, these numbers reflect the environment during the period of all the other tables from the CPS, including the tables on health insurance and poverty in sections A, B, and C. The unemployment rate ranges from 3 percent in Nebraska and Hawaii to 8 percent in Michigan, West Virginia, and Mississippi.

Tables G11 through G13 provide data, respectively, on the working population by firm size (less than 25 workers, 25–99 workers, 100–499 workers, and 500-plus workers) and sector (private, government, and self-employed), and on the private-sector working population by industry (manufacturing, wholesale/retail, services, and other). The percentage of workers who work for small firms (100 workers or less) may be important in understanding the number of uninsured for a state, because workers in small firms tend to have lower rates of insurance. The same is true for self-employed workers, nonunionized workers, and workers in the service and wholesale/retail trade industries. Thus, these data may be useful in integrating the health insurance status of workers described earlier in section B.

ESTABLISHMENT CHARACTERISTICS

Tables G14 through G16 provide information on the number of establishments, the number of workers by establishment size, and the annualized payroll per worker by establishment size from the County Business Patterns data. Establishment size, characterized by the number of workers within each establishment, is broken into size categories: 1–4 workers, 5–9 workers, 10–19 workers, 20–99 workers, 100–499 workers, and 500-plus workers. The data in table G15 show that 26 percent of workers are employed by establishments with less than 20 employees, 29 percent of workers are in establishments with 20–99 workers, and 44 percent of workers are employed by establishments with more than 100 employees. As stated in section A, firms with fewer than 25 workers are less likely to provide health insurance to their employees, whereas firms with over a 100 workers are more likely to provide health insurance to their employees. These data show that there is not wide variation in the distribution of workers by establishment size across the states with few exceptions. Some states in the West North Central, Mountain, and Pacific regions have higher-than-average concentration of workers in small establishments. For example, the percentage of establishments with fewer than 20 workers is 44 percent in Montana, about 38 percent in each of the Dakotas, and 35 percent in New Mexico, compared to the national average of 26 percent.

Table G16 shows that the variation in average annual salary by establishment size is quite large. Nationally, persons working in large establishments (500 or more employees) have an average salary of $24,599. This is substantially higher than the salaries of workers in smaller establishments, which range from $18,442 (20–99 workers) to $16,247 (5–9 workers). Since large establishments are more likely to provide comprehensive health insurance for their workers, total compensation including health benefits is even higher. These data may be useful in evaluating pay or play employer mandates, because businesses with lower pay would be more likely to choose the tax option than provide insurance.[1]

STATE FINANCES

Tables G17 and G18 provide information on general revenue per capita and sources of general revenue including the federal government and taxes. The data in G17 show that there is large variation in the amount of general revenue per capita among the states. For example, general revenue per capita ranges from $2,368 in Arkansas to $11,317 in Alaska.

In almost all of the states, 50 percent or more of general revenue comes from state and local taxes. Many health care reform proposals at the state level depend on raising additional tax revenue. What form of tax to levy and how much revenue can be raised are important questions for implementation of reforms.

The percent of funds raised from different types of taxes varies greatly across states (table G18). While the majority of state and local taxes are raised from a combination of property, sales/gross, and individual income taxes, there is considerable variety in the importance of these sources across states. Several states such as Washington and Wyoming have no individual income tax and raise a greater percent of income from sales taxes. The percent of tax revenue raised from corporate taxes is relatively small, 4 percent on average, ranging between 0 percent and 9 percent.

Table G19 shows expenditure per capita data followed by the percentage of general expenditures spent on education, welfare, health and hospitals, police protection and corrections, highways, and other areas.[2] General expenditures per capita show the same variation found in the general revenue per capita data. The data do show variation among the states in specific expenditure groups. For example, education expenditures range from 23.5 percent in Alaska to 42 percent in Vermont, and health and hospital expenditures range from 3 percent in Vermont to 15 percent in Georgia.

Notes, Section G
1. Sheila Zedlewski, Greg Acs, Laura Wheaton, and Colin Winterbottom, 1992, "Exploring the Effects of Play or Pay Employer Mandates: Effects on Insurance Coverage and Costs," in U.S. Department of Labor, *Health Benefits and the Workforce* (Washington, D.C.: U.S. Department of Labor), 231-69.

2. Outlays for Medicaid are included in general expenditures on welfare.

TABLE G1
TOTAL POPULATION UNDER AGE 65: BY AGE

	Number (000s)	Ages under 18	Ages 18-34	Ages 35-53	Ages 54-64
UNITED STATES	213,580	30% (0.15)	31% (0.16)	28% (0.15)	11% (0.11)
NEW ENGLAND	11,157	27% (0.51)	33% (0.54)	29% (0.53)	11% (0.36)
Connecticut	2,761	27% (1.43)	32% (1.50)	30% (1.48)	11% (1.01)
Maine	1,055	29% (1.31)	28% (1.29)	30% (1.32)	12% (0.95)
Massachusetts	5,062	26% (0.67)	34% (0.72)	29% (0.69)	11% (0.48)
New Hampshire	972	28% (1.41)	34% (1.49)	28% (1.42)	10% (0.95)
Rhode Island	823	26% (1.40)	34% (1.51)	27% (1.42)	12% (1.04)
Vermont	485	27% (1.38)	32% (1.45)	32% (1.45)	10% (0.94)
MIDDLE ATLANTIC	32,415	28% (0.36)	31% (0.37)	29% (0.36)	12% (0.26)
New Jersey	6,631	27% (0.66)	33% (0.69)	29% (0.67)	11% (0.46)
New York	15,507	29% (0.54)	32% (0.55)	28% (0.53)	12% (0.38)
Pennsylvania	10,277	29% (0.65)	30% (0.66)	29% (0.65)	13% (0.49)
SOUTH ATLANTIC	36,005	28% (0.37)	31% (0.39)	29% (0.38)	12% (0.27)
Delaware	574	27% (1.37)	33% (1.44)	29% (1.38)	11% (0.95)
District of Columbia	493	25% (1.43)	36% (1.58)	28% (1.47)	11% (1.02)
Florida	10,334	27% (0.64)	32% (0.67)	27% (0.64)	13% (0.49)
Georgia	5,475	29% (1.26)	32% (1.29)	29% (1.25)	10% (0.83)
Maryland	3,977	26% (1.33)	33% (1.42)	30% (1.38)	11% (0.94)
North Carolina	5,469	27% (0.65)	32% (0.68)	29% (0.66)	12% (0.48)
South Carolina	2,932	29% (1.16)	30% (1.17)	29% (1.17)	12% (0.84)
Virginia	5,166	29% (1.15)	30% (1.16)	30% (1.16)	11% (0.79)
West Virginia	1,586	30% (1.29)	29% (1.27)	30% (1.29)	12% (0.90)
EAST SOUTH CENTRAL	13,214	30% (0.65)	31% (0.65)	27% (0.62)	11% (0.45)
Alabama	3,570	31% (1.28)	31% (1.28)	26% (1.21)	13% (0.92)
Kentucky	3,123	29% (1.29)	32% (1.33)	28% (1.29)	11% (0.90)
Mississippi	2,285	34% (1.25)	32% (1.23)	24% (1.13)	10% (0.80)
Tennessee	4,236	29% (1.23)	31% (1.24)	28% (1.21)	12% (0.86)
WEST SOUTH CENTRAL	23,455	32% (0.51)	32% (0.51)	26% (0.48)	10% (0.33)
Arkansas	2,103	33% (1.29)	29% (1.25)	26% (1.20)	12% (0.89)
Louisiana	3,701	32% (1.35)	31% (1.35)	26% (1.27)	11% (0.91)
Oklahoma	2,679	30% (1.29)	29% (1.27)	29% (1.28)	12% (0.93)
Texas	14,973	32% (0.66)	33% (0.67)	26% (0.62)	9% (0.41)

	Number (000s)	Ages under 18	Ages 18-34	Ages 35-53	Ages 54-64
EAST NORTH CENTRAL	**36,786**	**30%** **(0.37)**	**31%** **(0.37)**	**28%** **(0.36)**	**11%** **(0.25)**
Illinois	10,171	29% (0.67)	31% (0.69)	28% (0.67)	11% (0.46)
Indiana	4,773	29% (1.32)	32% (1.36)	27% (1.30)	12% (0.93)
Michigan	8,201	30% (0.67)	31% (0.68)	27% (0.65)	12% (0.47)
Ohio	9,537	31% (0.66)	30% (0.66)	28% (0.65)	11% (0.45)
Wisconsin	4,104	29% (1.22)	31% (1.23)	29% (1.21)	11% (0.83)
WEST NORTH CENTRAL	**15,279**	**31%** **(0.59)**	**32%** **(0.59)**	**27%** **(0.56)**	**11%** **(0.39)**
Iowa	2,386	31% (1.27)	30% (1.27)	27% (1.22)	12% (0.89)
Kansas	2,078	31% (1.27)	31% (1.27)	28% (1.24)	11% (0.87)
Minnesota	3,849	31% (1.32)	33% (1.34)	26% (1.25)	9% (0.83)
Missouri	4,475	31% (1.34)	32% (1.36)	26% (1.27)	11% (0.90)
Nebraska	1,361	32% (1.25)	30% (1.24)	27% (1.19)	11% (0.83)
North Dakota	546	33% (1.25)	27% (1.19)	28% (1.20)	11% (0.84)
South Dakota	585	32% (1.19)	29% (1.16)	27% (1.14)	12% (0.81)
MOUNTAIN	**11,712**	**33%** **(0.57)**	**30%** **(0.56)**	**27%** **(0.54)**	**10%** **(0.36)**
Arizona	3,016	31% (1.34)	32% (1.36)	26% (1.27)	11% (0.89)
Colorado	2,836	32% (1.39)	30% (1.37)	30% (1.37)	8% (0.82)
Idaho	896	35% (1.26)	28% (1.18)	27% (1.17)	10% (0.80)
Montana	711	32% (1.28)	27% (1.21)	29% (1.24)	11% (0.86)
Nevada	1,010	28% (1.32)	31% (1.36)	30% (1.34)	11% (0.90)
New Mexico	1,302	33% (1.28)	30% (1.25)	26% (1.20)	11% (0.85)
Utah	1,525	40% (1.32)	30% (1.23)	21% (1.10)	9% (0.75)
Wyoming	414	32% (1.50)	26% (1.42)	31% (1.48)	11% (1.00)
PACIFIC	**33,556**	**30%** **(0.45)**	**32%** **(0.46)**	**28%** **(0.44)**	**10%** **(0.29)**
Alaska	435	32% (1.27)	29% (1.22)	31% (1.26)	8% (0.73)
California	25,588	30% (0.53)	33% (0.55)	28% (0.52)	9% (0.34)
Hawaii	850	26% (1.37)	28% (1.40)	30% (1.43)	15% (1.11)
Oregon	2,464	30% (1.40)	29% (1.38)	30% (1.39)	10% (0.92)
Washington	4,219	29% (1.27)	29% (1.27)	31% (1.29)	11% (0.86)

Source: Three-year merged March CPS, 1989, 1990, and 1991.

TABLE G2
TOTAL POPULATION UNDER AGE 65: BY RACE AND SEX

	Number (000s)	White	Nonwhite	Male	Female
UNITED STATES	213,580	83% (0.08)	17% (0.08)	50% (0.11)	50% (0.11)
NEW ENGLAND	11,157	93% (0.19)	7% (0.20)	50% (0.37)	50% (0.37)
Connecticut	2,761	88% (0.67)	12% (0.70)	50% (1.04)	50% (1.04)
Maine	1,055	99% (0.20)	1% (0.20)	50% (0.93)	50% (0.93)
Massachusetts	5,062	93% (0.26)	7% (0.27)	50% (0.49)	50% (0.49)
New Hampshire	972	98% (0.28)	2% (0.28)	50% (1.02)	50% (1.02)
Rhode Island	823	93% (0.51)	7% (0.53)	51% (1.03)	49% (1.03)
Vermont	485	99% (0.19)	1% (0.19)	50% (1.01)	50% (1.01)
MIDDLE ATLANTIC	32,415	84% (0.19)	16% (0.20)	49% (0.26)	51% (0.26)
New Jersey	6,631	82% (0.37)	18% (0.38)	50% (0.48)	50% (0.48)
New York	15,507	81% (0.30)	19% (0.31)	49% (0.38)	51% (0.38)
Pennsylvania	10,277	89% (0.29)	11% (0.30)	49% (0.47)	51% (0.47)
SOUTH ATLANTIC	36,005	74% (0.24)	26% (0.24)	49% (0.27)	51% (0.27)
Delaware	574	79% (0.81)	21% (0.84)	49% (0.99)	51% (0.99)
District of Columbia	493	32% (0.99)	68% (1.03)	48% (1.06)	52% (1.06)
Florida	10,334	81% (0.36)	19% (0.38)	49% (0.46)	51% (0.46)
Georgia	5,475	63% (0.86)	37% (0.89)	49% (0.89)	51% (0.89)
Maryland	3,977	70% (0.89)	30% (0.93)	48% (0.97)	52% (0.97)
North Carolina	5,469	76% (0.41)	24% (0.42)	50% (0.47)	50% (0.47)
South Carolina	2,932	67% (0.78)	33% (0.81)	50% (0.83)	50% (0.83)
Virginia	5,166	76% (0.70)	24% (0.72)	49% (0.82)	51% (0.82)
West Virginia	1,586	96% (0.37)	4% (0.38)	49% (0.91)	51% (0.91)
EAST SOUTH CENTRAL	13,214	77% (0.38)	23% (0.39)	49% (0.45)	51% (0.45)
Alabama	3,570	71% (0.81)	29% (0.85)	48% (0.90)	52% (0.90)
Kentucky	3,123	94% (0.43)	6% (0.45)	49% (0.92)	51% (0.92)
Mississippi	2,285	60% (0.83)	40% (0.87)	49% (0.85)	51% (0.85)
Tennessee	4,236	80% (0.70)	20% (0.73)	49% (0.87)	51% (0.87)
WEST SOUTH CENTRAL	23,455	82% (0.27)	18% (0.28)	50% (0.35)	50% (0.35)
Arkansas	2,103	82% (0.67)	18% (0.70)	50% (0.89)	50% (0.89)
Louisiana	3,701	69% (0.87)	31% (0.90)	48% (0.94)	52% (0.94)
Oklahoma	2,679	83% (0.68)	17% (0.71)	51% (0.91)	49% (0.91)
Texas	14,973	86% (0.32)	14% (0.33)	50% (0.46)	50% (0.46)

	Number (000s)	White	Nonwhite	Male	Female
EAST NORTH CENTRAL	**36,786**	**86%** (0.18)	**14%** (0.19)	**50%** (0.26)	**50%** (0.26)
Illinois	10,171	81% (0.37)	19% (0.39)	50% (0.48)	50% (0.48)
Indiana	4,773	90% (0.57)	10% (0.59)	49% (0.94)	51% (0.94)
Michigan	8,201	84% (0.35)	16% (0.36)	50% (0.47)	50% (0.47)
Ohio	9,537	88% (0.31)	12% (0.32)	49% (0.47)	51% (0.47)
Wisconsin	4,104	94% (0.42)	6% (0.44)	50% (0.86)	50% (0.86)
WEST NORTH CENTRAL	**15,279**	**92%** (0.23)	**8%** (0.24)	**50%** (0.41)	**50%** (0.41)
Iowa	2,386	97% (0.29)	3% (0.31)	50% (0.89)	50% (0.89)
Kansas	2,078	90% (0.53)	10% (0.55)	49% (0.89)	51% (0.89)
Minnesota	3,849	93% (0.47)	7% (0.49)	50% (0.92)	50% (0.92)
Missouri	4,475	86% (0.64)	14% (0.67)	49% (0.93)	51% (0.93)
Nebraska	1,361	95% (0.38)	5% (0.39)	50% (0.87)	50% (0.87)
North Dakota	546	94% (0.41)	6% (0.43)	51% (0.86)	49% (0.86)
South Dakota	585	91% (0.47)	9% (0.49)	50% (0.82)	50% (0.82)
MOUNTAIN	**11,712**	**94%** (0.19)	**6%** (0.20)	**50%** (0.39)	**50%** (0.39)
Arizona	3,016	96% (0.38)	4% (0.39)	50% (0.94)	50% (0.94)
Colorado	2,836	93% (0.51)	7% (0.53)	49% (0.97)	51% (0.97)
Idaho	896	97% (0.28)	3% (0.29)	50% (0.85)	50% (0.85)
Montana	711	92% (0.48)	8% (0.50)	51% (0.88)	49% (0.88)
Nevada	1,010	89% (0.59)	11% (0.61)	51% (0.94)	49% (0.94)
New Mexico	1,302	90% (0.54)	10% (0.56)	50% (0.88)	50% (0.88)
Utah	1,525	96% (0.32)	4% (0.34)	50% (0.87)	50% (0.87)
Wyoming	414	99% (0.24)	1% (0.24)	51% (1.04)	49% (1.04)
PACIFIC	**33,556**	**83%** (0.24)	**17%** (0.25)	**50%** (0.32)	**50%** (0.32)
Alaska	435	75% (0.75)	25% (0.78)	52% (0.87)	48% (0.87)
California	25,588	83% (0.28)	17% (0.30)	50% (0.38)	50% (0.38)
Hawaii	850	28% (0.90)	72% (0.93)	51% (1.00)	49% (1.00)
Oregon	2,464	95% (0.44)	5% (0.46)	50% (0.98)	50% (0.98)
Washington	4,219	91% (0.51)	9% (0.53)	50% (0.90)	50% (0.90)

Source: Three-year merged March CPS, 1989, 1990, and 1991.

TABLE G3
TOTAL POPULATION UNDER AGE 65: BY FAMILY TYPE

	Number (000s)	Married No Children	Married with Children	Single Parent	Single
UNITED STATES	213,580	20% (0.14)	50% (0.17)	13% (0.11)	17% (0.13)
NEW ENGLAND	11,157	22% (0.48)	49% (0.58)	11% (0.36)	18% (0.45)
Connecticut	2,761	23% (1.35)	50% (1.61)	11% (0.99)	17% (1.22)
Maine	1,055	22% (1.19)	53% (1.43)	11% (0.88)	15% (1.02)
Massachusetts	5,062	21% (0.62)	47% (0.76)	12% (0.50)	20% (0.61)
New Hampshire	972	23% (1.32)	53% (1.57)	9% (0.91)	15% (1.12)
Rhode Island	823	25% (1.38)	47% (1.59)	9% (0.90)	18% (1.24)
Vermont	485	19% (1.23)	52% (1.56)	10% (0.92)	19% (1.23)
MIDDLE ATLANTIC	32,415	21% (0.32)	50% (0.40)	13% (0.26)	16% (0.29)
New Jersey	6,631	22% (0.61)	50% (0.74)	12% (0.49)	16% (0.54)
New York	15,507	19% (0.47)	49% (0.59)	14% (0.42)	18% (0.46)
Pennsylvania	10,277	23% (0.61)	53% (0.72)	11% (0.46)	14% (0.50)
SOUTH ATLANTIC	36,005	22% (0.35)	46% (0.42)	14% (0.29)	18% (0.32)
Delaware	574	21% (1.25)	44% (1.52)	14% (1.07)	20% (1.23)
District of Columbia	493	14% (1.14)	22% (1.36)	25% (1.42)	39% (1.60)
Florida	10,334	24% (0.61)	43% (0.71)	14% (0.50)	19% (0.55)
Georgia	5,475	21% (1.12)	47% (1.38)	15% (0.99)	17% (1.04)
Maryland	3,977	22% (1.25)	42% (1.49)	15% (1.09)	21% (1.23)
North Carolina	5,469	23% (0.62)	47% (0.73)	12% (0.48)	17% (0.55)
South Carolina	2,932	25% (1.11)	48% (1.28)	14% (0.88)	13% (0.88)
Virginia	5,166	21% (1.03)	49% (1.27)	13% (0.85)	17% (0.94)
West Virginia	1,586	21% (1.15)	56% (1.40)	11% (0.89)	12% (0.90)
EAST SOUTH CENTRAL	13,214	22% (0.58)	49% (0.70)	15% (0.51)	14% (0.49)
Alabama	3,570	22% (1.16)	49% (1.39)	15% (0.99)	14% (0.95)
Kentucky	3,123	23% (1.21)	51% (1.43)	12% (0.94)	13% (0.98)
Mississippi	2,285	18% (1.02)	48% (1.32)	19% (1.04)	15% (0.93)
Tennessee	4,236	22% (1.11)	49% (1.35)	16% (0.98)	14% (0.93)
WEST SOUTH CENTRAL	23,455	19% (0.43)	53% (0.54)	13% (0.37)	15% (0.39)
Arkansas	2,103	20% (1.11)	49% (1.37)	16% (1.01)	14% (0.95)
Louisiana	3,701	19% (1.14)	51% (1.45)	17% (1.08)	14% (1.00)
Oklahoma	2,679	22% (1.17)	52% (1.40)	12% (0.90)	14% (0.98)
Texas	14,973	19% (0.56)	54% (0.71)	12% (0.46)	15% (0.51)

TOTAL POPULATION UNDER AGE 65: BY FAMILY TYPE

	Number (000s)	Married No Children	Married with Children	Single Parent	Single
EAST NORTH CENTRAL	**36,786**	**21%** **(0.33)**	**50%** **(0.40)**	**14%** **(0.28)**	**15%** **(0.29)**
Illinois	10,171	20% (0.59)	49% (0.74)	15% (0.53)	17% (0.55)
Indiana	4,773	22% (1.21)	50% (1.46)	14% (1.00)	14% (1.01)
Michigan	8,201	21% (0.60)	48% (0.73)	15% (0.52)	16% (0.53)
Ohio	9,537	20% (0.58)	52% (0.72)	13% (0.48)	15% (0.51)
Wisconsin	4,104	21% (1.10)	53% (1.33)	10% (0.81)	15% (0.96)
WEST NORTH CENTRAL	**15,279**	**19%** **(0.50)**	**54%** **(0.63)**	**11%** **(0.40)**	**15%** **(0.46)**
Iowa	2,386	19% (1.08)	56% (1.37)	10% (0.81)	15% (1.00)
Kansas	2,078	21% (1.12)	53% (1.38)	12% (0.89)	15% (0.98)
Minnesota	3,849	18% (1.10)	54% (1.42)	12% (0.92)	16% (1.06)
Missouri	4,475	20% (1.16)	54% (1.44)	11% (0.92)	15% (1.02)
Nebraska	1,361	20% (1.08)	56% (1.33)	9% (0.77)	15% (0.96)
North Dakota	546	19% (1.03)	61% (1.30)	8% (0.71)	13% (0.90)
South Dakota	585	20% (1.02)	54% (1.27)	12% (0.83)	13% (0.87)
MOUNTAIN	**11,712**	**18%** **(0.47)**	**53%** **(0.60)**	**12%** **(0.40)**	**16%** **(0.44)**
Arizona	3,016	21% (1.17)	49% (1.45)	13% (0.96)	18% (1.11)
Colorado	2,836	18% (1.14)	50% (1.50)	15% (1.06)	18% (1.14)
Idaho	896	18% (1.03)	59% (1.30)	9% (0.77)	13% (0.89)
Montana	711	20% (1.08)	54% (1.36)	12% (0.88)	14% (0.95)
Nevada	1,010	20% (1.16)	44% (1.45)	14% (1.01)	22% (1.21)
New Mexico	1,302	17% (1.03)	56% (1.35)	13% (0.90)	15% (0.96)
Utah	1,525	14% (0.94)	65% (1.28)	10% (0.80)	10% (0.82)
Wyoming	414	21% (1.31)	57% (1.59)	10% (0.98)	12% (1.04)
PACIFIC	**33,556**	**19%** **(0.38)**	**49%** **(0.49)**	**13%** **(0.33)**	**19%** **(0.39)**
Alaska	435	16% (1.00)	52% (1.35)	13% (0.90)	19% (1.06)
California	25,588	18% (0.45)	49% (0.58)	13% (0.39)	20% (0.46)
Hawaii	850	26% (1.36)	46% (1.55)	10% (0.95)	18% (1.19)
Oregon	2,464	20% (1.22)	51% (1.52)	12% (0.97)	17% (1.14)
Washington	4,219	21% (1.14)	49% (1.39)	12% (0.89)	18% (1.08)

Source: Three-year merged March CPS, 1989, 1990, and 1991.

TABLE G4
UPPER LIMIT OF QUARTILES, FAMILY INCOME (1990 DOLLARS)

	Number (000s)	PERCENTILES		
		25th	Median	75th
UNITED STATES	82,664	$14,000 (87)	$28,167 (112)	$47,229 (173)
NEW ENGLAND	**4,433**	**19,000 (371)**	**34,066 (415)**	**56,251 (687)**
Connecticut	1,093	23,435 (951)	38,472 (1,198)	62,896 (1,562)
Maine	406	14,135 (725)	26,410 (1,064)	43,845 (1,145)
Massachusetts	2,027	18,500 (514)	34,029 (566)	57,025 (1,052)
New Hampshire	380	21,827 (951)	36,820 (1,300)	55,453 (1,424)
Rhode Island	324	16,275 (842)	31,719 (1,011)	52,632 (1,247)
Vermont	203	15,420 (628)	27,801 (1,056)	46,245 (1,309)
MIDDLE ATLANTIC	**12,154**	**16,314 (240)**	**31,800 (300)**	**52,850 (416)**
New Jersey	2,491	20,024 (516)	38,629 (669)	61,743 (923)
New York	5,930	14,600 (368)	30,200 (449)	51,730 (667)
Pennsylvania	3,733	16,720 (416)	30,541 (507)	48,326 (729)
SOUTH ATLANTIC	**14,416**	**13,729 (201)**	**27,060 (271)**	**46,025 (416)**
Delaware	238	16,472 (698)	29,513 (860)	48,689 (1,276)
District of Columbia	247	11,515 (595)	24,072 (919)	40,100 (1,758)
Florida	4,276	13,066 (300)	25,142 (444)	42,617 (581)
Georgia	2,165	12,813 (633)	25,910 (876)	45,385 (1,312)
Maryland	1,681	17,500 (960)	32,780 (1,224)	53,700 (1,807)
North Carolina	2,191	13,166 (342)	25,910 (459)	43,352 (599)
South Carolina	1,054	13,165 (704)	27,829 (977)	45,392 (1,275)
Virginia	1,993	16,479 (770)	32,300 (846)	54,257 (1,403)
West Virginia	571	11,516 (620)	23,643 (800)	38,972 (1,168)
EAST SOUTH CENTRAL	**4,901**	**10,796 (293)**	**22,907 (467)**	**38,999 (513)**
Alabama	1,293	10,800 (556)	22,225 (967)	39,033 (974)
Kentucky	1,194	11,310 (582)	24,329 (928)	39,632 (902)
Mississippi	818	8,600 (470)	18,585 (750)	35,339 (1,045)
Tennessee	1,596	12,003 (632)	24,100 (867)	40,807 (1,148)
WEST SOUTH CENTRAL	**8,733**	**12,000 (251)**	**24,537 (336)**	**42,331 (517)**
Arkansas	772	11,000 (624)	21,591 (679)	36,321 (1,252)
Louisiana	1,331	8,924 (571)	22,658 (1,235)	39,125 (1,169)
Oklahoma	1,060	12,000 (650)	24,770 (835)	42,640 (1,244)
Texas	5,570	12,667 (325)	25,299 (485)	43,560 (639)

	Number (000s)	PERCENTILES		
		25th	Median	75th
EAST NORTH CENTRAL	13,990	$14,756 (231)	$29,526 (267)	$48,000 (364)
Illinois	3,862	15,335 (469)	31,053 (531)	50,172 (733)
Indiana	1,839	14,017 (676)	26,901 (822)	43,388 (1,169)
Michigan	3,142	13,473 (441)	29,355 (506)	49,215 (679)
Ohio	3,550	14,777 (439)	29,678 (513)	47,932 (663)
Wisconsin	1,597	15,404 (769)	30,000 (876)	46,161 (1,168)
WEST NORTH CENTRAL	5,917	14,157 (296)	27,128 (412)	44,516 (563)
Iowa	939	13,765 (558)	26,185 (871)	40,826 (1,340)
Kansas	813	14,756 (674)	28,282 (879)	46,000 (1,472)
Minnesota	1,507	15,099 (667)	28,892 (858)	48,125 (1,266)
Missouri	1,724	13,892 (641)	26,253 (1,038)	45,551 (1,218)
Nebraska	516	14,202 (734)	26,956 (856)	42,161 (801)
North Dakota	199	12,895 (673)	25,624 (922)	42,013 (961)
South Dakota	218	11,764 (545)	23,856 (767)	37,878 (872)
MOUNTAIN	4,562	13,000 (283)	25,959 (373)	43,440 (519)
Arizona	1,212	12,953 (664)	26,091 (782)	42,935 (1,090)
Colorado	1,177	13,702 (750)	28,291 (956)	47,693 (1,126)
Idaho	324	12,000 (559)	23,812 (681)	39,344 (1,080)
Montana	272	11,197 (595)	23,400 (883)	39,658 (1,134)
Nevada	447	14,143 (633)	26,000 (776)	42,274 (1,112)
New Mexico	497	10,817 (504)	21,000 (802)	37,069 (1,316)
Utah	480	15,900 (737)	29,034 (1,035)	44,290 (880)
Wyoming	154	14,195 (926)	28,114 (1,009)	46,533 (1,231)
PACIFIC	13,559	14,000 (233)	28,510 (327)	48,393 (537)
Alaska	179	15,676 (835)	31,848 (1,029)	56,451 (1,675)
California	10,299	13,749 (269)	28,626 (389)	49,300 (665)
Hawaii	326	16,843 (1,179)	31,621 (1,410)	55,050 (1,936)
Oregon	999	13,377 (762)	26,869 (944)	42,129 (1,236)
Washington	1,756	15,497 (637)	28,654 (951)	46,636 (1,372)

Source: Three-year merged March CPS, 1989, 1990, and 1991.

TABLE G5
TOTAL POPULATION UNDER AGE 65: BY INCOME AS PERCENTAGE OF POVERTY

	Number (000s)	< 100% of Poverty	100-149% of Poverty	150-199% of Poverty	200-399% of Poverty	400+% of Poverty
UNITED STATES	213,580	14% (0.17)	8% (0.13)	9% (0.13)	34% (0.22)	34% (0.22)
NEW ENGLAND	11,157	8% (0.44)	5% (0.36)	6% (0.38)	33% (0.75)	48% (0.80)
Connecticut	2,761	5% (0.94)	4% (0.87)	5% (0.96)	31% (2.08)	55% (2.23)
Maine	1,055	12% (1.32)	9% (1.16)	9% (1.13)	39% (1.95)	30% (1.84)
Massachusetts	5,062	9% (0.62)	6% (0.48)	5% (0.47)	31% (0.98)	49% (1.06)
New Hampshire	972	7% (1.09)	3% (0.78)	6% (1.07)	36% (2.10)	48% (2.19)
Rhode Island	823	9% (1.26)	6% (1.04)	9% (1.27)	34% (2.09)	43% (2.19)
Vermont	485	9% (1.25)	6% (1.06)	8% (1.20)	40% (2.12)	37% (2.09)
MIDDLE ATLANTIC	32,415	12% (0.36)	7% (0.28)	8% (0.29)	34% (0.52)	40% (0.54)
New Jersey	6,631	9% (0.58)	4% (0.42)	5% (0.43)	31% (0.95)	52% (1.03)
New York	15,507	14% (0.58)	7% (0.43)	8% (0.44)	33% (0.77)	38% (0.80)
Pennsylvania	10,277	11% (0.64)	7% (0.53)	9% (0.58)	38% (0.98)	35% (0.96)
SOUTH ATLANTIC	36,005	14% (0.41)	9% (0.33)	9% (0.33)	33% (0.55)	35% (0.55)
Delaware	574	9% (1.25)	6% (1.01)	8% (1.14)	37% (2.06)	40% (2.09)
District of Columbia	493	20% (1.82)	7% (1.20)	9% (1.31)	27% (2.04)	37% (2.21)
Florida	10,334	15% (0.71)	10% (0.59)	9% (0.58)	34% (0.94)	31% (0.92)
Georgia	5,475	17% (1.44)	8% (1.06)	10% (1.15)	33% (1.80)	32% (1.79)
Maryland	3,977	10% (1.27)	7% (1.05)	5% (0.94)	30% (1.93)	48% (2.10)
North Carolina	5,469	14% (0.70)	9% (0.59)	9% (0.59)	37% (0.98)	31% (0.94)
South Carolina	2,932	16% (1.32)	10% (1.07)	8% (0.99)	35% (1.70)	30% (1.64)
Virginia	5,166	12% (1.13)	8% (0.94)	7% (0.93)	29% (1.59)	45% (1.75)
West Virginia	1,586	19% (1.52)	11% (1.23)	12% (1.28)	37% (1.89)	21% (1.58)
EAST SOUTH CENTRAL	13,214	20% (0.79)	11% (0.62)	10% (0.60)	34% (0.93)	24% (0.83)
Alabama	3,570	21% (1.57)	11% (1.21)	11% (1.19)	35% (1.84)	22% (1.61)
Kentucky	3,123	17% (1.49)	12% (1.28)	11% (1.26)	34% (1.88)	26% (1.75)
Mississippi	2,285	27% (1.63)	12% (1.20)	10% (1.11)	32% (1.71)	19% (1.43)
Tennessee	4,236	19% (1.47)	10% (1.15)	9% (1.09)	36% (1.80)	26% (1.64)
WEST SOUTH CENTRAL	23,455	19% (0.60)	10% (0.46)	10% (0.45)	32% (0.71)	28% (0.68)
Arkansas	2,103	20% (1.53)	13% (1.30)	12% (1.26)	34% (1.81)	20% (1.53)
Louisiana	3,701	25% (1.74)	10% (1.20)	9% (1.16)	33% (1.89)	24% (1.71)
Oklahoma	2,679	16% (1.45)	11% (1.21)	11% (1.22)	32% (1.82)	30% (1.79)
Texas	14,973	18% (0.77)	10% (0.59)	10% (0.58)	32% (0.92)	30% (0.90)

	Number (000s)	< 100% of Poverty	100-149% of Poverty	150-199% of Poverty	200-399% of Poverty	400+% of Poverty
EAST NORTH CENTRAL	**36,786**	**14%** **(0.38)**	**7%** **(0.29)**	**8%** **(0.30)**	**36%** **(0.54)**	**35%** **(0.54)**
Illinois	10,171	14% (0.72)	6% (0.50)	8% (0.55)	34% (0.98)	38% (1.00)
Indiana	4,773	14% (1.42)	9% (1.13)	9% (1.16)	39% (1.98)	29% (1.84)
Michigan	8,201	15% (0.73)	7% (0.51)	7% (0.52)	33% (0.96)	37% (0.98)
Ohio	9,537	13% (0.67)	8% (0.54)	8% (0.56)	36% (0.96)	35% (0.95)
Wisconsin	4,104	9% (1.06)	6% (0.90)	8% (1.01)	42% (1.84)	35% (1.77)
WEST NORTH CENTRAL	**15,279**	**13%** **(0.59)**	**9%** **(0.50)**	**10%** **(0.53)**	**38%** **(0.86)**	**31%** **(0.82)**
Iowa	2,386	11% (1.21)	8% (1.07)	11% (1.18)	44% (1.90)	26% (1.69)
Kansas	2,078	12% (1.23)	9% (1.08)	9% (1.08)	36% (1.85)	35% (1.83)
Minnesota	3,849	13% (1.35)	7% (1.00)	9% (1.12)	37% (1.91)	34% (1.87)
Missouri	4,475	13% (1.34)	10% (1.21)	10% (1.23)	35% (1.92)	32% (1.88)
Nebraska	1,361	12% (1.21)	8% (1.03)	11% (1.15)	40% (1.83)	29% (1.69)
North Dakota	546	14% (1.30)	8% (1.00)	12% (1.21)	42% (1.83)	24% (1.57)
South Dakota	585	15% (1.28)	11% (1.09)	12% (1.16)	40% (1.74)	22% (1.47)
MOUNTAIN	**11,712**	**15%** **(0.60)**	**10%** **(0.50)**	**10%** **(0.52)**	**36%** **(0.81)**	**29%** **(0.76)**
Arizona	3,016	16% (1.48)	9% (1.13)	10% (1.20)	35% (1.92)	30% (1.86)
Colorado	2,836	14% (1.45)	8% (1.11)	9% (1.22)	33% (1.96)	36% (1.99)
Idaho	896	14% (1.26)	13% (1.25)	14% (1.29)	36% (1.77)	22% (1.53)
Montana	711	17% (1.43)	11% (1.19)	10% (1.16)	39% (1.85)	23% (1.58)
Nevada	1,010	11% (1.29)	8% (1.09)	8% (1.12)	40% (1.99)	33% (1.91)
New Mexico	1,302	22% (1.57)	12% (1.24)	11% (1.21)	33% (1.78)	21% (1.55)
Utah	1,525	9% (1.09)	13% (1.27)	12% (1.22)	41% (1.84)	24% (1.59)
Wyoming	414	12% (1.47)	8% (1.22)	10% (1.33)	38% (2.18)	31% (2.08)
PACIFIC	**33,556**	**14%** **(0.47)**	**9%** **(0.40)**	**8%** **(0.37)**	**33%** **(0.64)**	**36%** **(0.65)**
Alaska	435	15% (1.36)	10% (1.12)	8% (1.03)	35% (1.80)	31% (1.75)
California	25,588	15% (0.57)	10% (0.48)	8% (0.44)	31% (0.74)	36% (0.77)
Hawaii	850	14% (1.50)	8% (1.20)	8% (1.19)	33% (2.03)	36% (2.08)
Oregon	2,464	13% (1.42)	9% (1.23)	8% (1.12)	39% (2.06)	31% (1.95)
Washington	4,219	10% (1.16)	6% (0.95)	8% (1.05)	38% (1.88)	37% (1.88)

Source: Three-year merged March CPS, 1989, 1990, and 1991.

TABLE G6
PERSONS UNDER AGE 65 IN MARRIED-COUPLE-WITH-CHILDREN FAMILIES:
BY INCOME AS PERCENTAGE OF POVERTY

	Number (000s)	< 100% of Poverty	100-149% of Poverty	150-199% of Poverty	200-399% of Poverty	400+% of Poverty
UNITED STATES	106,567	9% (0.19)	8% (0.19)	9% (0.19)	40% (0.33)	33% (0.31)
NEW ENGLAND	5,482	3% (0.39)	5% (0.48)	6% (0.56)	39% (1.12)	47% (1.15)
Connecticut	1,370	0% (0.37)	3% (0.99)	5% (1.38)	38% (3.10)	54% (3.18)
Maine	554	7% (1.37)	9% (1.60)	9% (1.58)	46% (2.75)	29% (2.51)
Massachusetts	2,401	3% (0.56)	5% (0.64)	6% (0.71)	35% (1.47)	51% (1.54)
New Hampshire	516	3% (1.02)	3% (1.04)	8% (1.58)	43% (2.97)	44% (2.98)
Rhode Island	390	4% (1.29)	6% (1.53)	10% (1.93)	40% (3.15)	40% (3.15)
Vermont	250	5% (1.35)	6% (1.39)	9% (1.71)	44% (3.00)	37% (2.92)
MIDDLE ATLANTIC	16,295	7% (0.39)	6% (0.37)	9% (0.43)	41% (0.76)	38% (0.75)
New Jersey	3,346	3% (0.50)	3% (0.49)	4% (0.59)	36% (1.39)	54% (1.45)
New York	7,552	8% (0.63)	7% (0.58)	9% (0.67)	41% (1.16)	36% (1.13)
Pennsylvania	5,397	8% (0.76)	7% (0.73)	11% (0.86)	43% (1.38)	30% (1.28)
SOUTH ATLANTIC	16,496	8% (0.45)	8% (0.48)	10% (0.51)	39% (0.84)	35% (0.82)
Delaware	253	4% (1.31)	3% (1.16)	8% (1.72)	45% (3.20)	39% (3.14)
District of Columbia	107	7% (2.56)	6% (2.32)	8% (2.60)	32% (4.58)	47% (4.90)
Florida	4,477	9% (0.87)	10% (0.92)	11% (0.94)	40% (1.48)	30% (1.39)
Georgia	2,568	7% (1.47)	9% (1.61)	12% (1.82)	38% (2.72)	34% (2.66)
Maryland	1,654	2% (0.83)	6% (1.58)	5% (1.44)	36% (3.13)	51% (3.26)
North Carolina	2,587	8% (0.79)	7% (0.78)	10% (0.89)	44% (1.47)	31% (1.37)
South Carolina	1,416	9% (1.49)	9% (1.49)	10% (1.55)	42% (2.54)	29% (2.33)
Virginia	2,548	6% (1.20)	6% (1.22)	7% (1.27)	34% (2.38)	47% (2.50)
West Virginia	886	14% (1.80)	11% (1.66)	13% (1.74)	44% (2.60)	18% (2.02)
EAST SOUTH CENTRAL	6,489	13% (0.93)	11% (0.89)	11% (0.88)	42% (1.38)	23% (1.18)
Alabama	1,740	13% (1.87)	12% (1.80)	11% (1.76)	42% (2.73)	21% (2.27)
Kentucky	1,586	11% (1.75)	13% (1.89)	13% (1.86)	39% (2.72)	24% (2.40)
Mississippi	1,102	16% (1.92)	12% (1.72)	12% (1.69)	41% (2.60)	20% (2.12)
Tennessee	2,061	12% (1.74)	9% (1.56)	10% (1.59)	44% (2.66)	26% (2.34)
WEST SOUTH CENTRAL	12,331	14% (0.73)	11% (0.66)	10% (0.64)	36% (1.01)	28% (0.94)
Arkansas	1,037	11% (1.68)	16% (2.00)	15% (1.92)	40% (2.66)	19% (2.11)
Louisiana	1,871	14% (1.98)	11% (1.78)	10% (1.70)	40% (2.78)	24% (2.43)
Oklahoma	1,388	11% (1.69)	13% (1.80)	11% (1.72)	36% (2.61)	29% (2.47)
Texas	8,034	15% (0.97)	11% (0.83)	10% (0.80)	35% (1.28)	30% (1.23)

TABLE G6 (continued)
PERSONS UNDER AGE 65 IN MARRIED-COUPLE-WITH-CHILDREN FAMILIES:
BY INCOME AS PERCENTAGE OF POVERTY

	Number (000s)	< 100% of Poverty	100-149% of Poverty	150-199% of Poverty	200-399% of Poverty	400+% of Poverty
EAST NORTH CENTRAL	**18,448**	**7%** (0.40)	**7%** (0.40)	**8%** (0.43)	**44%** (0.79)	**34%** (0.75)
Illinois	4,936	7% (0.73)	6% (0.70)	8% (0.82)	42% (1.46)	37% (1.42)
Indiana	2,393	9% (1.62)	8% (1.59)	9% (1.64)	49% (2.86)	25% (2.47)
Michigan	3,950	8% (0.78)	7% (0.75)	8% (0.77)	41% (1.44)	37% (1.41)
Ohio	4,981	6% (0.65)	8% (0.74)	9% (0.80)	44% (1.38)	33% (1.30)
Wisconsin	2,189	5% (1.11)	6% (1.19)	6% (1.24)	51% (2.55)	32% (2.37)
WEST NORTH CENTRAL	**8,313**	**8%** (0.66)	**9%** (0.67)	**10%** (0.73)	**44%** (1.19)	**29%** (1.09)
Iowa	1,338	7% (1.27)	8% (1.42)	10% (1.54)	52% (2.56)	23% (2.17)
Kansas	1,095	5% (1.20)	9% (1.48)	9% (1.51)	43% (2.62)	34% (2.50)
Minnesota	2,061	11% (1.68)	7% (1.41)	10% (1.60)	40% (2.65)	32% (2.52)
Missouri	2,410	8% (1.49)	9% (1.60)	11% (1.73)	40% (2.69)	31% (2.54)
Nebraska	759	8% (1.38)	9% (1.41)	11% (1.54)	47% (2.50)	25% (2.17)
North Dakota	331	10% (1.45)	8% (1.31)	13% (1.60)	48% (2.38)	21% (1.92)
South Dakota	318	9% (1.36)	10% (1.47)	13% (1.60)	49% (2.40)	19% (1.88)
MOUNTAIN	**6,221**	**10%** (0.70)	**11%** (0.71)	**13%** (0.77)	**41%** (1.14)	**25%** (1.01)
Arizona	1,477	11% (1.78)	10% (1.73)	12% (1.89)	41% (2.84)	26% (2.52)
Colorado	1,419	9% (1.72)	7% (1.46)	12% (1.94)	38% (2.86)	33% (2.77)
Idaho	531	11% (1.47)	14% (1.67)	17% (1.81)	38% (2.32)	20% (1.90)
Montana	386	12% (1.67)	12% (1.64)	13% (1.71)	44% (2.56)	20% (2.05)
Nevada	449	6% (1.40)	8% (1.70)	8% (1.67)	47% (3.05)	31% (2.83)
New Mexico	725	20% (2.03)	14% (1.75)	12% (1.66)	36% (2.44)	18% (1.97)
Utah	997	4% (0.95)	15% (1.63)	15% (1.64)	45% (2.30)	21% (1.87)
Wyoming	237	9% (1.69)	7% (1.54)	11% (1.89)	45% (2.95)	28% (2.65)
PACIFIC	**16,492**	**11%** (0.61)	**10%** (0.57)	**9%** (0.55)	**38%** (0.94)	**33%** (0.91)
Alaska	228	10% (1.53)	9% (1.50)	8% (1.41)	42% (2.57)	31% (2.42)
California	12,562	13% (0.76)	10% (0.70)	9% (0.66)	36% (1.10)	32% (1.07)
Hawaii	391	11% (2.01)	9% (1.84)	10% (1.94)	37% (3.08)	33% (2.99)
Oregon	1,255	7% (1.47)	11% (1.84)	7% (1.53)	48% (2.96)	27% (2.63)
Washington	2,056	5% (1.26)	5% (1.23)	7% (1.46)	43% (2.75)	39% (2.70)

Source: Three-year merged March CPS, 1989, 1990, and 1991.

TABLE G7
PERSONS UNDER AGE 65 IN MARRIED-COUPLE-NO-CHILDREN FAMILIES:
BY INCOME AS PERCENTAGE OF POVERTY

	Number (000s)	< 100% of Poverty	100-149% of Poverty	150-199% of Poverty	200-399% of Poverty	400+% of Poverty
UNITED STATES	43,682	4% (0.21)	4% (0.21)	5% (0.24)	28% (0.47)	58% (0.51)
NEW ENGLAND	2,435	2% (0.49)	2% (0.51)	3% (0.60)	20% (1.39)	72% (1.54)
Connecticut	626	1% (1.08)	2% (1.18)	3% (1.65)	12% (3.08)	82% (3.64)
Maine	232	5% (1.82)	4% (1.62)	7% (2.11)	34% (4.05)	50% (4.26)
Massachusetts	1,053	2% (0.65)	2% (0.71)	2% (0.67)	21% (1.87)	73% (2.06)
New Hampshire	222	3% (1.43)	2% (1.27)	1% (1.03)	20% (3.66)	74% (4.00)
Rhode Island	208	1% (0.96)	2% (1.11)	6% (2.08)	25% (3.79)	67% (4.15)
Vermont	94	2% (1.31)	3% (1.73)	3% (1.60)	32% (4.61)	60% (4.83)
MIDDLE ATLANTIC	6,720	3% (0.39)	3% (0.40)	4% (0.46)	26% (1.05)	65% (1.15)
New Jersey	1,428	2% (0.65)	2% (0.61)	2% (0.64)	20% (1.78)	74% (1.96)
New York	2,958	4% (0.71)	3% (0.65)	4% (0.75)	23% (1.59)	66% (1.79)
Pennsylvania	2,334	2% (0.57)	3% (0.73)	4% (0.85)	32% (1.97)	59% (2.08)
SOUTH ATLANTIC	8,049	4% (0.50)	5% (0.54)	6% (0.57)	29% (1.11)	56% (1.22)
Delaware	122	1% (0.69)	2% (1.27)	6% (2.13)	26% (4.04)	66% (4.38)
District of Columbia	69	7% (3.09)	4% (2.37)	5% (2.64)	25% (5.28)	59% (5.99)
Florida	2,451	5% (0.91)	5% (0.91)	7% (1.01)	30% (1.87)	53% (2.04)
Georgia	1,136	3% (1.51)	5% (1.82)	7% (2.17)	35% (4.01)	50% (4.22)
Maryland	869	1% (1.09)	2% (1.39)	1% (1.03)	20% (3.57)	75% (3.89)
North Carolina	1,256	5% (0.88)	5% (0.97)	6% (0.99)	32% (1.98)	53% (2.12)
South Carolina	723	6% (1.77)	6% (1.75)	5% (1.53)	32% (3.34)	51% (3.60)
Virginia	1,085	4% (1.45)	6% (1.80)	4% (1.58)	20% (3.08)	66% (3.64)
West Virginia	338	7% (2.21)	8% (2.35)	11% (2.70)	35% (4.04)	38% (4.11)
EAST SOUTH CENTRAL	2,872	8% (1.15)	7% (1.08)	9% (1.22)	34% (1.99)	41% (2.07)
Alabama	803	8% (2.19)	8% (2.22)	9% (2.27)	36% (3.90)	40% (3.99)
Kentucky	731	7% (2.08)	8% (2.17)	10% (2.43)	32% (3.82)	44% (4.08)
Mississippi	415	11% (2.64)	9% (2.43)	10% (2.54)	35% (4.10)	36% (4.14)
Tennessee	923	8% (2.22)	5% (1.81)	9% (2.35)	35% (3.83)	42% (3.96)
WEST SOUTH CENTRAL	4,562	6% (0.83)	7% (0.87)	7% (0.89)	33% (1.61)	47% (1.72)
Arkansas	431	7% (2.20)	6% (2.01)	9% (2.37)	37% (4.07)	41% (4.14)
Louisiana	704	6% (2.27)	9% (2.69)	8% (2.50)	34% (4.37)	43% (4.57)
Oklahoma	602	5% (1.81)	7% (2.04)	9% (2.36)	31% (3.82)	48% (4.12)
Texas	2,825	6% (1.09)	7% (1.12)	6% (1.12)	32% (2.12)	49% (2.27)

	Number (000s)	< 100% of Poverty	100-149% of Poverty	150-199% of Poverty	200-399% of Poverty	400+% of Poverty
EAST NORTH CENTRAL	**7,651**	**3%** (0.42)	**3%** (0.41)	**6%** (0.57)	**28%** (1.10)	**61%** (1.20)
Illinois	2,028	2% (0.71)	3% (0.74)	5% (1.01)	24% (1.97)	66% (2.19)
Indiana	1,053	4% (1.63)	3% (1.53)	8% (2.30)	33% (4.05)	53% (4.31)
Michigan	1,757	3% (0.80)	2% (0.59)	5% (0.94)	29% (1.98)	61% (2.14)
Ohio	1,933	4% (0.86)	4% (0.83)	6% (1.05)	26% (1.96)	60% (2.18)
Wisconsin	879	1% (0.87)	3% (1.38)	5% (1.82)	31% (3.73)	59% (3.95)
WEST NORTH CENTRAL	**2,978**	**4%** (0.81)	**5%** (0.85)	**5%** (0.91)	**31%** (1.85)	**55%** (2.00)
Iowa	453	4% (1.77)	6% (2.02)	8% (2.41)	32% (4.09)	50% (4.40)
Kansas	430	3% (1.52)	3% (1.32)	4% (1.65)	29% (3.82)	61% (4.11)
Minnesota	701	3% (1.52)	1% (0.97)	4% (1.71)	33% (4.37)	59% (4.56)
Missouri	903	5% (1.97)	8% (2.37)	6% (2.08)	28% (4.02)	54% (4.47)
Nebraska	273	5% (1.74)	5% (1.74)	4% (1.66)	34% (3.95)	53% (4.17)
North Dakota	101	8% (2.39)	5% (1.80)	7% (2.25)	35% (4.12)	44% (4.27)
South Dakota	117	7% (1.98)	8% (2.16)	10% (2.33)	34% (3.75)	42% (3.91)
MOUNTAIN	**2,161**	**5%** (0.85)	**4%** (0.79)	**5%** (0.84)	**31%** (1.82)	**55%** (1.95)
Arizona	623	6% (2.04)	3% (1.49)	4% (1.77)	31% (4.12)	56% (4.41)
Colorado	505	3% (1.79)	4% (1.87)	3% (1.77)	26% (4.31)	64% (4.74)
Idaho	166	4% (1.69)	6% (2.00)	6% (2.09)	39% (4.18)	44% (4.25)
Montana	139	6% (2.08)	5% (1.85)	6% (2.11)	36% (4.12)	46% (4.26)
Nevada	199	5% (1.92)	3% (1.61)	2% (1.35)	31% (4.22)	59% (4.50)
New Mexico	224	9% (2.56)	8% (2.49)	9% (2.63)	32% (4.27)	42% (4.52)
Utah	220	3% (1.70)	4% (2.01)	6% (2.31)	36% (4.72)	50% (4.91)
Wyoming	86	5% (2.07)	4% (1.93)	5% (2.14)	29% (4.47)	57% (4.86)
PACIFIC	**6,255**	**3%** (0.57)	**4%** (0.62)	**5%** (0.70)	**25%** (1.36)	**62%** (1.52)
Alaska	71	6% (2.23)	4% (1.85)	5% (1.99)	32% (4.36)	53% (4.66)
California	4,566	3% (0.68)	4% (0.77)	5% (0.86)	23% (1.60)	64% (1.83)
Hawaii	218	5% (1.88)	3% (1.56)	3% (1.36)	29% (3.88)	60% (4.19)
Oregon	501	4% (1.73)	3% (1.56)	5% (2.00)	33% (4.40)	56% (4.65)
Washington	898	3% (1.49)	4% (1.55)	5% (1.81)	29% (3.83)	59% (4.13)

Source: Three-year merged March CPS, 1989, 1990, and 1991.

TABLE G8
PERSONS UNDER AGE 65 IN SINGLE-PARENT-WITH-CHILDREN FAMILIES:
BY INCOME AS PERCENTAGE OF POVERTY

	Number (000s)	< 100% of Poverty	100-149% of Poverty	150-199% of Poverty	200-399% of Poverty	400+% of Poverty
UNITED STATES	28,004	47% (0.65)	14% (0.45)	10% (0.39)	22% (0.54)	7% (0.34)
NEW ENGLAND	1,223	38% (2.36)	14% (1.67)	8% (1.34)	29% (2.21)	11% (1.53)
Connecticut	292	27% (6.12)	14% (4.81)	7% (3.53)	40% (6.76)	12% (4.42)
Maine	111	48% (6.14)	19% (4.81)	11% (3.87)	16% (4.49)	6% (2.99)
Massachusetts	610	42% (3.01)	13% (2.08)	7% (1.54)	26% (2.68)	12% (1.97)
New Hampshire	89	32% (6.73)	7% (3.75)	13% (4.93)	31% (6.68)	17% (5.47)
Rhode Island	73	44% (7.39)	16% (5.42)	12% (4.91)	24% (6.35)	4% (2.88)
Vermont	47	32% (6.51)	10% (4.15)	11% (4.32)	36% (6.68)	12% (4.52)
MIDDLE ATLANTIC	4,176	44% (1.52)	14% (1.07)	8% (0.85)	24% (1.30)	9% (0.88)
New Jersey	814	39% (2.87)	12% (1.90)	8% (1.57)	28% (2.63)	14% (2.01)
New York	2,218	47% (2.17)	14% (1.53)	9% (1.22)	22% (1.79)	8% (1.20)
Pennsylvania	1,144	44% (2.99)	15% (2.18)	9% (1.70)	25% (2.61)	7% (1.58)
SOUTH ATLANTIC	5,079	47% (1.54)	14% (1.08)	10% (0.93)	21% (1.26)	7% (0.79)
Delaware	82	37% (5.45)	17% (4.21)	10% (3.35)	25% (4.90)	11% (3.56)
District of Columbia	122	45% (4.58)	12% (3.01)	14% (3.21)	19% (3.59)	9% (2.69)
Florida	1,492	47% (2.61)	15% (1.89)	10% (1.60)	23% (2.19)	4% (1.07)
Georgia	834	60% (4.82)	9% (2.83)	7% (2.56)	18% (3.77)	6% (2.26)
Maryland	616	39% (5.22)	14% (3.66)	8% (2.90)	26% (4.71)	13% (3.54)
North Carolina	681	44% (2.87)	19% (2.28)	11% (1.80)	20% (2.30)	5% (1.31)
South Carolina	399	49% (4.84)	17% (3.61)	9% (2.82)	22% (4.01)	3% (1.72)
Virginia	674	42% (4.81)	13% (3.23)	14% (3.42)	18% (3.77)	13% (3.31)
West Virginia	178	58% (5.75)	16% (4.28)	8% (3.17)	14% (4.09)	3% (2.12)
EAST SOUTH CENTRAL	2,031	56% (2.48)	15% (1.80)	9% (1.45)	16% (1.81)	4% (0.99)
Alabama	537	54% (4.96)	12% (3.29)	13% (3.29)	17% (3.70)	4% (1.94)
Kentucky	385	51% (5.66)	18% (4.35)	9% (3.24)	19% (4.45)	3% (1.97)
Mississippi	437	70% (3.83)	13% (2.84)	5% (1.85)	9% (2.44)	2% (1.13)
Tennessee	671	50% (4.71)	17% (3.56)	10% (2.77)	17% (3.51)	6% (2.26)
WEST SOUTH CENTRAL	3,090	55% (2.08)	12% (1.35)	11% (1.31)	18% (1.61)	4% (0.84)
Arkansas	343	55% (4.70)	14% (3.28)	13% (3.17)	14% (3.27)	4% (1.79)
Louisiana	613	73% (4.41)	7% (2.51)	6% (2.28)	12% (3.22)	3% (1.61)
Oklahoma	312	53% (5.72)	13% (3.87)	12% (3.74)	19% (4.47)	3% (1.88)
Texas	1,822	49% (2.83)	13% (1.90)	12% (1.85)	21% (2.30)	5% (1.24)

TABLE G8 (continued)
PERSONS UNDER AGE 65 IN SINGLE-PARENT-WITH-CHILDREN FAMILIES:
BY INCOME AS PERCENTAGE OF POVERTY

	Number (000s)	<100% of Poverty	100-149% of Poverty	150-199% of Poverty	200-399% of Poverty	400+% of Poverty
EAST NORTH CENTRAL	**4,991**	**50%** (1.52)	**13%** (1.01)	**10%** (0.89)	**21%** (1.25)	**6%** (0.75)
Illinois	1,511	53% (2.67)	11% (1.66)	10% (1.57)	20% (2.13)	7% (1.35)
Indiana	654	49% (5.48)	16% (4.05)	11% (3.38)	22% (4.52)	2% (1.66)
Michigan	1,194	51% (2.66)	13% (1.79)	8% (1.44)	20% (2.12)	8% (1.43)
Ohio	1,217	49% (2.81)	13% (1.89)	9% (1.59)	23% (2.35)	6% (1.36)
Wisconsin	416	37% (5.64)	12% (3.78)	15% (4.21)	28% (5.27)	8% (3.15)
WEST NORTH CENTRAL	**1,675**	**44%** (2.66)	**14%** (1.87)	**14%** (1.86)	**23%** (2.24)	**5%** (1.17)
Iowa	228	42% (6.13)	11% (3.87)	16% (4.55)	28% (5.57)	4% (2.29)
Kansas	247	48% (5.56)	15% (3.96)	10% (3.32)	23% (4.66)	5% (2.40)
Minnesota	453	44% (5.72)	12% (3.74)	12% (3.75)	29% (5.22)	4% (2.22)
Missouri	513	44% (5.92)	19% (4.65)	15% (4.28)	16% (4.32)	6% (2.80)
Nebraska	122	39% (6.08)	10% (3.75)	21% (5.05)	22% (5.20)	8% (3.28)
North Dakota	42	42% (6.58)	10% (4.08)	14% (4.59)	25% (5.77)	9% (3.76)
South Dakota	70	50% (5.12)	14% (3.54)	14% (3.53)	17% (3.89)	5% (2.25)
MOUNTAIN	**1,460**	**46%** (2.38)	**13%** (1.63)	**9%** (1.37)	**24%** (2.04)	**7%** (1.25)
Arizona	379	54% (5.67)	11% (3.49)	8% (3.00)	21% (4.67)	7% (2.85)
Colorado	415	43% (5.39)	14% (3.74)	9% (3.09)	23% (4.58)	11% (3.46)
Idaho	84	38% (5.83)	16% (4.43)	13% (4.06)	29% (5.44)	3% (2.06)
Montana	84	52% (5.49)	15% (3.91)	9% (3.11)	21% (4.46)	3% (2.00)
Nevada	140	37% (5.29)	12% (3.53)	11% (3.47)	32% (5.12)	8% (2.94)
New Mexico	163	47% (5.36)	14% (3.75)	11% (3.29)	23% (4.51)	5% (2.28)
Utah	151	45% (5.90)	18% (4.59)	7% (3.03)	24% (5.06)	5% (2.66)
Wyoming	43	38% (6.75)	12% (4.56)	10% (4.17)	31% (6.44)	9% (3.95)
PACIFIC	**4,279**	**42%** (1.88)	**14%** (1.32)	**9%** (1.09)	**25%** (1.65)	**10%** (1.16)
Alaska	55	47% (5.27)	14% (3.62)	13% (3.55)	19% (4.11)	8% (2.79)
California	3,359	43% (2.20)	14% (1.53)	8% (1.24)	24% (1.90)	11% (1.38)
Hawaii	88	46% (6.71)	17% (5.11)	7% (3.40)	22% (5.54)	8% (3.69)
Oregon	286	45% (6.17)	16% (4.50)	10% (3.71)	23% (5.24)	6% (2.99)
Washington	491	32% (5.28)	14% (3.97)	12% (3.63)	32% (5.32)	10% (3.45)

Source: Three-year merged March CPS, 1989, 1990, and 1991.

TABLE G9
PERSONS UNDER AGE 65 IN SINGLE-PERSON FAMILIES:
BY INCOME AS PERCENTAGE OF POVERTY

	Number (000s)	< 100% of Poverty	100-149% of Poverty	150-199% of Poverty	200-399% of Poverty	400+% of Poverty
UNITED STATES	35,327	17% (0.44)	9% (0.34)	9% (0.34)	33% (0.54)	31% (0.54)
NEW ENGLAND	2,018	12% (1.21)	6% (0.92)	7% (0.94)	33% (1.79)	42% (1.87)
Connecticut	473	8% (2.86)	5% (2.27)	6% (2.48)	32% (5.04)	51% (5.42)
Maine	157	19% (4.08)	11% (3.18)	10% (3.09)	39% (5.06)	21% (4.26)
Massachusetts	998	12% (1.54)	6% (1.16)	6% (1.11)	32% (2.23)	44% (2.37)
New Hampshire	145	11% (3.50)	4% (2.19)	6% (2.67)	37% (5.49)	43% (5.61)
Rhode Island	152	15% (3.64)	6% (2.53)	9% (2.98)	34% (4.90)	35% (4.93)
Vermont	93	15% (3.55)	10% (2.96)	12% (3.16)	39% (4.82)	25% (4.26)
MIDDLE ATLANTIC	5,224	15% (0.98)	8% (0.74)	8% (0.76)	32% (1.27)	37% (1.32)
New Jersey	1,043	12% (1.68)	6% (1.26)	7% (1.31)	31% (2.40)	44% (2.58)
New York	2,779	18% (1.48)	8% (1.06)	8% (1.06)	30% (1.77)	37% (1.87)
Pennsylvania	1,403	13% (1.84)	9% (1.54)	10% (1.65)	36% (2.62)	32% (2.54)
SOUTH ATLANTIC	6,382	18% (1.05)	9% (0.80)	9% (0.80)	34% (1.30)	30% (1.26)
Delaware	117	10% (2.86)	8% (2.62)	9% (2.65)	39% (4.62)	34% (4.47)
District of Columbia	194	15% (2.58)	6% (1.79)	8% (1.96)	31% (3.37)	40% (3.58)
Florida	1,914	17% (1.73)	9% (1.31)	9% (1.35)	37% (2.23)	28% (2.07)
Georgia	937	21% (3.78)	9% (2.68)	10% (2.83)	32% (4.32)	28% (4.16)
Maryland	838	14% (3.22)	7% (2.30)	8% (2.42)	31% (4.25)	40% (4.48)
North Carolina	945	19% (1.92)	12% (1.57)	11% (1.53)	37% (2.36)	22% (2.02)
South Carolina	394	27% (4.32)	13% (3.24)	8% (2.65)	29% (4.43)	23% (4.13)
Virginia	859	14% (3.03)	10% (2.60)	8% (2.30)	32% (4.04)	36% (4.13)
West Virginia	184	25% (4.99)	10% (3.49)	15% (4.08)	31% (5.32)	18% (4.44)
EAST SOUTH CENTRAL	1,822	28% (2.36)	13% (1.74)	10% (1.59)	31% (2.43)	19% (2.07)
Alabama	489	33% (4.92)	11% (3.27)	10% (3.09)	29% (4.75)	16% (3.85)
Kentucky	420	26% (4.76)	8% (2.99)	12% (3.48)	33% (5.09)	21% (4.44)
Mississippi	332	28% (4.34)	15% (3.48)	13% (3.27)	30% (4.39)	13% (3.28)
Tennessee	581	24% (4.32)	15% (3.62)	7% (2.65)	31% (4.66)	23% (4.26)
WEST SOUTH CENTRAL	3,472	23% (1.67)	10% (1.19)	11% (1.24)	31% (1.82)	24% (1.70)
Arkansas	292	31% (4.76)	13% (3.49)	10% (3.01)	31% (4.72)	15% (3.67)
Louisiana	512	31% (4.99)	9% (3.14)	12% (3.55)	29% (4.91)	19% (4.26)
Oklahoma	376	25% (4.49)	8% (2.88)	12% (3.36)	29% (4.74)	26% (4.59)
Texas	2,291	20% (2.03)	10% (1.54)	11% (1.59)	32% (2.35)	27% (2.23)

PERSONS UNDER AGE 65 IN SINGLE-PERSON FAMILIES: BY INCOME AS PERCENTAGE OF POVERTY

	Number (000s)	< 100% of Poverty	100-149% of Poverty	150-199% of Poverty	200-399% of Poverty	400+% of Poverty
EAST NORTH CENTRAL	**5,696**	**18%** (1.09)	**8%** (0.77)	**9%** (0.82)	**33%** (1.34)	**32%** (1.32)
Illinois	1,696	16% (1.84)	7% (1.27)	8% (1.34)	35% (2.40)	35% (2.40)
Indiana	673	16% (4.00)	10% (3.20)	10% (3.24)	32% (5.03)	32% (5.04)
Michigan	1,301	22% (2.10)	8% (1.35)	8% (1.41)	30% (2.35)	32% (2.38)
Ohio	1,406	19% (2.03)	9% (1.48)	10% (1.56)	34% (2.47)	29% (2.37)
Wisconsin	620	15% (3.40)	9% (2.67)	12% (3.13)	35% (4.58)	29% (4.36)
WEST NORTH CENTRAL	**2,313**	**16%** (1.66)	**10%** (1.35)	**11%** (1.45)	**36%** (2.19)	**27%** (2.02)
Iowa	367	18% (3.77)	11% (3.02)	12% (3.17)	38% (4.76)	21% (3.98)
Kansas	305	15% (3.62)	12% (3.30)	13% (3.40)	34% (4.75)	25% (4.33)
Minnesota	635	12% (3.17)	8% (2.62)	10% (2.89)	37% (4.70)	34% (4.61)
Missouri	650	15% (3.82)	9% (3.10)	11% (3.26)	37% (5.12)	27% (4.70)
Nebraska	206	18% (3.71)	11% (2.98)	13% (3.22)	34% (4.55)	24% (4.10)
North Dakota	72	24% (4.37)	9% (2.97)	15% (3.64)	34% (4.84)	17% (3.84)
South Dakota	79	24% (4.11)	12% (3.09)	13% (3.20)	34% (4.56)	19% (3.77)
MOUNTAIN	**1,870**	**17%** (1.58)	**11%** (1.31)	**10%** (1.28)	**34%** (1.99)	**28%** (1.90)
Arizona	537	16% (3.54)	10% (2.83)	11% (3.00)	32% (4.46)	31% (4.40)
Colorado	497	14% (3.49)	10% (2.98)	8% (2.71)	33% (4.69)	34% (4.72)
Idaho	116	22% (4.25)	18% (3.93)	13% (3.40)	29% (4.63)	18% (3.93)
Montana	101	22% (4.16)	15% (3.60)	9% (2.89)	36% (4.82)	17% (3.81)
Nevada	222	13% (2.91)	8% (2.32)	12% (2.80)	39% (4.23)	28% (3.92)
New Mexico	190	24% (4.28)	10% (2.96)	12% (3.27)	32% (4.63)	22% (4.09)
Utah	157	16% (4.24)	13% (3.97)	8% (3.19)	36% (5.58)	27% (5.14)
Wyoming	49	19% (5.15)	15% (4.68)	10% (3.93)	31% (6.07)	24% (5.60)
PACIFIC	**6,530**	**14%** (1.06)	**11%** (0.95)	**9%** (0.88)	**31%** (1.43)	**35%** (1.47)
Alaska	81	19% (3.39)	14% (3.06)	8% (2.34)	31% (4.02)	29% (3.94)
California	5,101	13% (1.20)	11% (1.14)	9% (1.01)	30% (1.66)	37% (1.74)
Hawaii	153	16% (3.72)	8% (2.76)	12% (3.33)	35% (4.87)	29% (4.63)
Oregon	422	21% (4.19)	8% (2.81)	11% (3.13)	32% (4.75)	28% (4.58)
Washington	773	16% (3.35)	8% (2.48)	10% (2.77)	38% (4.40)	27% (4.02)

Source: Three-year merged March CPS, 1989, 1990, and 1991.

TABLE G10
ADULTS AGES 18-64: BY LABOR FORCE STATUS

	Adults Ages 18-64 (000s)	Labor Force Participation Rate	Employment Rate	Adults Ages 18-64 in Labor Force (000s)	Unemployment Rate in Labor Force
UNITED STATES	150,318	77% (0.12)	73% (0.13)	116,464	6% (0.07)
NEW ENGLAND	8,163	81% (0.38)	76% (0.41)	6,637	6% (0.25)
Connecticut	2,022	84% (1.01)	79% (1.10)	1,688	5% (0.64)
Maine	747	78% (1.01)	73% (1.09)	585	6% (0.66)
Massachusetts	3,731	80% (0.51)	75% (0.55)	2,996	6% (0.34)
New Hampshire	701	84% (0.99)	79% (1.08)	587	5% (0.62)
Rhode Island	607	80% (1.07)	74% (1.17)	485	7% (0.75)
Vermont	355	83% (0.98)	79% (1.07)	296	5% (0.62)
MIDDLE ATLANTIC	23,262	75% (0.29)	71% (0.30)	17,491	5% (0.17)
New Jersey	4,855	79% (0.51)	75% (0.54)	3,847	5% (0.30)
New York	11,077	73% (0.45)	69% (0.47)	8,089	5% (0.26)
Pennsylvania	7,330	76% (0.53)	72% (0.56)	5,555	5% (0.31)
SOUTH ATLANTIC	25,967	78% (0.29)	75% (0.31)	20,382	5% (0.16)
Delaware	417	81% (1.02)	77% (1.09)	337	5% (0.59)
District of Columbia	369	79% (1.12)	75% (1.19)	291	5% (0.68)
Florida	7,518	78% (0.50)	74% (0.53)	5,850	5% (0.29)
Georgia	3,865	78% (0.98)	74% (1.04)	3,020	5% (0.58)
Maryland	2,936	82% (0.97)	79% (1.04)	2,407	4% (0.53)
North Carolina	3,998	79% (0.50)	76% (0.52)	3,176	4% (0.26)
South Carolina	2,087	78% (0.91)	75% (0.95)	1,628	4% (0.48)
Virginia	3,669	80% (0.87)	76% (0.92)	2,931	4% (0.48)
West Virginia	1,110	67% (1.14)	61% (1.18)	742	8% (0.80)
EAST SOUTH CENTRAL	9,213	73% (0.54)	69% (0.56)	6,766	6% (0.33)
Alabama	2,469	72% (1.07)	68% (1.12)	1,787	7% (0.68)
Kentucky	2,233	74% (1.07)	70% (1.12)	1,655	6% (0.65)
Mississippi	1,513	73% (1.04)	67% (1.10)	1,102	8% (0.72)
Tennessee	2,997	74% (1.01)	70% (1.05)	2,221	5% (0.58)
WEST SOUTH CENTRAL	15,962	76% (0.41)	71% (0.43)	12,107	6% (0.26)
Arkansas	1,410	76% (1.03)	70% (1.11)	1,075	8% (0.74)
Louisiana	2,528	69% (1.17)	65% (1.21)	1,744	6% (0.72)
Oklahoma	1,882	76% (1.04)	71% (1.10)	1,423	6% (0.64)
Texas	10,142	78% (0.52)	73% (0.55)	7,866	6% (0.33)

	Adults Ages 18-64 (000s)	Labor Force Participation Rate	Employment Rate	Adults Ages 18-64 in Labor Force (000s)	Unemployment Rate in Labor Force
EAST NORTH CENTRAL	**25,836**	**78%** **(0.29)**	**73%** **(0.31)**	**20,139**	**7%** **(0.19)**
Illinois	7,174	78% (0.52)	73% (0.56)	5,604	6% (0.34)
Indiana	3,391	79% (1.02)	74% (1.09)	2,677	6% (0.67)
Michigan	5,755	75% (0.54)	69% (0.58)	4,310	8% (0.38)
Ohio	6,617	77% (0.52)	72% (0.56)	5,110	6% (0.34)
Wisconsin	2,898	84% (0.84)	79% (0.93)	2,439	6% (0.57)
WEST NORTH CENTRAL	**10,548**	**82%** **(0.42)**	**78%** **(0.46)**	**8,680**	**5%** **(0.26)**
Iowa	1,655	83% (0.90)	79% (0.97)	1,372	5% (0.53)
Kansas	1,444	82% (0.91)	79% (0.97)	1,190	4% (0.51)
Minnesota	2,657	85% (0.89)	80% (0.99)	2,250	6% (0.61)
Missouri	3,100	80% (1.01)	76% (1.07)	2,474	5% (0.60)
Nebraska	927	83% (0.88)	80% (0.93)	769	3% (0.44)
North Dakota	366	82% (0.90)	78% (0.98)	299	5% (0.56)
South Dakota	399	82% (0.86)	78% (0.92)	325	5% (0.50)
MOUNTAIN	**7,871**	**79%** **(0.43)**	**74%** **(0.46)**	**6,205**	**6%** **(0.27)**
Arizona	2,078	78% (1.04)	74% (1.10)	1,618	5% (0.60)
Colorado	1,938	81% (1.02)	77% (1.10)	1,570	5% (0.62)
Idaho	582	79% (0.95)	75% (1.03)	463	6% (0.61)
Montana	480	80% (0.96)	74% (1.05)	383	7% (0.68)
Nevada	725	82% (0.96)	78% (1.03)	595	5% (0.59)
New Mexico	878	72% (1.07)	67% (1.12)	634	7% (0.69)
Utah	909	79% (1.02)	75% (1.08)	720	5% (0.60)
Wyoming	281	79% (1.14)	74% (1.24)	222	7% (0.78)
PACIFIC	**23,495**	**77%** **(0.36)**	**73%** **(0.38)**	**18,059**	**6%** **(0.22)**
Alaska	295	77% (1.00)	71% (1.07)	227	7% (0.69)
California	17,870	76% (0.43)	72% (0.45)	13,650	6% (0.26)
Hawaii	626	78% (1.07)	76% (1.11)	491	3% (0.47)
Oregon	1,714	79% (1.08)	74% (1.15)	1,346	6% (0.69)
Washington	2,990	78% (0.98)	74% (1.05)	2,344	6% (0.62)

Source: Three-year merged March CPS, 1989, 1990, and 1991.

TABLE G11
WORKERS AGES 18-64: BY FIRM SIZE

	Number (000s)	< 25 Workers	25-99 Workers	100-499 Workers	500+ Workers
UNITED STATES	122,769	29% (0.15)	13% (0.11)	14% (0.11)	43% (0.16)
NEW ENGLAND	7,003	29% (0.48)	14% (0.36)	17% (0.39)	41% (0.52)
Connecticut	1,783	27% (1.29)	14% (1.00)	16% (1.06)	43% (1.43)
Maine	622	33% (1.27)	16% (0.98)	16% (0.98)	35% (1.29)
Massachusetts	3,165	27% (0.61)	14% (0.47)	17% (0.52)	42% (0.69)
New Hampshire	614	32% (1.33)	14% (0.98)	15% (1.02)	40% (1.39)
Rhode Island	506	28% (1.32)	15% (1.05)	17% (1.09)	40% (1.43)
Vermont	312	40% (1.37)	13% (0.95)	16% (1.02)	31% (1.29)
MIDDLE ATLANTIC	18,444	27% (0.34)	14% (0.26)	16% (0.28)	42% (0.37)
New Jersey	4,027	27% (0.61)	14% (0.48)	17% (0.51)	42% (0.68)
New York	8,528	28% (0.52)	14% (0.40)	15% (0.42)	43% (0.57)
Pennsylvania	5,889	26% (0.61)	14% (0.48)	18% (0.52)	42% (0.68)
SOUTH ATLANTIC	21,401	28% (0.35)	12% (0.25)	12% (0.26)	48% (0.39)
Delaware	356	25% (1.21)	11% (0.87)	13% (0.93)	52% (1.40)
District of Columbia	302	22% (1.25)	12% (0.98)	13% (1.02)	54% (1.51)
Florida	6,122	33% (0.63)	13% (0.45)	11% (0.41)	43% (0.66)
Georgia	3,168	27% (1.15)	11% (0.82)	13% (0.88)	49% (1.31)
Maryland	2,513	25% (1.19)	12% (0.90)	11% (0.87)	51% (1.37)
North Carolina	3,354	26% (0.59)	12% (0.44)	14% (0.47)	48% (0.67)
South Carolina	1,697	26% (1.06)	12% (0.78)	14% (0.85)	49% (1.22)
Virginia	3,102	26% (1.03)	11% (0.73)	13% (0.78)	51% (1.18)
West Virginia	787	32% (1.34)	13% (0.98)	12% (0.95)	42% (1.42)
EAST SOUTH CENTRAL	7,097	28% (0.62)	11% (0.44)	14% (0.48)	47% (0.69)
Alabama	1,852	27% (1.24)	12% (0.89)	13% (0.94)	48% (1.39)
Kentucky	1,722	31% (1.28)	11% (0.86)	14% (0.97)	44% (1.38)
Mississippi	1,164	29% (1.21)	11% (0.83)	15% (0.96)	45% (1.32)
Tennessee	2,359	25% (1.13)	12% (0.84)	14% (0.90)	49% (1.30)
WEST SOUTH CENTRAL	12,767	31% (0.49)	12% (0.34)	12% (0.35)	44% (0.53)
Arkansas	1,140	33% (1.26)	12% (0.87)	14% (0.94)	41% (1.32)
Louisiana	1,826	32% (1.38)	13% (1.01)	11% (0.92)	44% (1.48)
Oklahoma	1,522	32% (1.25)	13% (0.91)	12% (0.87)	43% (1.33)
Texas	8,278	31% (0.64)	11% (0.43)	13% (0.46)	45% (0.69)

	Number (000s)	< 25 Workers	25-99 Workers	100-499 Workers	500+ Workers
EAST NORTH CENTRAL	**21,194**	**26%** **(0.34)**	**14%** **(0.27)**	**16%** **(0.28)**	**44%** **(0.38)**
Illinois	5,825	26% (0.62)	14% (0.49)	17% (0.53)	43% (0.70)
Indiana	2,847	26% (1.19)	14% (0.95)	16% (0.99)	44% (1.35)
Michigan	4,556	28% (0.63)	13% (0.48)	14% (0.49)	45% (0.70)
Ohio	5,398	25% (0.60)	14% (0.47)	16% (0.51)	45% (0.69)
Wisconsin	2,568	29% (1.10)	15% (0.88)	17% (0.93)	39% (1.19)
WEST NORTH CENTRAL	**9,236**	**32%** **(0.55)**	**14%** **(0.41)**	**14%** **(0.41)**	**39%** **(0.58)**
Iowa	1,456	33% (1.19)	15% (0.90)	15% (0.91)	38% (1.23)
Kansas	1,270	33% (1.19)	15% (0.91)	12% (0.83)	40% (1.25)
Minnesota	2,395	33% (1.22)	15% (0.92)	14% (0.91)	38% (1.26)
Missouri	2,633	28% (1.23)	13% (0.92)	14% (0.95)	45% (1.35)
Nebraska	811	35% (1.19)	14% (0.87)	15% (0.91)	36% (1.20)
North Dakota	322	44% (1.24)	14% (0.88)	12% (0.82)	30% (1.14)
South Dakota	350	43% (1.17)	16% (0.86)	13% (0.81)	28% (1.07)
MOUNTAIN	**6,585**	**33%** **(0.55)**	**12%** **(0.38)**	**12%** **(0.37)**	**43%** **(0.58)**
Arizona	1,695	32% (1.30)	13% (0.94)	12% (0.91)	43% (1.38)
Colorado	1,651	30% (1.30)	10% (0.85)	13% (0.95)	47% (1.41)
Idaho	508	39% (1.23)	14% (0.87)	12% (0.81)	36% (1.21)
Montana	413	45% (1.28)	13% (0.88)	11% (0.79)	30% (1.19)
Nevada	617	27% (1.20)	14% (0.92)	11% (0.84)	49% (1.35)
New Mexico	693	38% (1.31)	12% (0.88)	10% (0.80)	40% (1.32)
Utah	766	31% (1.26)	10% (0.83)	10% (0.80)	49% (1.36)
Wyoming	242	40% (1.48)	11% (0.96)	13% (1.03)	35% (1.45)
PACIFIC	**19,042**	**33%** **(0.44)**	**14%** **(0.33)**	**13%** **(0.32)**	**40%** **(0.46)**
Alaska	249	36% (1.24)	11% (0.82)	12% (0.85)	40% (1.27)
California	14,320	33% (0.53)	14% (0.39)	13% (0.37)	40% (0.55)
Hawaii	514	27% (1.28)	14% (1.01)	13% (0.98)	45% (1.43)
Oregon	1,439	34% (1.35)	13% (0.95)	17% (1.08)	36% (1.38)
Washington	2,520	31% (1.21)	13% (0.88)	13% (0.87)	42% (1.28)

Source: Three-year merged March CPS, 1989, 1990, and 1991.

TABLE G12
WORKERS AGES 18-64: BY SECTOR

	Number (000s)	Private	Government	Self-Employed
UNITED STATES	122,769	75% (0.14)	15% (0.12)	10% (0.10)
NEW ENGLAND	7,003	77% (0.44)	13% (0.36)	10% (0.31)
Connecticut	1,783	78% (1.19)	13% (0.96)	9% (0.81)
Maine	622	71% (1.22)	15% (0.96)	14% (0.93)
Massachusetts	3,165	78% (0.58)	14% (0.48)	9% (0.39)
New Hampshire	614	78% (1.18)	10% (0.86)	11% (0.90)
Rhode Island	506	79% (1.19)	12% (0.95)	9% (0.82)
Vermont	312	70% (1.28)	15% (0.99)	14% (0.98)
MIDDLE ATLANTIC	18,444	76% (0.32)	15% (0.27)	9% (0.21)
New Jersey	4,027	77% (0.58)	14% (0.48)	9% (0.39)
New York	8,528	73% (0.51)	17% (0.44)	9% (0.33)
Pennsylvania	5,889	79% (0.56)	12% (0.45)	8% (0.38)
SOUTH ATLANTIC	21,401	74% (0.34)	17% (0.29)	9% (0.23)
Delaware	356	78% (1.17)	14% (0.97)	8% (0.78)
District of Columbia	302	61% (1.47)	32% (1.41)	7% (0.75)
Florida	6,122	73% (0.59)	15% (0.48)	12% (0.43)
Georgia	3,168	78% (1.09)	15% (0.93)	8% (0.69)
Maryland	2,513	70% (1.26)	22% (1.14)	8% (0.74)
North Carolina	3,354	77% (0.57)	14% (0.47)	9% (0.38)
South Carolina	1,697	76% (1.03)	15% (0.88)	8% (0.66)
Virginia	3,102	71% (1.07)	20% (0.95)	8% (0.66)
West Virginia	787	75% (1.25)	16% (1.05)	9% (0.81)
EAST SOUTH CENTRAL	7,097	75% (0.60)	16% (0.50)	9% (0.40)
Alabama	1,852	73% (1.23)	17% (1.05)	9% (0.80)
Kentucky	1,722	75% (1.20)	14% (0.97)	10% (0.84)
Mississippi	1,164	74% (1.17)	16% (0.98)	10% (0.79)
Tennessee	2,359	76% (1.11)	15% (0.93)	9% (0.74)
WEST SOUTH CENTRAL	12,767	73% (0.47)	15% (0.39)	11% (0.33)
Arkansas	1,140	72% (1.20)	14% (0.95)	12% (0.88)
Louisiana	1,826	73% (1.32)	16% (1.10)	10% (0.90)
Oklahoma	1,522	68% (1.25)	18% (1.04)	13% (0.89)
Texas	8,278	75% (0.60)	15% (0.49)	10% (0.42)

	Number (000s)	Private	Government	Self-Employed
EAST NORTH CENTRAL	**21,194**	**77%** **(0.32)**	**14%** **(0.26)**	**8%** **(0.21)**
Illinois	5,825	78% (0.58)	13% (0.48)	8% (0.39)
Indiana	2,847	80% (1.09)	12% (0.89)	7% (0.70)
Michigan	4,556	77% (0.59)	14% (0.49)	9% (0.40)
Ohio	5,398	77% (0.58)	14% (0.49)	8% (0.38)
Wisconsin	2,568	74% (1.07)	15% (0.87)	10% (0.74)
WEST NORTH CENTRAL	**9,236**	**72%** **(0.53)**	**15%** **(0.42)**	**12%** **(0.39)**
Iowa	1,456	70% (1.17)	16% (0.93)	14% (0.88)
Kansas	1,270	71% (1.16)	16% (0.94)	12% (0.84)
Minnesota	2,395	74% (1.13)	13% (0.87)	12% (0.85)
Missouri	2,633	77% (1.15)	13% (0.93)	10% (0.81)
Nebraska	811	68% (1.17)	17% (0.94)	15% (0.90)
North Dakota	322	61% (1.22)	20% (1.01)	18% (0.95)
South Dakota	350	62% (1.15)	18% (0.91)	19% (0.94)
MOUNTAIN	**6,585**	**71%** **(0.53)**	**17%** **(0.43)**	**12%** **(0.38)**
Arizona	1,695	75% (1.20)	13% (0.93)	12% (0.89)
Colorado	1,651	71% (1.28)	17% (1.07)	11% (0.90)
Idaho	508	69% (1.17)	16% (0.93)	14% (0.87)
Montana	413	62% (1.25)	21% (1.04)	17% (0.96)
Nevada	617	80% (1.09)	12% (0.88)	8% (0.74)
New Mexico	693	63% (1.30)	22% (1.12)	14% (0.94)
Utah	766	69% (1.27)	19% (1.07)	12% (0.88)
Wyoming	242	63% (1.47)	22% (1.26)	15% (1.07)
PACIFIC	**19,042**	**73%** **(0.42)**	**15%** **(0.33)**	**12%** **(0.30)**
Alaska	249	59% (1.27)	28% (1.16)	13% (0.87)
California	14,320	74% (0.49)	14% (0.39)	12% (0.36)
Hawaii	514	69% (1.33)	21% (1.17)	10% (0.85)
Oregon	1,439	71% (1.29)	15% (1.03)	13% (0.96)
Washington	2,520	71% (1.17)	17% (0.97)	12% (0.84)

Source: Three-year merged March CPS, 1989, 1990, and 1991.

TABLE G13
PRIVATE-SECTOR WORKERS AGES 18-64: BY INDUSTRY

	Number (000s)	Manufacturing	Wholesale/ Retail	Services	Other
UNITED STATES	91,950	24% (0.16)	25% (0.16)	28% (0.17)	24% (0.16)
NEW ENGLAND	5,416	26% (0.53)	21% (0.49)	30% (0.55)	23% (0.50)
Connecticut	1,403	29% (1.48)	19% (1.28)	28% (1.47)	24% (1.39)
Maine	445	25% (1.38)	26% (1.39)	27% (1.42)	22% (1.32)
Massachusetts	2,463	24% (0.67)	21% (0.64)	32% (0.73)	22% (0.65)
New Hampshire	482	31% (1.49)	23% (1.35)	23% (1.36)	23% (1.35)
Rhode Island	401	29% (1.49)	24% (1.39)	27% (1.45)	21% (1.34)
Vermont	221	21% (1.36)	22% (1.38)	32% (1.55)	25% (1.45)
MIDDLE ATLANTIC	14,039	23% (0.36)	23% (0.36)	30% (0.40)	25% (0.37)
New Jersey	3,097	24% (0.66)	22% (0.65)	29% (0.71)	26% (0.68)
New York	6,264	20% (0.54)	23% (0.57)	31% (0.62)	25% (0.58)
Pennsylvania	4,678	25% (0.67)	22% (0.64)	29% (0.70)	23% (0.66)
SOUTH ATLANTIC	15,852	22% (0.38)	25% (0.39)	27% (0.40)	26% (0.40)
Delaware	277	25% (1.38)	21% (1.30)	27% (1.42)	27% (1.40)
District of Columbia	185	5% (0.87)	19% (1.53)	53% (1.93)	22% (1.61)
Florida	4,495	14% (0.54)	28% (0.70)	30% (0.71)	29% (0.71)
Georgia	2,462	24% (1.26)	27% (1.31)	25% (1.28)	25% (1.28)
Maryland	1,757	15% (1.18)	23% (1.37)	35% (1.57)	26% (1.44)
North Carolina	2,578	36% (0.74)	22% (0.64)	21% (0.62)	21% (0.63)
South Carolina	1,300	35% (1.33)	20% (1.12)	23% (1.16)	22% (1.15)
Virginia	2,204	22% (1.15)	25% (1.20)	28% (1.25)	26% (1.23)
West Virginia	594	19% (1.30)	27% (1.47)	24% (1.41)	30% (1.51)
EAST SOUTH CENTRAL	5,323	31% (0.74)	24% (0.69)	22% (0.67)	22% (0.67)
Alabama	1,363	31% (1.49)	26% (1.41)	22% (1.34)	21% (1.32)
Kentucky	1,301	27% (1.42)	26% (1.40)	23% (1.34)	24% (1.37)
Mississippi	861	30% (1.43)	25% (1.35)	21% (1.26)	23% (1.31)
Tennessee	1,798	34% (1.41)	22% (1.22)	23% (1.25)	22% (1.23)
WEST SOUTH CENTRAL	9,434	19% (0.49)	26% (0.54)	28% (0.55)	27% (0.55)
Arkansas	834	28% (1.41)	27% (1.39)	22% (1.29)	23% (1.33)
Louisiana	1,341	13% (1.17)	27% (1.54)	30% (1.59)	30% (1.59)
Oklahoma	1,050	20% (1.30)	24% (1.38)	27% (1.44)	29% (1.46)
Texas	6,209	19% (0.63)	25% (0.69)	28% (0.71)	27% (0.71)

	Number (000s)	Manufacturing	Wholesale/ Retail	Services	Other
EAST NORTH CENTRAL	**16,468**	**29%** **(0.39)**	**24%** **(0.37)**	**26%** **(0.38)**	**21%** **(0.35)**
Illinois	4,566	24% (0.68)	25% (0.69)	27% (0.71)	24% (0.68)
Indiana	2,296	32% (1.41)	24% (1.30)	24% (1.28)	21% (1.23)
Michigan	3,520	31% (0.74)	25% (0.70)	25% (0.70)	18% (0.62)
Ohio	4,169	29% (0.71)	24% (0.67)	26% (0.69)	20% (0.63)
Wisconsin	1,919	32% (1.32)	23% (1.19)	25% (1.21)	20% (1.12)
WEST NORTH CENTRAL	**6,723**	**22%** **(0.57)**	**26%** **(0.61)**	**28%** **(0.62)**	**24%** **(0.59)**
Iowa	1,024	23% (1.29)	27% (1.35)	27% (1.34)	22% (1.27)
Kansas	906	23% (1.27)	26% (1.32)	27% (1.34)	24% (1.28)
Minnesota	1,795	23% (1.26)	25% (1.30)	29% (1.37)	23% (1.26)
Missouri	2,024	23% (1.30)	26% (1.37)	27% (1.38)	24% (1.32)
Nebraska	554	20% (1.21)	27% (1.35)	28% (1.37)	24% (1.30)
North Dakota	200	10% (0.93)	30% (1.45)	31% (1.47)	29% (1.44)
South Dakota	221	17% (1.12)	28% (1.34)	30% (1.37)	25% (1.29)
MOUNTAIN	**4,690**	**16%** **(0.50)**	**27%** **(0.61)**	**29%** **(0.63)**	**28%** **(0.62)**
Arizona	1,279	17% (1.22)	27% (1.43)	29% (1.46)	26% (1.41)
Colorado	1,181	17% (1.27)	25% (1.45)	27% (1.49)	30% (1.54)
Idaho	356	20% (1.21)	29% (1.36)	25% (1.31)	27% (1.34)
Montana	259	9% (0.93)	33% (1.53)	29% (1.48)	28% (1.46)
Nevada	491	7% (0.79)	23% (1.27)	43% (1.50)	27% (1.34)
New Mexico	440	14% (1.16)	30% (1.55)	27% (1.50)	29% (1.54)
Utah	530	20% (1.32)	25% (1.43)	30% (1.50)	24% (1.40)
Wyoming	153	7% (0.99)	28% (1.71)	23% (1.59)	42% (1.88)
PACIFIC	**14,005**	**22%** **(0.45)**	**25%** **(0.47)**	**28%** **(0.49)**	**25%** **(0.47)**
Alaska	146	8% (0.92)	26% (1.47)	31% (1.55)	35% (1.61)
California	10,663	22% (0.54)	25% (0.56)	28% (0.58)	25% (0.56)
Hawaii	358	7% (0.90)	29% (1.56)	33% (1.62)	31% (1.60)
Oregon	1,036	26% (1.49)	25% (1.46)	29% (1.53)	20% (1.35)
Washington	1,801	22% (1.28)	26% (1.35)	28% (1.38)	23% (1.30)

Source: Three-year merged March CPS, 1989, 1990, and 1991.

TABLE G14
NUMBER OF ESTABLISHMENTS: BY ESTABLISHMENT SIZE, 1989

	1-4 Workers	5-9 Workers	10-19 Workers	20-99 Workers	100-499 Workers	500+ Workers
NEW ENGLAND	**203,370**	**75,274**	**46,704**	**40,830**	**7,838**	**995**
Connecticut	51,390	18,793	11,640	10,118	1,997	240
Maine	20,657	7,113	4,142	3,210	504	69
Massachuetts	84,731	33,007	21,030	19,179	3,953	531
New Hampshire	19,112	7,013	4,244	3,464	618	65
Rhode Island	15,591	5,469	3,395	3,137	530	69
Vermont	11,889	3,879	2,253	1,722	236	21
MIDDLE ATLANTIC	**542,955**	**180,819**	**112,073**	**99,683**	**19,424**	**2,791**
New Jersey	121,679	39,621	24,908	22,618	4,662	548
New York	274,032	84,737	51,884	46,159	8,503	1,391
Pennsylvania	147,244	56,461	35,281	30,906	6,259	852
SOUTH ATLANTIC	**584,010**	**223,654**	**135,346**	**118,609**	**21,201**	**2,608**
Delaware	9,630	3,665	2,318	1,996	366	61
District of Columbia	9,786	4,000	2,842	2,724	540	86
Florida	199,774	71,788	41,189	35,570	5,832	576
Georgia	81,644	32,242	19,823	18,139	3,520	418
Maryland	56,677	23,582	15,841	13,638	2,318	264
North Carolina	87,029	33,563	19,618	17,876	3,435	508
South Carolina	42,096	16,411	9,490	8,228	1,617	251
Virginia	76,499	30,658	19,734	16,721	3,013	375
West Virginia	20,875	7,745	4,491	3,717	560	69
EAST SOUTH CENTRAL	**177,450**	**67,658**	**39,916**	**36,211**	**6,867**	**876**
Alabama	45,957	18,025	10,580	9,578	1,718	245
Kentucky	41,938	16,139	9,602	8,728	1,557	177
Mississippi	29,662	10,718	5,926	4,989	989	113
Tennessee	59,893	22,776	13,808	12,916	2,603	341
EAST NORTH CENTRAL	**500,686**	**200,622**	**127,452**	**115,009**	**21,364**	**2,744**
Illinois	141,922	52,609	34,697	31,875	6,271	823
Indiana	64,125	26,870	16,675	15,234	2,861	333
Michigan	106,246	44,030	27,772	24,223	4,109	542
Ohio	125,069	52,413	32,947	29,797	5,520	703
Wisconsin	63,324	24,700	15,361	13,880	2,603	343
WEST SOUTH CENTRAL	**332,734**	**122,319**	**72,486**	**63,823**	**10,970**	**1,306**
Arkansas	30,277	10,434	6,117	4,841	992	138
Louisiana	47,123	18,655	10,869	9,716	1,603	163
Oklahoma	42,186	14,670	8,602	7,297	1,042	117
Texas	213,148	78,560	46,898	41,969	7,333	888
WEST NORTH CENTRAL	**251,608**	**93,148**	**56,642**	**48,426**	**8,215**	**1,025**
Iowa	39,861	15,006	8,805	7,252	1,152	156
Kansas	36,471	13,327	8,047	6,713	1,027	107
Minnesota	57,494	22,484	14,617	12,844	2,358	294
Missouri	70,293	25,580	15,764	14,124	2,571	338
Nebraska	24,174	9,123	5,081	4,182	646	96
North Dakota	11,302	3,769	2,086	1,614	228	16
South Dakota	12,013	3,859	2,242	1,697	233	18
MOUNTAIN	**193,104**	**70,227**	**41,584**	**34,925**	**5,287**	**625**
Arizona	46,181	17,645	10,747	9,619	1,521	164
Colorado	54,758	18,660	10,593	9,410	1,470	164
Idaho	14,458	5,346	3,120	2,261	298	40
Montana	15,132	4,845	2,735	1,851	198	18
Nevada	15,352	5,852	3,702	3,233	514	118
New Mexico	19,934	7,172	4,276	3,484	472	38
Utah	18,518	7,800	4,868	3,906	686	77
Wyoming	8,771	2,907	1,543	1,161	128	6
PACIFIC	**540,071**	**191,128**	**122,267**	**110,485**	**18,013**	**1,956**
Alaska	9,028	2,884	1,638	1,135	188	15
California	400,873	140,666	91,314	85,097	14,238	1,567
Hawaii	14,736	6,006	3,805	3,317	513	66
Oregon	44,332	16,258	9,842	8,076	1,209	117
Washington	71,102	25,314	15,668	12,860	1,865	191
UNITED STATES	**3,325,988**	**1,224,849**	**754,470**	**668,001**	**119,179**	**14,926**

Source: County Business Patterns, 1989.

	Total Workers	1-4 Workers	5-9 Workers	10-19 Workers	20-99 Workers	100-499 Workers	500+ Workers
NEW ENGLAND	**5,925,599**	**6%**	**8%**	**11%**	**28%**	**25%**	**22%**
Connecticut	1,497,491	6%	8%	10%	27%	25%	23%
Maine	438,331	8%	11%	13%	29%	22%	18%
Massachuetts	2,896,456	5%	8%	10%	27%	26%	25%
New Hampshire	464,198	7%	10%	12%	30%	25%	15%
Rhode Island	409,914	7%	9%	11%	31%	24%	19%
Vermont	219,209	9%	12%	14%	31%	21%	14%
MIDDLE ATLANTIC	**14,885,173**	**6%**	**8%**	**10%**	**27%**	**25%**	**24%**
New Jersey	3,248,244	6%	8%	10%	28%	27%	20%
New York	7,097,310	7%	8%	10%	26%	23%	27%
Pennsylvania	4,539,619	6%	8%	10%	28%	26%	22%
SOUTH ATLANTIC	**16,018,642**	**6%**	**9%**	**11%**	**30%**	**25%**	**19%**
Delaware	301,759	5%	8%	10%	26%	23%	27%
District of Columbia	427,179	4%	6%	9%	26%	25%	29%
Florida	4,499,372	8%	10%	12%	32%	23%	15%
Georgia	2,468,390	6%	9%	11%	30%	27%	18%
Maryland	1,771,672	6%	9%	12%	31%	24%	18%
North Carolina	2,596,312	6%	8%	10%	28%	26%	21%
South Carolina	1,219,341	6%	9%	10%	27%	26%	21%
Virginia	2,266,834	6%	9%	12%	30%	25%	19%
West Virginia	467,783	8%	11%	13%	31%	22%	15%
EAST SOUTH CENTRAL	**4,990,734**	**6%**	**9%**	**11%**	**29%**	**26%**	**19%**
Alabama	1,301,249	6%	9%	11%	29%	25%	19%
Kentucky	1,154,424	7%	9%	11%	30%	26%	17%
Mississippi	705,690	8%	10%	11%	28%	27%	16%
Tennessee	1,829,371	6%	8%	10%	28%	27%	21%
EAST NORTH CENTRAL	**16,077,166**	**6%**	**8%**	**11%**	**29%**	**25%**	**22%**
Illinois	4,535,494	5%	8%	10%	29%	26%	22%
Indiana	2,108,821	6%	8%	11%	29%	25%	21%
Michigan	3,363,850	6%	9%	11%	29%	23%	23%
Ohio	4,179,287	5%	8%	11%	29%	25%	22%
Wisconsin	1,889,714	6%	9%	11%	30%	26%	19%
WEST SOUTH CENTRAL	**8,514,851**	**7%**	**9%**	**11%**	**30%**	**24%**	**18%**
Arkansas	727,073	7%	9%	11%	27%	26%	19%
Louisiana	1,223,543	7%	10%	12%	32%	25%	14%
Oklahoma	912,193	8%	10%	13%	32%	21%	15%
Texas	5,652,042	7%	9%	11%	30%	24%	19%
WEST NORTH CENTRAL	**6,572,885**	**7%**	**9%**	**12%**	**29%**	**23%**	**20%**
Iowa	978,584	7%	10%	12%	29%	22%	19%
Kansas	865,859	8%	10%	13%	31%	22%	17%
Minnesota	1,786,575	6%	8%	11%	29%	25%	21%
Missouri	1,982,329	6%	9%	11%	28%	24%	22%
Nebraska	564,125	8%	11%	12%	29%	22%	19%
North Dakota	190,767	10%	13%	15%	33%	22%	7%
South Dakota	204,646	10%	12%	15%	33%	21%	10%
MOUNTAIN	**4,485,483**	**7%**	**10%**	**12%**	**31%**	**22%**	**18%**
Arizona	1,219,822	6%	9%	12%	31%	23%	18%
Colorado	1,213,527	8%	10%	12%	31%	22%	18%
Idaho	285,610	9%	12%	15%	30%	19%	15%
Montana	212,417	12%	15%	17%	33%	16%	7%
Nevada	500,449	5%	8%	10%	26%	20%	32%
New Mexico	401,665	9%	12%	14%	34%	21%	11%
Utah	541,541	6%	10%	12%	28%	24%	21%
Wyoming	110,452	0%	17%	19%	40%	21%	3%
PACIFIC	**14,144,417**	**6%**	**9%**	**12%**	**31%**	**24%**	**18%**
Alaska	145,317	10%	13%	15%	30%	23%	9%
California	10,959,450	6%	8%	11%	31%	24%	19%
Hawaii	410,745	6%	10%	13%	32%	22%	17%
Oregon	976,920	8%	11%	14%	33%	23%	12%
Washington	1,651,985	7%	10%	13%	31%	21%	19%
UNITED STATES	**91,614,950**	**6%**	**9%**	**11%**	**29%**	**24%**	**20%**

Source: County Business Patterns, 1989.

TABLE G16
ANNUALIZED PAYROLL PER WORKER: BY ESTABLISHMENT SIZE, 1989

	1-4 Workers	5-9 Workers	10-19 Workers	20-99 Workers	100-499 Workers	500+ Workers
NEW ENGLAND	**$18,468**	**$18,069**	**$19,031**	**$20,352**	**$22,948**	**$29,350**
Connecticut	$21,025	$20,498	$21,501	$22,968	$25,679	$34,009
Maine	$13,501	$13,709	$15,146	$15,650	$17,685	$27,294
Massachuetts	$19,514	$18,713	$19,375	$20,853	$23,258	$28,370
New Hampshire	$16,393	$16,539	$17,668	$18,596	$20,200	$26,952
Rhode Island	$16,595	$16,368	$17,000	$17,488	$20,316	$23,706
Vermont	$13,527	$13,938	$15,868	$16,736	$18,802	$25,225
MIDDLE ATLANTIC	**$18,268**	**$18,383**	**$19,749**	**$21,351**	**$24,208**	**$20,278**
New Jersey	$20,019	$19,869	$20,784	$22,775	$25,268	$29,808
New York	$19,440	$19,671	$21,171	$22,743	$25,941	$13,480
Pennsylvania	$14,839	$15,415	$16,925	$18,254	$21,033	$27,086
SOUTH ATLANTIC	**$16,120**	**$15,729**	**$16,591**	**$17,090**	**$19,434**	**$25,741**
Delaware	$16,034	$15,761	$17,044	$17,854	$20,528	$37,306
District of Columbia	$28,869	$24,652	$25,043	$25,988	$28,422	$22,849
Florida	$16,988	$16,264	$16,745	$16,571	$17,793	$24,436
Georgia	$16,787	$16,176	$17,163	$17,523	$20,259	$26,183
Maryland	$18,607	$16,927	$17,461	$18,786	$21,306	$27,998
North Carolina	$13,487	$14,144	$15,334	$15,568	$18,057	$24,163
South Carolina	$13,127	$13,457	$14,457	$14,635	$17,520	$24,396
Virginia	$15,671	$15,497	$16,504	$17,740	$20,478	$25,630
West Virginia	$11,709	$13,161	$14,396	$16,570	$21,592	$34,987
EAST SOUTH CENTRAL	**$12,775**	**$13,701**	**$14,616**	**$15,605**	**$18,004**	**$24,432**
Alabama	$12,749	$13,697	$14,737	$15,514	$17,846	$24,552
Kentucky	$12,430	$13,381	$13,981	$15,337	$19,147	$25,838
Mississippi	$11,546	$12,623	$13,647	$14,297	$15,950	$21,779
Tennessee	$13,652	$14,435	$15,377	$16,346	$18,215	$24,422
EAST NORTH CENTRAL	**$15,797**	**$15,529**	**$16,720**	**$18,306**	**$21,841**	**$30,960**
Illinois	$18,390	$17,502	$18,425	$20,325	$23,735	$29,810
Indiana	$13,662	$13,869	$14,970	$16,322	$19,462	$29,620
Michigan	$16,212	$15,840	$17,387	$18,919	$22,745	$36,132
Ohio	$14,890	$14,945	$16,120	$17,567	$21,106	$29,917
Wisconsin	$13,440	$13,809	$14,853	$16,344	$20,068	$27,243
WEST SOUTH CENTRAL	**$15,907**	**$15,516**	**$16,212**	**$17,067**	**$20,461**	**$27,194**
Arkansas	$12,385	$13,126	$14,011	$14,278	$16,830	$20,386
Louisiana	$15,139	$14,373	$15,361	$16,159	$19,955	$26,130
Oklahoma	$14,164	$14,707	$14,922	$15,670	$20,583	$27,556
Texas	$16,930	$16,254	$16,932	$17,846	$21,059	$28,190
WEST NORTH CENTRAL	**$13,404**	**$13,867**	**$15,208**	**$16,305**	**$19,442**	**$26,742**
Iowa	$12,053	$12,620	$14,225	$14,759	$18,074	$24,074
Kansas	$13,261	$14,047	$15,333	$16,098	$19,231	$27,950
Minnesota	$14,822	$14,612	$16,003	$17,477	$20,869	$28,654
Missouri	$14,336	$14,531	$15,691	$17,091	$19,975	$27,420
Nebraska	$11,937	$13,253	$14,419	$14,792	$17,549	$21,108
North Dakota	$11,726	$12,627	$13,748	$14,602	$16,299	$24,971
South Dakota	$10,889	$11,985	$13,129	$13,470	$14,952	$21,776
WEST REGION	**$15,816**	**$14,935**	**$15,559**	**$16,466**	**$19,814**	**$25,662**
Arizona	$17,739	$15,767	$16,124	$16,240	$19,249	$26,728
Colorado	$16,191	$16,134	$16,894	$17,868	$21,142	$30,488
Idaho	$12,571	$13,048	$13,454	$14,843	$18,764	$26,363
Montana	$12,024	$12,429	$13,429	$14,555	$18,880	$20,650
Nevada	$19,640	$16,515	$17,447	$17,313	$18,165	$19,445
New Mexico	$13,493	$13,475	$14,292	$14,881	$19,078	$28,230
Utah	$15,114	$13,592	$14,110	$16,269	$19,417	$22,373
Wyoming	N/A	$13,844	$14,011	$15,806	$27,083	$33,918
PACIFIC	**$20,116**	**$17,876**	**$18,381**	**$19,950**	**$23,418**	**$15,259**
Alaska	$20,001	$19,410	$20,464	$22,649	$28,539	$48,714
California	$21,641	$18,679	$19,125	$20,574	$23,966	$11,843
Hawaii	$17,805	$16,579	$16,692	$17,292	$19,709	$23,352
Oregon	$14,681	$14,365	$14,983	$17,117	$20,418	$25,705
Washington	$15,533	$15,795	$16,353	$17,972	$21,624	$30,787
UNITED STATES	**$16,754**	**$16,247**	**$17,224**	**$18,442**	**$21,511**	**$24,599**

Source: County Business Patterns, 1989.

TABLE G17
GENERAL REVENUE AND REVENUE SOURCES, FISCAL YEAR 1990

	State/Local General Revenue Per Capita	Percent from Federal Government	Percent from Other Sources	Percent from State/Local Taxes
NEW ENGLAND	**$3,653**	**13%**	**24%**	**63%**
Connecticut	$3,969	10%	23%	67%
Maine	$3,294	15%	25%	60%
Massachusetts	$3,764	12%	25%	63%
New Hampshire	$2,767	14%	25%	61%
Rhode Island	$3,430	17%	24%	59%
Vermont	$3,587	16%	28%	56%
MIDDLE ATLANTIC	**$4,167**	**10%**	**26%**	**64%**
New Jersey	$3,904	9%	26%	65%
New York	$5,022	9%	26%	65%
Pennsylvania	$3,062	15%	24%	61%
SOUTH ATLANTIC	**$3,081**	**13%**	**28%**	**59%**
Delaware	$3,913	9%	38%	53%
District of Columbia	N/A	N/A	N/A	N/A
Florida	$3,096	11%	33%	56%
Georgia	$3,110	14%	28%	58%
Maryland	$3,545	11%	24%	65%
North Carolina	$2,816	16%	25%	59%
South Carolina	$2,863	18%	27%	55%
Virginia	$3,065	12%	27%	62%
West Virginia	$2,798	19%	25%	56%
EAST SOUTH CENTRAL	**$2,688**	**22%**	**27%**	**51%**
Alabama	$2,719	20%	31%	49%
Kentucky	$2,697	20%	25%	55%
Mississippi	$2,677	25%	28%	47%
Tennessee	$2,661	22%	26%	53%
EAST NORTH CENTRAL	**$3,186**	**13%**	**25%**	**61%**
Illinois	$3,227	12%	22%	65%
Indiana	$2,958	14%	31%	55%
Michigan	$3,373	12%	27%	61%
Ohio	$3,001	15%	24%	60%
Wisconsin	$3,412	12%	26%	61%
WEST SOUTH CENTRAL	**$2,877**	**16%**	**29%**	**56%**
Arkansas	$2,368	25%	21%	54%
Louisiana	$3,222	17%	35%	48%
Oklahoma	$2,817	16%	28%	56%
Texas	$2,872	14%	28%	58%
WEST NORTH CENTRAL	**$3,218**	**14%**	**29%**	**57%**
Iowa	$3,279	13%	29%	57%
Kansas	$3,103	12%	29%	60%
Minnesota	$4,032	11%	32%	57%
Missouri	$2,550	17%	22%	61%
Nebraska	$3,254	13%	32%	56%
North Dakota	$3,486	17%	38%	45%
South Dakota	$2,911	23%	27%	50%
MOUNTAIN	**$3,322**	**13%**	**32%**	**55%**
Arizona	$3,171	12%	28%	61%
Colorado	$3,382	11%	32%	57%
Idaho	$2,836	19%	26%	55%
Montana	$3,495	17%	31%	51%
Nevada	$3,304	10%	32%	58%
New Mexico	$3,497	14%	38%	48%
Utah	$3,023	18%	29%	52%
Wyoming	$5,335	11%	47%	41%
PACIFIC	**$3,931**	**11%**	**32%**	**57%**
Alaska	$11,317	3%	61%	36%
California	$3,870	11%	31%	58%
Hawaii	$4,545	8%	35%	57%
Oregon	$3,565	15%	31%	54%
Washington	$3,556	12%	29%	60%
UNITED STATES	**$3,416**	**16%**	**25%**	**59%**

Source: United States Bureau of the Census, 1991, "Government Finances in 89-90, GF-90 No. 5".

TABLE G18
TAX REVENUE AND TAX REVENUE SOURCES, FISCAL YEAR 1990

	State/Local Taxes Per Capita	Percent from Property Taxes	Percent from Sales/Gross Taxes	Percent from Individual Income Taxes	Percent from Corporate Income Taxes	Percent from Other Taxes
NEW ENGLAND	**$2,305**	**39%**	**27%**	**22%**	**6%**	**6%**
Connecticut	$2,675	39%	40%	7%	8%	6%
Maine	$1,974	37%	32%	24%	2%	5%
Massachusetts	$2,360	33%	20%	35%	6%	6%
New Hampshire	$1,690	68%	14%	2%	7%	8%
Rhode Island	$2,037	40%	32%	21%	3%	5%
Vermont	$2,009	41%	28%	22%	2%	6%
MIDDLE ATLANTIC	**$2,664**	**33%**	**28%**	**26%**	**4%**	**8%**
New Jersey	$2,519	46%	28%	15%	6%	5%
New York	$3,267	31%	27%	33%	3%	5%
Pennsylvania	$1,859	28%	30%	23%	5%	14%
SOUTH ATLANTIC	**$1,808**	**28%**	**40%**	**20%**	**4%**	**8%**
Delaware	$2,058	15%	12%	35%	9%	30%
District of Columbia	N/A	N/A	N/A	N/A	N/A	N/A
Florida	$1,746	35%	53%	0%	3%	9%
Georgia	$1,801	27%	40%	25%	4%	4%
Maryland	$2,305	26%	26%	38%	3%	7%
North Carolina	$1,675	21%	37%	31%	6%	6%
South Carolina	$1,562	26%	40%	25%	3%	6%
Virginia	$1,896	32%	31%	26%	3%	9%
West Virginia	$1,562	16%	43%	18%	8%	14%
EAST SOUTH CENTRAL	**$1,380**	**19%**	**50%**	**15%**	**4%**	**11%**
Alabama	$1,328	12%	50%	22%	3%	12%
Kentucky	$1,496	17%	37%	28%	5%	13%
Mississippi	$1,264	27%	49%	13%	4%	7%
Tennessee	$1,399	23%	61%	2%	5%	10%
EAST NORTH CENTRAL	**$1,956**	**34%**	**32%**	**24%**	**5%**	**5%**
Illinois	$2,102	36%	37%	18%	4%	5%
Indiana	$1,631	29%	38%	26%	4%	4%
Michigan	$2,068	40%	23%	22%	9%	5%
Ohio	$1,813	28%	32%	30%	3%	6%
Wisconsin	$2,090	35%	30%	26%	4%	5%
WEST SOUTH CENTRAL	**$1,601**	**31%**	**49%**	**6%**	**2%**	**12%**
Arkansas	$1,273	18%	47%	25%	4%	6%
Louisiana	$1,562	17%	51%	11%	6%	15%
Oklahoma	$1,575	18%	43%	20%	2%	17%
Texas	$1,663	39%	50%	0%	0%	11%
WEST NORTH CENTRAL	**$1,849**	**31%**	**36%**	**23%**	**4%**	**7%**
Iowa	$1,881	35%	29%	25%	4%	8%
Kansas	$1,848	36%	34%	19%	5%	7%
Minnesota	$2,305	31%	30%	29%	5%	6%
Missouri	$1,551	22%	44%	25%	3%	7%
Nebraska	$1,815	42%	33%	17%	3%	5%
North Dakota	$1,568	30%	40%	11%	5%	15%
South Dakota	$1,447	40%	48%	0%	3%	9%
MOUNTAIN	**$1,829**	**30%**	**41%**	**17%**	**3%**	**9%**
Arizona	$1,921	33%	44%	15%	3%	5%
Colorado	$1,925	36%	36%	21%	2%	6%
Idaho	$1,560	27%	36%	26%	5%	7%
Montana	$1,795	46%	13%	19%	6%	16%
Nevada	$1,926	22%	64%	0%	0%	14%
New Mexico	$1,690	13%	53%	14%	2%	18%
Utah	$1,582	27%	41%	24%	3%	5%
Wyoming	$2,204	41%	26%	0%	0%	33%
PACIFIC	**$2,228**	**28%**	**36%**	**22%**	**6%**	**8%**
Alaska	$4,069	31%	8%	0%	8%	53%
California	$2,226	27%	34%	25%	7%	6%
Hawaii	$2,596	15%	54%	24%	3%	4%
Oregon	$1,934	44%	9%	33%	3%	11%
Washington	$2,123	28%	62%	0%	0%	10%
UNITED STATES	**$2,017**	**31%**	**35%**	**21%**	**4%**	**8%**

Source: United States Bureau of the Census, 1991, "Government Finances in 89-90, GF-90 No. 5".

TABLE G19
GENERAL EXPENDITURES, FISCAL YEAR 1990

	State/Local General Expenditures Per Capita	Percent of General Expenditures on Education	Percent of General Expenditures on Welfare	Percent of General Expenditures on Health/Hospitals	Percent of General Expenditures on Police/Correction	Percent of General Expenditures on Highways	Percent of General Expenditures on Other
NEW ENGLAND	**$3,752**	**30.42%**	**16.26%**	**7.46%**	**5.89%**	**6.88%**	**33.09%**
Connecticut	$4,083	30.33%	13.35%	6.98%	5.82%	9.30%	34.22%
Maine	$3,265	36.47%	17.20%	4.34%	4.32%	9.10%	28.57%
Massachusetts	$3,845	26.56%	19.16%	9.46%	6.50%	4.27%	34.05%
New Hampshire	$2,963	37.10%	11.22%	4.52%	6.00%	9.91%	31.26%
Rhode Island	$3,663	32.53%	14.65%	6.52%	5.50%	6.85%	33.94%
Vermont	$3,600	41.98%	13.11%	3.03%	3.68%	9.92%	28.28%
MIDDLE ATLANTIC	**$4,134**	**32.12%**	**15.32%**	**7.20%**	**6.59%**	**6.36%**	**32.40%**
New Jersey	$3,864	33.55%	11.96%	5.13%	6.74%	6.68%	35.94%
New York	$4,999	28.25%	17.35%	9.49%	7.48%	5.33%	32.09%
Pennsylvania	$2,998	37.06%	14.44%	5.09%	5.14%	7.71%	30.56%
SOUTH ATLANTIC	**$3,086**	**36.20%**	**10.02%**	**9.46%**	**7.01%**	**7.91%**	**29.41%**
Delaware	$3,865	37.09%	8.86%	4.92%	6.11%	9.16%	33.87%
District of Columbia	N/A	N/A	N/A	N/A	N/A	N/A	N/A
Florida	$3,160	32.76%	9.12%	8.59%	8.24%	6.75%	34.53%
Georgia	$3,033	35.59%	10.99%	15.20%	6.81%	7.35%	24.06%
Maryland	$3,479	34.09%	11.43%	3.90%	7.77%	9.07%	33.74%
North Carolina	$2,823	40.26%	10.25%	10.00%	6.29%	8.07%	25.12%
South Carolina	$2,859	39.64%	10.83%	13.06%	5.92%	5.78%	24.78%
Virginia	$3,151	38.78%	8.16%	8.30%	6.74%	10.17%	27.86%
West Virginia	$2,590	37.83%	13.63%	6.42%	2.93%	10.40%	28.79%
EAST SOUTH CENTRAL	**$2,621**	**36.07%**	**11.58%**	**11.79%**	**5.33%**	**8.60%**	**26.63%**
Alabama	$2,690	38.07%	9.87%	14.29%	4.87%	8.05%	24.84%
Kentucky	$2,607	35.19%	14.91%	6.93%	5.18%	8.40%	29.40%
Mississippi	$2,562	38.20%	10.78%	14.76%	4.14%	8.49%	23.63%
Tennessee	$2,605	33.94%	10.90%	11.84%	6.45%	9.28%	27.60%
EAST NORTH CENTRAL	**$3,086**	**37.23%**	**14.69%**	**7.58%**	**6.17%**	**7.28%**	**27.04%**
Illinois	$3,021	34.27%	13.13%	5.71%	6.56%	8.74%	31.58%
Indiana	$2,757	41.00%	12.92%	8.82%	5.23%	6.86%	25.18%
Michigan	$3,349	38.03%	14.78%	9.93%	6.84%	5.97%	24.45%
Ohio	$2,954	37.06%	16.73%	7.75%	5.86%	6.67%	25.91%
Wisconsin	$3,397	38.76%	15.62%	5.72%	5.72%	8.17%	26.01%
WEST SOUTH CENTRAL	**$2,769**	**39.20%**	**10.29%**	**8.44%**	**6.18%**	**8.86%**	**27.03%**
Arkansas	$2,276	40.48%	14.75%	8.47%	4.59%	9.14%	22.57%
Louisiana	$3,063	31.97%	10.46%	10.37%	5.89%	8.00%	33.32%
Oklahoma	$2,679	37.88%	13.08%	9.32%	5.49%	9.22%	25.02%
Texas	$2,780	41.06%	9.11%	7.80%	6.60%	8.97%	26.46%
WEST NORTH CENTRAL	**$3,107**	**37.95%**	**12.39%**	**8.60%**	**4.88%**	**10.08%**	**26.10%**
Iowa	$3,178	38.90%	13.59%	9.77%	4.05%	10.85%	22.85%
Kansas	$3,024	39.38%	10.12%	7.79%	5.85%	10.94%	25.93%
Minnesota	$3,914	33.69%	14.96%	8.49%	4.03%	9.59%	29.24%
Missouri	$2,441	39.70%	11.52%	9.13%	6.08%	8.70%	24.88%
Nebraska	$3,051	40.74%	10.94%	9.99%	4.38%	10.88%	23.08%
North Dakota	$3,396	39.15%	11.53%	3.58%	2.77%	11.51%	31.46%
South Dakota	$2,799	35.58%	10.08%	5.00%	4.25%	14.14%	30.96%
MOUNTAIN	**$3,303**	**36.41%**	**9.23%**	**6.42%**	**6.85%**	**10.93%**	**30.15%**
Arizona	$3,558	34.18%	9.85%	4.12%	7.79%	13.10%	30.96%
Colorado	$3,250	37.54%	9.59%	7.22%	7.26%	9.23%	29.16%
Idaho	$2,632	37.63%	9.44%	8.06%	5.38%	12.29%	27.21%
Montana	$3,144	37.60%	11.62%	5.19%	3.92%	12.37%	29.29%
Nevada	$3,428	29.70%	6.09%	6.83%	9.26%	10.81%	37.30%
New Mexico	$3,276	37.62%	9.26%	7.57%	6.70%	9.90%	28.95%
Utah	$2,879	41.37%	9.27%	6.98%	5.28%	8.46%	28.64%
Wyoming	$4,754	36.31%	5.06%	10.81%	4.79%	13.26%	29.76%
PACIFIC	**$3,749**	**32.77%**	**12.88%**	**7.68%**	**7.70%**	**5.10%**	**33.86%**
Alaska	$9,644	23.48%	5.71%	3.38%	4.20%	10.11%	53.12%
California	$3,721	31.95%	13.47%	8.02%	8.38%	4.55%	33.63%
Hawaii	$3,974	25.29%	9.75%	6.17%	4.95%	6.00%	47.85%
Oregon	$3,397	38.21%	9.94%	6.27%	6.11%	7.13%	32.35%
Washington	$3,410	37.41%	12.54%	7.26%	5.47%	6.52%	30.80%
UNITED STATES	**$3,343**	**34.65%**	**12.90%**	**8.16%**	**6.64%**	**7.34%**	**30.30%**

Source: United States Bureau of the Census, 1991, "Government Finances in 89-90, GF-90 No.5".

Notes for tables G3–G19

G3, G6–G9	The distribution listed is the number of individuals in families of a given type. One family of the type "Single" will have fewer persons than one family of the type "Married with Children."
G4	Income levels are for families. Unrelated individuals are included as a family. The income quartiles listed are the highest income for the given quartile. That is, 25 percent of families have incomes lower than the 25th quartile income level listed.
G5, G6–G9	Poverty is defined using the federal poverty guidelines from the U.S. Department of Health and Human Services.
G10	The worker and unemployed populations are defined as individuals who reported working or being unemployed, respectively, in the week before the interview. Workers are furthermore defined as individuals who reported a positive number of usual hours of work per week in the previous year. The labor force participation rate is defined as the number of individuals in the labor force divided by the population ages 18 to 64. The labor force is defined as workers plus unemployed. The employment rate is defined as the number of employed workers divided by the population ages 18 to 64. The unemployment rate is divided as the number of individuals who reported themselves as unemployed divided by the number of individuals in the labor force.
G11–G13	Workers are defined as individuals who reported a positive number of usual hours of work per week in the previous year.
G12	Sector is based on the longest job held in the previous year.
G13	Private sector includes self-employed.
G14	Private-sector workers are individuals who reported working a positive number of usual hours of work per week in the previous year and reported working in either the private sector or were self-employed on their longest job of the previous year. Industry is based on the longest job in the previous year. The category "Other" includes agriculture, forestry, fisheries, mining, construction, transportation, communication, other public utilities, finance, insurance, and real estate.
G16	In County Business Patterns, average payroll is reported for the first quarter of the year. We report an annualized figure defined as the first quarter payroll multiplied by 4.
G17–19	State finance data from the U.S. Department of Commerce are reproduced in the publication "States in Profile, 1991 Second Edition." Data for the District of Columbia are not included.
G17	General revenues exclude employee retirement fund revenue and revenue of certain utility operations.
G18	Other taxes include severance tax, parimutual tax, lottery tax, alcohol tax, tobacco tax, and motor fuel tax.
G19	General expenditures exclude expenditures on utilities, liquor stores, and employee retirement funds. Outlays for Medicaid are included in general expenditures on welfare.

The Three–Year Merged March Current Population Survey

The estimates in sections A, B, C, and G of this report are from a sample constructed from three years of the March Current Population Survey (CPS): 1989, 1990, and 1991.[1] The purpose of merging three years of data was to produce more reliable estimates, particularly estimates calculated using relatively small subsamples of the data. Three-year merged CPS samples have also been used to calculate state-level poverty rates.[2]

The March CPS sample used for this monograph does not include individuals who were in the military at the time of the survey or their families. (This removed approximately 4,500 individuals from our three-year merged sample.) All estimates are for the population under age 65 or a subsample of this population.

THREE-YEAR MERGED SAMPLE

The estimates obtained using the merged sample are averages over the three years. Estimates from this merged sample are more meaningful if the true number remains relatively unchanged over the period of the merge. Merging more years would reduce the standard errors further, but would require assuming little change over a longer period. For this reason, we merged three years to balance this concern against gaining larger sample sizes.

Due to the CPS sampling frame, using three years of the March CPS only doubles the CPS sample size. In the CPS design, each sample household is surveyed in two consecutive years. In a given March survey, half of the households were interviewed the previous year and half of the households will be interviewed again in the next year. To ensure that all observations in the merged sample were independent, we included each household only once. For those that were interviewed in both 1989 and 1990, we kept the interview from 1990, and for households that were interviewed in 1990 and 1991 we kept the 1990 interview. In this way, one-quarter of the sample's observations are from 1989, one-half from 1990, and one-quarter are from 1991.

The population numbers cited in this report's tables reflect the weighted population for the appropriate subsample being used. There is an associated number of unweighted observations for every sample and subsample used. For example, the population in New Jersey under age 65 is 6,631,000. In the three-year merged CPS sample there are 10,729 unweighted observations under age 65 for New Jersey. There are too many tables to report the unweighted subsample size for each estimate. However, to give the reader an idea of the number of unweighted observations underlying population estimates, we reproduce here as table 1.1 the health insurance coverage for the population under age 65 (see also table A1 in section A), showing the unweighted counts in each cell. The first column shows the total number of unweighted observations from the three-year merged CPS under age 65 for each state. The total unweighted count varies from 2,189 for Vermont to 23,084 for California. This total is then broken down into six categories of health insurance coverage.

Even after doubling the sample size, some state subsamples of interest may have small numbers of unweighted observations. For this reason, we have included standard errors, which reflect the reliability of a given estimate. They are reported in parentheses under each estimate for tables from the three-year merged CPS. In addition, we do not report estimates based on a subsample of less than 100 unweighted observations. These estimates are replaced with a (—) in the tables.

CALCULATING STANDARD ERRORS

In calculating the standard errors of estimates from the CPS data, we need to make adjustments for the sample design of the CPS. The Census Bureau provides adjustment factors and formulas that can be used to calculate correct standard errors. There are two types of adjustment factors, one for the characteristic being estimated, such as marital status, and one for each state. The factors used in this monograph were obtained from the March CPS Technical Documentation from 1989, 1990, and 1991, as well as directly from the Bureau of the Census.

The formula used to calculate the standard error of a percentage is as follows[3]:

$$SE\,(p) = \sqrt{\frac{f^2 b}{x}\, p\,(100{-}p)}\,, \qquad (1.1)$$

where $SE\,(p)$ is the standard error of the percentage, b is the adjustment factor for the characteristic estimated, f^2 is the state adjustment factor, p is the estimated percentage, and x is the population base of the percentage. The base of the percentage, x, is two times larger for the three-year merged CPS sample than for a one-year sample. This translates into approximately a 30 percent reduction in standard errors.

USING STANDARD ERRORS

The standard error is a measure of the reliability of a given estimate. The numbers from the CPS are estimates, because only a sample of the entire population is surveyed each year. We do not know exactly how many people are, for example, working part-time, but we have an estimate based on a sample of the population. The CPS is one possible sample of the entire population, and gives one estimate of the percentage working part-time. These are the estimates presented in the monograph. It is also possible to draw other samples from the entire population, using the same general design as the CPS. We could then calculate other estimates of the percentage working part-time, which could be different from the first estimate. Standard errors allow us to construct a confidence interval around an estimate, and to state that the average estimated percentage from all samples falls within that interval with a specified probability, called the level of confidence.

For example, if the estimate of the percentage of part-time workers is p, and the standard error is s, then we can create an interval around p that contains the true percentage of part-time workers with 95 percent probability. The interval around p for the 95 percent confidence level would be:

$$p - (1.96 * s) \leq p \leq p + (1.96 * s). \qquad (1.2)$$

Using numbers, if we estimate 10 percent of the population works part-time with a standard error of 2, then the 95 percent confidence interval ranges from 6.1 to 13.9. With 95 percent confidence, we can report that the percentage of the population working part-time falls within this range.

Standard errors can also be used to distinguish whether two estimates are different from each other at a certain level of significance. Again, because these reported numbers are estimates, two estimates that appear to be different (for example 20 percent and 23 percent) may not be "significantly different" when we take into account that these numbers are calculated from one sample. If the difference between two estimates is greater than the standard error of the difference multiplied by 1.96, then the two estimates are different at the 95 percent confidence level.

To calculate this, the formula for the standard error of the difference of two estimates is as follows:

$$SE\,(X_1 - X_2) = \sqrt{SE\,(X_1)^2 + SE\,(X_2)^2} \qquad (1.3)$$

where SE stands for standard error, X_1 is one estimate, and X_2 is the other.

For example, the percentage uninsured in Connecticut is 11 with a standard error of .62, and the percentage uninsured in Vermont is 10 with a standard error of .64. We wanted to know if these two numbers are different at the 95 percent confidence level. We can check this by calculating the standard error of the difference between the two estimates. Using the preceding formula, the standard error of the difference is calculated as .89. The difference between the two estimates is 1 percent. The two estimates are considered significantly different at the 95 percent confidence level if

$$\frac{X_1 - X_2}{SE\,(X_1 - X_2)} \geq 1.96. \qquad (1.4)$$

In our example, 1 divided by .89 is not greater than 1.96. Therefore, these two estimates are not significantly different at the 95 percent level.

In general, it is important to remember that small differences in estimates, even if statistically significant, should be used with caution. Any comparison of a certain characteristic across states or rank-ordering of states when the differences are small should be viewed with caution.

Notes, Appendix One

1. The March CPS collects information from the previous year, so the period covered by this sample is 1988, 1989, and 1990.

2. For other examples using three years of CPS data, see Jon Haveman, Sheldon Danziger, and Robert Plotnick, 1991, "State Poverty Rates for Whites, Blacks, and Hispanics in the Late 1980s," *Focus* 13 (Spring):1–7; and U.S. Department of Commerce, Bureau of the Census, 1991, "Poverty in the United States: 1991," Current Population Reports, ser. P-60 (Washington, D.C.: U.S. Government Printing Office). For more information on the Current Population Survey design and reliability of estimates see Bureau of the Census Technical Paper 40, "The Current Population Survey: Design and Methodology" (Washington, D.C.: Author).

3. This formula and the parameters for various characteristics and for states can be found in the Current Population Survey March "Technical Documentation" in the "Source and Accuracy Statement" appendix.

TABLE 1.1
UNWEIGHTED COUNTS OF POPULATION UNDER AGE 65: BY TYPE OF HEALTH INSURANCE COVERAGE

	Total	Employer (own)	Employer (other)	Medicaid	Other Government	Other Private	Uninsured
NEW ENGLAND	**21,474**	**7,798**	**7,882**	**1,617**	**275**	**1,556**	**2,346**
Connecticut	2,325	940	883	117	21	135	229
Maine	2,695	893	982	257	53	218	292
Massachusetts	9,863	3,592	3,597	882	120	671	1,001
New Hampshire	2,208	764	813	65	31	185	350
Rhode Island	2,194	830	812	149	22	148	233
Vermont	2,189	779	795	147	28	199	241
MIDDLE ATLANTIC	**39,903**	**13,933**	**13,952**	**4,087**	**368**	**2,695**	**4,868**
New Jersey	10,729	4,154	3,802	742	77	785	1,169
New York	18,217	5,862	5,954	2,470	175	1,169	2,587
Pennsylvania	10,957	3,917	4,196	875	116	741	1,112
SOUTH ATLANTIC	**43,529**	**15,029**	**13,436**	**3,492**	**1,018**	**3,088**	**7,466**
Delaware	2,388	909	817	132	36	150	344
District of Columbia	2,247	824	405	353	35	175	455
Florida	12,575	3,925	3,571	877	325	1,065	2,812
Georgia	3,069	1,011	991	293	68	191	515
Maryland	2,537	981	908	197	35	140	276
North Carolina	10,194	3,829	3,146	742	251	758	1,468
South Carolina	3,529	1,264	1,164	254	101	196	550
Virginia	3,811	1,359	1,306	219	91	229	607
West Virginia	3,179	927	1,128	425	76	184	439
EAST SOUTH CENTRAL	**13,004**	**3,801**	**4,235**	**1,506**	**374**	**880**	**2,208**
Alabama	3,284	992	1,101	255	106	198	632
Kentucky	2,927	897	991	357	85	196	401
Mississippi	3,624	893	1,076	568	120	267	700
Tennessee	3,169	1,019	1,067	326	63	219	475
EAST NORTH CENTRAL	**40,409**	**13,737**	**15,398**	**3,862**	**512**	**2,699**	**4,201**
Illinois	11,360	3,864	4,052	1,204	126	834	1,280
Indiana	2,995	978	1,158	144	64	235	416
Michigan	10,995	3,674	4,212	1,265	126	663	1,055
Ohio	11,510	3,963	4,534	1,018	158	691	1,146
Wisconsin	3,549	1,258	1,442	231	38	276	304
WEST SOUTH CENTRAL	**24,763**	**6,643**	**7,278**	**2,222**	**675**	**1,759**	**6,186**
Arkansas	3,450	961	1,112	307	128	270	672
Louisiana	2,775	680	864	363	85	197	586
Oklahoma	3,001	827	941	253	99	259	622
Texas	15,537	4,175	4,361	1,299	363	1,033	4,306
WEST NORTH CENTRAL	**22,441**	**6,667**	**8,129**	**1,450**	**376**	**3,224**	**2,595**
Iowa	3,201	981	1,211	196	46	492	275
Kansas	3,141	1,011	1,235	219	35	320	321
Minnesota	2,852	931	993	247	35	325	321
Missouri	2,951	966	1,068	214	61	242	400
Nebraska	3,331	1,014	1,212	182	49	479	395
North Dakota	3,434	844	1,206	210	69	768	337
South Dakota	3,531	920	1,204	182	81	598	546
MOUNTAIN	**26,311**	**7,515**	**9,230**	**1,703**	**594**	**2,320**	**4,949**
Arizona	3,156	963	988	254	85	207	659
Colorado	2,963	931	1,039	191	72	204	526
Idaho	3,663	991	1,334	156	73	426	683
Montana	3,509	931	1,123	289	80	471	615
Nevada	2,947	1,094	920	116	63	201	553
New Mexico	4,119	955	1,260	332	122	271	1,179
Utah	3,475	953	1,602	217	42	290	371
Wyoming	2,479	697	964	148	57	250	363
PACIFIC	**35,087**	**10,549**	**10,334**	**4,184**	**590**	**2,334**	**7,096**
Alaska	3,791	1,098	1,213	270	147	230	833
California	23,084	6,516	6,320	3,236	272	1,528	5,212
Hawaii	2,295	898	749	216	47	137	248
Oregon	2,705	919	970	192	38	181	405
Washington	3,212	1,118	1,082	270	86	258	398
UNITED STATES	**266,921**	**85,672**	**89,874**	**24,123**	**4,782**	**20,555**	**41,915**

Source: Three-year merged March CPS, 1989, 1990, and 1991.

Issues in Using the CPS to Measure Health Insurance Coverage

The March Current Population Survey (CPS) is an important source of information on the health insurance coverage of Americans. Administered annually by the U.S. Bureau of the Census, the survey covers a representative sample of about 60,000 households including over 150,000 people. In addition to questions about household composition and income, the survey has included questions related to health insurance coverage since 1980. A great deal of the current discussion related to health insurance coverage and the reorganization of the U.S. health care system is framed with reference to data from the CPS. This appendix discusses the CPS health insurance questions and general issues related to these data.

The interpretation of survey-based data requires careful consideration of the survey itself and the comparison of results to other sources of data. Such scrutiny of health insurance data from the CPS has raised a few concerns about the data. These include concerns about whether all possible forms of coverage are represented, the apparent underreporting of Medicaid coverage, the handling of inconsistent answers to different questions, and the possibility that information provided by survey respondents reflects their health insurance coverage at the time of the interview rather than during the previous year. Before discussing each of these concerns individually, we review the questions as they appear in the CPS.

Appendix table 2.1 shows the questions as they appear on the CPS questionnaire. The first set of questions (74 through 75F) inquires about coverage of household members under the major forms of public and private health coverage during the previous calendar year. Question 74 asks which members, if any, were covered under the major forms of public coverage—Medicare, Medicaid, CHAMPUS, Veteran's Administration (VA), and military health care. Questions 75A through 75F ask about private sources of health coverage, including whether coverage is employment-related. Dependent coverage is captured through question 75F, which asks which other family members are covered under the private plan or plans. The second set of questions (80 through 81A) asks directly about the coverage status of children under 15. These questions try to capture children's coverage overlooked during the interview—in particular, children's coverage as dependents on policies of persons outside the household (question 81A) and to confirm coverage of children under public programs.

It is important to note that at no point in the CPS are respondents asked if any members of the household were uninsured for either part or all of the previous year. Estimates of the uninsured from the CPS reflect the number of persons for whom none of the specified types of coverage are reported for the year. Therefore, if survey respondents are answering the questions as intended, a person reported as uninsured on the CPS is without insurance for the entire year. For example, if a person has coverage under an employer-sponsored plan for six months of the previous year and is uninsured for the remainder of the year, the person's accurate response to the CPS questions would indicate coverage under employment-related insurance for some part of the year, but the period without insurance would not be captured. When respondents answer the questions accurately, we capture any type of coverage held for even part of the year, but only capture as uninsured those who were without insurance for the entire year.

COVERAGE UNDER OTHER GOVERNMENT PROGRAMS

Note also that the CPS questions do not offer respondents the opportunity to report coverage under government programs other than those specified. Coverage under state-funded programs for the ill and medically indigent, for example, are not represented by the questions on the CPS. In response to growing concerns about the uninsured, a number of states have introduced state-funded programs to extend coverage

APPENDIX TABLE 2.1

CPS Health Insurance Questions

74. There are several government programs which provide medical care or help pay medical bills.

    During *[previous year]* was anyone in this household covered by:

    74A. Medicare *(for the disabled and elderly)*?

    　　　74B. [if yes. . .] Who was that? *(Anyone else?)*

    74C. Medicaid *(for the needy)*?

    　　　74D. [if yes. . .] Who was that? *(Anyone else?)*

    74E. CHAMPUS, VA, or military health care?

    　　　74F. [if yes. . .] Who was that? *(Anyone else?)*

75A. Other than government sponsored policies, health insurance can be obtained privately or through a current of former employer or union. Was anyone in this household covered by health insurance of this type at any time during *[previous year]*?

    [if yes. . .]

    75B. Who was that? *(Anyone else?)*

    [for each person with such coverage . . .]

    75C. Was . . .'s health insurance coverage from a plan in . . .'s own name?

    75D. Was this health insurance plan offered through . . .'s current or former employer or union?

    75E. Did . . .'s employer or union pay for all, part, or none of the cost of this plan?

    75F. What other persons were covered by this health insurance policy? *(Mark all that apply)*

    - Spouse
    - Child(ren) in the household
    - Child(ren) not in the household
    - Other
    - No one

TABLE 2.1 *(continued)*

Supplemental Question
if Children Under 15

80. During *[previous year]*, how many of the children under age 15 in this household were covered by Medicare or Medicaid?

   - All
   - Some, but not all *(indicate number)*
   - None

81. During *[previous year]*, how many children under age 15 in this household were covered by a health insurance plan *(excluding Medicaid or Medicare)*?

   - All
   - Some, but not all *(indicate number)*
   - None

[if all or some . . .]

   81A. How many of these children were covered by the health insurance plan of someone not residing in this household?

   - All
   - Some, but not all *(indicate number)*
   - None

to those in need. California and Vermont, for example, are providing coverage to pregnant women whose incomes are just over the Medicaid limits. In addition to programs covering poor and near-poor families who do not qualify for Medicaid, a number of states have developed and funded programs targeted to persons with specific medical conditions, such as those with mental retardation or persons infected with HIV.

The CPS questions, however, do not directly capture coverage under special state-funded programs. A person with coverage under such a state program may mistakenly report coverage as Medicaid, or if he or she is aware of the distinction and reports no form of private coverage, may fall into the residual uninsured category. Still other states—21 states as of 1991—have facilitated state-sponsored "pools" to help persons who are considered "uninsurable" owing to high medical risks;[1] it is unclear how a person with such coverage would report it on the CPS. Although coverage under such programs should be captured as private, nongroup coverage, survey respondents may mistakenly believe that the opening to question 75, which asks about coverage that is *not* "government sponsored" and is "obtained privately" precludes this type of coverage.

Few good estimates are currently available for the number of people who obtain coverage through these state-funded programs. In 1983, the Health Care Financing Administration (HCFA) estimated that at least 875,000 persons were covered through state-only programs for the indigent in 29 states at a cost of $1.7 billion.[2] Programs of this sort have been considered and adopted in an increasing number of states in recent years and are expected to grow further. The U.S. General Accounting Office estimates that only 77,000 persons gained access to private insurance through state-sponsored high-risk pools in 1989.[3] A systematic collection of data from states on the extent of such programs, if any, was beyond the scope of this project. If your use of these data focuses on a few states, we suggest that it may be worthwhile to check if these states have such programs, and request estimates of the number of persons covered during 1988–91.

Medicaid reporting

The underreporting of Medicaid coverage on the CPS also raises some concerns. Participation in Medicaid and other income-related programs, such as Aid to Families with Dependent Children (AFDC) and Supplemental Security Income (SSI), is said to be underreported because the number of persons on the survey file reporting participation in these programs is significantly lower than the number of program participants shown in the programs' administrative data systems. For example, the number of nonelderly, noninstitutionalized persons reporting Medicaid coverage on the March 1991 CPS is about 21 percent lower than the "unduplicated" counts of nonelderly, noninstitutionalized persons reported in data from the HCFA.[4] Thus, relying completely on self-reported Medicaid coverage from the CPS understates the significance of Medicaid in providing coverage and overstates the number of uninsured. The enhanced version of the CPS used in this analysis, however, corrects for the underreporting of Medicaid coverage by imputing Medicaid coverage. The Urban Institute's Transfer Income Model (TRIM2), a microsimulation model, passes each person on the CPS through the various state rules for Medicaid eligibility to identify which persons are *eligible* for coverage. Statistical procedures are used to choose enough additional persons from the pool of eligibles who did not report coverage on the CPS to match the known enrollment figures.[5] The TRIM2 model aligns program enrollees to known enrollment figures in each state by age and disability group. Giannarelli provides further discussion of the methodology of these corrections.[6]

INCONSISTENT RESPONSES

There are also cases in which the reported coverage of children from the multipartite questions 74–75 conflicts with the information provided in the more direct questions 80 and 81. For example, survey respondents may report that their children are covered under their employer-sponsored plan in response to question 75F, but then report on question 81 that their children are without insurance. Likewise, the reverse may occur: a child may be categorized as uninsured based on the first set of questions, but categorized as insured under the second set. The 1991 CPS includes about 7 million weighted children with such conflicting information.[7] These discrepancies may be difficult to reconcile. Some analysts have employed a series of assumptions about children covered by plans outside the household to assign coverage status in these cases.[8] Others have counted children as covered if coverage is indicated under either set of questions.[9] Our analysis employs the latter assumption. This avoids overstating the number of children who are without insurance, but as a result may understate that figure.

TIMING OF COVERAGE

Finally, there is concern that persons responding to the CPS may be reporting their coverage status at the time of the interview, rather than their status during the previous calendar year, as requested. These concerns are based on comparisons of estimates of health insurance coverage based on the CPS to other surveys of health insurance coverage. For example, Swartz found that if the number of uninsured from the CPS is compared to counts of persons uninsured for the entire year from other surveys (e.g., the Health Interview Survey and the National Medical Care Utilization and Expenditure Survey), the CPS number is considerably larger.[10] If, however, comparisons of the CPS estimates are made to "point-in-time" estimates of the uninsured from other surveys—estimates of the number who are without insurance at a particular time (a given month, for example)—the CPS numbers are a much closer match. Similarly, Swartz found CPS estimates of persons with Medicaid and private coverage more similar to point-in-time estimates than annual estimates from other surveys. The Census Bureau arrives at similar conclusions in comparing results from the Survey of Income and Program Participation (SIPP) to CPS data.[11] We believe the evidence suggests that there is at best a mix of responses among respondents to the CPS: some are reporting their current coverage while others are reporting coverage during the previous year, as requested.

Notes, Appendix Two

1. U.S. General Accounting Office, 1992, *Access to Health Care: States Respond to Growing Crisis*, GAO/HRD-92-70 (Washington, D.C.: Author), June.

2. Health Care Financing Administration, 1985, *Health Care Financing Program Statistics: Analysis of State Medicaid Program Characteristics, 1984* (Baltimore: U.S. Department of Health and Human Services).

3. U.S. General Accounting Office, *Access to Health Care*.

4. Institutionalized persons are not represented on the CPS. On the 1991 CPS, 19.6 million noninstitutionalized nonelderly persons reported Medicaid coverage. Comparable data from the Health Care Financing Administration indicate that 24.7 million were enrolled in Medicaid for that period.

5. For example, after correction, TRIM2 identified 24.3 million Medicaid enrollees on the March 1991 CPS, a figure significantly closer to the 24.7 million known to have been enrolled than the 19.6 million reporting coverage on the uncorrected CPS.

6. Linda Giannarelli, 1992, *An Analyst's Guide to TRIM2* (Washington, D.C.: Urban Institute Press).

7. Employee Benefits Research Institute, 1992, *Sources of Health Insurance and Characteristics of the Uninsured, Analysis of the March 1991 Current Population Survey* (Washington, D.C.: Author, February).

8. Ibid.

9. Richard Kronick, 1991, "Health Insurance, 1979–1989: The Frayed Connection between Employment and Insurance," *Inquiry* 28: 318–32.

10. Katherine Swartz, 1986, "Interpreting the Estimates from Four National Surveys of the Number of People without Health Insurance," *Journal of Economic and Social Measurement* 14:233–42.

11. U.S. Department of Commerce, Bureau of the Census, 1990, *Health Insurance Coverage: 1986–88*, Current Population Reports, ser. P-70, no. 17 (Washington, D.C.: U.S. Government Printing Office).